# Handbook of Pediatric Primary Care

# Handbook of Pediatric Primary Care

Edited by

**Raymond C. Baker, M.D.**

Professor of Clinical Pediatrics, University of Cincinnati College of Medicine; Pediatrician, Division of Pediatrics, Children's Hospital Medical Center, Cincinnati

Foreword by

**William K. Schubert, M.D.**

Chairman Emeritus and Professor of Pediatrics, University of Cincinnati College of Medicine; President and Chief Executive Officer, Children's Hospital Medical Center, Cincinnati

**Little, Brown and Company**

**Boston New York Toronto London**

**Library of Congress Cataloging-in-Publication Data**
Handbook of pediatric primary care / [edited by] Raymond C. Baker; foreword by William K. Schubert.
p. cm.
Includes bibliographical references and index.
ISBN 0-316-07825-5
1. Pediatrics—Handbooks, manuals, etc. I. Baker, Raymond C.
[DNLM: 1. Pediatrics—handbooks. 2. Primary Health Care—handbooks. WS 39 H2363 1995]
RJ48.H343 1995
618.92—dc20
DNLM/DLC
for Library of Congress 95-20030
CIP

Printed in the United States of America
RRD-VA

Editorial: Nancy E. Chorpenning
Production Editor: Katharine S. Mascaro
Editorial and Production Services: Silverchair Science + Communications
Production Supervisor: Mike Burggren
Cover Designer: Mike Burggren and Linda Dana Willis

*To my mother, Ruth Abigail Baker,*
*who taught me that learning is a lifelong process*

# Contents

Foreword — xi
*William K. Schubert*

Preface — xiii

Contributing Authors — xv

## I. The Well-Child Care Visit

1. Overview of Well-Child Care — 3
*Raymond C. Baker*
2. History — 8
*Christine L. McHenry*
3. Physical Examination — 14
*Paul S. Bellet*
4. Screening Tests — 21
*Omer G. Berger*
5. Immunizations — 24
*Robert M. Siegel*
6. Nutrition — 33
*Anita Cavallo and Mary Pat Alfaro*
7. Anticipatory Guidance — 41
*Julie Jaskiewicz*
8. Infant Dental Care — 61
*James F. Steiner*
9. Normal Speech and Language Development — 64
*Ann W. Kummer*
10. Normal Motor and Cognitive Development — 71
*Rosemary E. Schmidt and Sonya Oppenheimer*

## II. The Problem Visit—Medical

### A. Dermatologic Disorders

11. Atopic Dermatitis (Eczema) — 83
*Raymond C. Baker*
12. Diaper Dermatitis — 85
*Raymond C. Baker*
13. Impetigo — 87
*Raymond C. Baker*
14. Lice and Scabies — 89
*Raymond C. Baker*
15. Tinea Capitis — 92
*Christine L. McHenry*

**B. HEENT Disorders**

16. Acute Otitis Media 97
*Raymond C. Baker*

17. Acute, Subacute, and Chronic Sinusitis 101
*Christine L. McHenry*

18. Pharyngitis and Tonsillitis 103
*Paul S. Bellet*

19. Upper Respiratory Tract Infection (The Common Cold) 105
*Paul S. Bellet*

20. Conjunctivitis 107
*Raymond C. Baker*

21. Common Oral Conditions in Infants and Children 110
*James F. Steiner*

**C. Lower Respiratory Tract Disorders**

22. Asthma 117
*Christine L. McHenry*

23. Bronchiolitis 120
*Robert M. Siegel*

24. Croup (Acute Viral Laryngotracheobronchitis) 123
*Raymond C. Baker*

25. Pertussis 125
*Raymond C. Baker*

26. Pneumonia in Infants and Children 127
*Raymond C. Baker*

**D. Gastrointestinal Disorders**

27. Acute Gastroenteritis 133
*Raymond C. Baker*

28. Chronic Abdominal Pain in Children 136
*Michael K. Farrell*

29. Encopresis 139
*Raymond C. Baker*

30. Hyperbilirubinemia in the Term Infant 142
*Christine L. McHenry*

31. Infantile Colic 145
*Raymond C. Baker*

**E. Genitourinary Disorders**

32. Primary Nocturnal Enuresis 151
*Raymond C. Baker*

33. Urinary Tract Infections in Children 153
*Robert M. Siegel*

34. Sexually Transmitted Diseases 156
*Robert M. Siegel*

**F. Endocrine/Growth Disorders**

35. Assessment of Pubertal Development Variations 163
*Anita Cavallo*

36. Assessment of Abnormal Linear Growth 170
*Anita Cavallo*

37. Failure to Thrive 174
*Julie Jaskiewicz*

38. Obesity 180
*Julie Jaskiewicz*

39. Contraception 185
*Julie Jaskiewicz*

**G. Neuromusculoskeletal Disorders**

40. Genu Varum and Genu Valgum 193
*Raymond C. Baker*

41. Congenital Hip Dislocation 196
*Raymond C. Baker*

42. Evaluation of the Patient with Intoeing 199
*Raymond C. Baker*

43. Evaluation and Management of Headaches in Children 203
*David N. Franz*

44. Febrile Seizures 212
*Julie Jaskiewicz*

**H. Hematologic Disorders**

45. Iron Deficiency 217
*Omer G. Berger*

46. Lead Poisoning in Childhood: Screening and Evaluation 219
*Omer G. Berger*

47. Sickle Cell Disease Episodes and Infections 221
*Paul S. Bellet*

**I. Medicolegal Issues**

48. Physical Abuse 227
*Robert A. Shapiro*

49. Sexual Abuse 231
*Robert A. Shapiro*

50. Ethical Issues in the Outpatient Setting 235
*Christine L. McHenry*

**J. Miscellaneous Topics**

51. The Evaluation of Fever in Infancy 241
*Sherman J. Alter*

52. Antibiotic Selection and Compliance 245
*Raymond C. Baker*

53. Symptomatic Therapy of Children 249
*Raymond C. Baker*

54. Management of the Infant Born to an HIV-Positive Mother 255
*Raymond C. Baker*

## III. The Problem Visit—Behavioral

55. Behavior Management and Discipline 263
*Janet R. Schultz*

56. Sleep and Bedtime Behavior 273
*Janet R. Schultz*

57. Eating and Mealtime Behavior 278
*Janet R. Schultz*

58. School-Related Problems 281
*Janet R. Schultz*

59. Temper Tantrums 287
*Janet R. Schultz*

60. Toilet Training 289
*Janet R. Schultz*

61. Sibling Rivalry 292
*Janet R. Schultz*

62. Attention Deficit Hyperactivity Disorder 295
*Rosemary E. Schmidt*

63. School Failure 299
*Rosemary E. Schmidt*

## Appendixes

A. Drug Dosages 305
B. Infant Formula Composition 317
C. Oral Rehydration Solution Composition 319
D. Recommended Dietary Allowances 320
E. Growth Charts 322
F. Blood Pressure Norms 329
G. Clinical Stages of Pubertal Development (Tanner Stages) 333
H. Sequence of Sexual Maturity 334
I. Denver Developmental Screening Test-II 335
J. Surface Area Nomogram 336

Index 339

# Foreword

There are multiple large textbooks of pediatrics that include sections on growth and development and pediatric primary care. The need for a handbook of pediatric primary care that will fit into the pocket of a pediatric resident's or medical student's jacket has skyrocketed with recent changes in pediatric care. These changes include the shift from inpatient to outpatient treatment and the emphasis on pediatric primary care payment by multiple third parties.

The staff of Children's Hospital Medical Center, Division of General Pediatrics, has written this handbook that is particularly responsive to the challenges described above. Dr. Baker and his associates have produced, in *Handbook of Pediatric Primary Care*, a discussion not only of growth and development, behavior problems, immunizations, and history and physical taking, but a discussion of many of the common problems and disorders encountered in the practice of pediatrics.

Having been in pediatric private practice for 7 years, I would like to emphasize that this compact volume encompasses, in a readily accessible format, much of what is needed by the pediatric practitioner, the pediatric resident, and the medical student in an outpatient pediatrics rotation. I recommend *Handbook of Pediatric Primary Care* as a book that is comprehensive in its subject and that provides references in each chapter to lead the reader to more definitive and longer texts.

William K. Schubert, M.D.

# Preface

*Handbook of Pediatric Primary Care* is written for physicians and nurses providing primary care to infants, children, and adolescents. Its content is geared toward students, residents, and fellows learning about primary care of children and toward recent graduates of pediatric or family medicine residencies who are entering into private practice. I hope it will find a special purpose in pediatric and family medicine continuity clinics, which have become such an important part of the training for primary care physicians in this new age of ambulatory medicine.

The book is divided into three main parts. Part I provides a discussion of the different parameters of health maintenance supervision of infants, children, and adolescents (well-child care). Part II offers a series of shorter chapters addressing everyday illnesses and problems the primary care physician encounters in the care of children. Part II also emphasizes the diagnosis and management of these illnesses and problems *by the primary care physician,* in a cost-effective manner, without undue dependence on subspecialties. Part III covers common topics in behavioral pediatrics.

As in any handbook, the task of compressing a large amount of information into a useable and readable format is difficult. My goal is for this handbook to provide easy access to practical information on well-child care and management of common diseases and problems rather than definitive descriptions of diseases and disease processes. Up-to-date references and reviews are provided at the end of each chapter for the reader who seeks more information about any of the topics discussed.

R.C.B.

# Contributing Authors

**Mary Pat Alfaro, R.D., L.D.**
Research Dietitian, Clinical Research Center, Children's Hospital Medical Center, Cincinnati

**Sherman J. Alter, M.D.**
Associate Professor of Pediatrics, Wright State University School of Medicine; Pediatrician, Division of Infectious Diseases, Dayton Children's Hospital, Dayton, Ohio

**Raymond C. Baker, M.D.**
Professor of Clinical Pediatrics, University of Cincinnati College of Medicine; Pediatrician, Division of General Pediatrics, Children's Hospital Medical Center, Cincinnati

**Paul S. Bellet, M.D.**
Professor of Clinical Pediatrics, University of Cincinnati College of Medicine; Pediatrician, Division of General Pediatrics, Children's Hospital Medical Center, Cincinnati

**Omer G. Berger, M.D.**
Professor of Clinical Pediatrics, University of Cincinnati College of Medicine; Pediatrician, Division of General Pediatrics, Children's Hospital Medical Center, Cincinnati

**Anita Cavallo, M.D.**
Associate Professor of Clinical Pediatrics, University of Cincinnati College of Medicine; Pediatrician, Division of General Pediatrics, Children's Hospital Medical Center, Cincinnati

**Michael K. Farrell, M.D.**
Professor of Pediatrics, University of Cincinnati College of Medicine; Gastroenterologist, Division of Gastroenterology, Children's Hospital Medical Center, Cincinnati

**David N. Franz, M.D.**
Assistant Professor of Pediatrics and Neurology, University of Cincinnati College of Medicine; Neurologist, Division of Neurology, Children's Hospital Medical Center, Cincinnati

**Julie Jaskiewicz, M.D.**
Assistant Professor of Clinical Pediatrics, University of Cincinnati College of Medicine; Pediatrician, Division of General Pediatrics, Children's Hospital Medical Center, Cincinnati

**Ann W. Kummer, Ph.D.**
Field Service Associate Professor, University of Cincinnati College of Medicine; Director, Speech Pathology Department, Children's Hospital Medical Center, Cincinnati

**Christine L. McHenry, M.D.**
Associate Professor of Clinical Pediatrics, University of Cincinnati College of Medicine; Director, Medical Ethics Program, Division of General Pediatrics, Children's Hospital Medical Center, Cincinnati

**Sonya Oppenheimer, M.D.**
Professor of Clinical Pediatrics, University of Cincinnati College of Medicine; Director of Pediatrics, Cincinnati Center for Developmental Disorders, Children's Hospital Medical Center, Cincinnati

**Rosemary E. Schmidt, M.D.**
Professor of Clinical Pediatrics, University of Cincinnati College of Medicine; Pediatrician, Division of General Pediatrics, Children's Hospital Medical Center, Cincinnati

**Janet R. Schultz, Ph.D.**
Associate Professor of Clinical Pediatrics, University of Cincinnati College of Medicine; Director, Division of Child Psychology, Children's Hospital Medical Center, Cincinnati

**Robert A. Shapiro, M.D.**
Associate Professor of Clinical Pediatrics, University of Cincinnati College of Medicine; Director, Child Abuse Program, Division of Emergency Medicine, Children's Hospital Medical Center, Cincinnati

**Robert M. Siegel, M.D.**
Assistant Professor of Clinical Pediatrics, University of Cincinnati College of Medicine; Pediatrician, Division of General Pediatrics, Children's Hospital Medical Center, Cincinnati

**James F. Steiner, D.D.S.**
Professor of Clinical Pediatrics, University of Cincinnati College of Medicine; Assistant Director, Division of Pediatric Dentistry, Children's Hospital Medical Center, Cincinnati

**Jennifer Walker**
Medical Illustrator

# The Well-Child Care Visit

**NOTICE**

The indications for and dosages of all drugs in this book have been recommended in the medical literature and conform to the practices of the general medical community. The medications described do not necessarily have specific approval by the Food and Drug Administration (FDA) for use in the diseases and dosages for which they are recommended. The package insert for each drug should be consulted for use and dosage as approved by the FDA. Because standards for usage change, it is advisable to keep abreast of revised recommendations, particularly those concerning new drugs.

1

# Overview of Well-Child Care

Raymond C. Baker

I. **Routine health maintenance supervision** is the most rewarding aspect of the care of infants, children, and adolescents. The opportunity to practice anticipatory and preventive medicine is greatest during routine well-child checkups and is the cornerstone of pediatric medicine. The importance of well-child care to the pediatrician is apparent if one examines the day-to-day activities of primary care physicians. A 1993 survey of Cincinnati community pediatricians showed that 40% of their time was spent performing well-child examinations, although this percentage varied somewhat with the time of year. Summer and fall are commonly peak times for well-child care, especially of school-age children, whereas during the winter months, there is often an increase in the number of ill-child visits, especially by younger children.

Integral to the provision of routine health maintenance supervision is understanding the concept of anticipatory guidance, which is somewhat unique to the field of pediatrics. Whereas other medical specialties, especially internal medicine, recommend regular health maintenance visits, chronic illness commonly occupies the majority of an internist's time. In pediatrics, on the other hand, the population tends to be healthier, and the routine provision of immunizations provides the opportunity for the physician to interact with patients more frequently and regularly and permits the formation of a bond with the caregiver. Furthermore, since vaccination is regulated and required by law, the caregiver *must* seek the services of the primary care physician. Therefore, pediatric medicine has evolved to incorporate extensive counseling of a preventive nature into routine visits.

The well-child visit in most settings is a combined effort of the physician and nursing or ancillary medical care providers. Growth parameters, vital signs, and the chief complaint usually are obtained during the initial nursing assessment prior to the physician's interaction with the child. With this information, the physician then can obtain the history, perform the physical examination, and counsel the parents (and child) regarding anticipatory guidance and behavioral issues. In many physicians' practices, some of the routine anticipatory guidance relating to safety, development, and nutrition is provided by nursing and ancillary personnel. Other services that may be performed by ancillary personnel with appropriate training may include developmental testing (e.g., the Denver Developmental Screening Test) and visiting children with educational and behavioral problems in the school setting.

Well-child care takes time; the amount of time depends on several factors including (1) the physician's level of training, (2) physician interests, (3) available space (number of exam rooms and support space), (4) number of nursing and ancillary medical providers available, (5) number of ill patients to be seen, and (6) prevalence of chronic illness and psychosocial disorders in the patient population. A lower socioeconomic, medically indigent population tends to have a higher prevalence of medical and psychosocial problems than a middle-class population. In a survey of Cincinnati private pediatricians, the average time spent during a well-child encounter was 15 minutes by the physician and 10 minutes by the nurse. This did not include registration time, waiting time, and checkout time. Ill-child care took somewhat less time—about 10 minutes per patient by the physician and 5 minutes by the nurse. The average number of patients seen in a typical pediatrician's day was about 40.

By contrast, in the pediatric residents' continuity clinic at Cincinnati Children's Hospital, where resident physicians of all levels see patients, four to six patients per 3- to 4-hour clinic is average, with well-child care requiring about 30 minutes and ill-child care 15–20 minutes. Nursing time is relatively less, since resident physicians are encouraged to do the majority of patient education.

Since the amount of time available for personal, one-to-one counseling of the patient may be limited, the physician must choose the topics to cover at each visit. In most instances, the history will provide a clue as to which areas require discussion. Sometimes, in patients with complicated psychosocial problems, reappointment at a later time is necessary so that a greater amount of time can be spent counseling. A physician nearly always can accomplish more during a return appointment scheduled specifically for counseling rather than during a hurried, one-sided discussion of the problem at the end of a routine visit. Written educational materials and a suggested reading list are especially helpful in counseling situations such as these.

**II. The well-child visit: an overview**

**A. Intake visit: first visit to office or clinic.** The first visit for well-child care is characteristically an **intake visit**, at which time extensive historical information is obtained. This should include, in addition to the historical information below (see sec. **II.B**), a detailed maternal, prenatal, and birth history, immunization history, dietary history, history of previous medical and surgical illnesses, family history, and social history. Typically, the first regular office or clinic visit is at 1–4 weeks of age, although whenever a child of any age presents for a first visit having received previous care elsewhere, obtaining an extended history is appropriate to establish a base of information about the child.

**B. Routine visit**. The purpose of the **routine well-child visit** is to monitor the overall physical growth, psychological and physical development, and health of the child and to guide the parent or guardian through the complexities of child rearing. The content of each visit is unique to the child's age and the circumstances of the child's current state of health. Each element of the encounter is geared toward the expected achievements and problems that are related to the particular age and developmental stage of the child.

The history at the routine well-child visit represents a chronicle of the child since the last well-child visit. It should include information concerning past and present problems or illnesses, immunization-related events, achievement of developmental milestones, and nutritional information, including feeding habits and diet content. The history should be elicited from the parent in an informal and empathetic way so the parent will be encouraged to share his or her concerns about the child's behavior and health. Open-ended questions should be used to maximize the parent's opportunity to discuss problems and concerns. The examiner should engage the child in interactive communication using an active question-and-answer approach in the verbal child and by gesture and imitative speech in the preverbal child. The child's active participation allows him or her some control over the encounter and encourages more cooperation and rapport with the physician.

**C.** The **prenatal visit** commonly occurs sometime during the third trimester of pregnancy when prospective parents are selecting their newborn's source of medical care. This visit is the opportunity for future parents to get to know a physician or practice and for the practitioner to advise and discuss with the parents information about breast-feeding and nutrition, circumcision, fee schedules, appointment times, on-call services, well-child schedule, and general philosophy of medical care delivery. Many practices offer prenatal classes supervised either by the physician or nursing personnel and written materials that confirm the information.

**D. Postpartum examination.** The first examination of the newborn by the primary care physician occurs in the hospital nursery—usually within 24 hours after delivery—barring intrapartum and postpartum complications. This examination is important to the physician as the opportunity to review the birth and maternal history and evaluate for congenital abnormalities and neonatal problems. It is important to new parents as an educational visit and an opportunity to ask questions. Many community pediatricians have nursing personnel who perform much of the educational services needed in the newborn setting.

**E. Postdischarge visit.** With the recent move to shorten the hospital stays of postpartum mothers and infants, it has become increasingly important to monitor the first few days home after discharge from the newborn nursery. Common problems that may develop during the first few days of the infant's life are poor weight gain due to difficulties with feeding (especially with breast-feeding), hyperbilirubinemia, and infection. Since it is sometimes difficult for parents to come to the physician's office the first few days after delivery, many hospitals and primary care physicians have initiated programs of routine home visits by nursing personnel. At these visits, the newborn is examined and weighed and may have blood drawn for measuring bilirubin, hematocrit, and hemoglobin levels, and for metabolic screening. A home visit is also an additional opportunity for new parents to ask questions regarding newborn care. Based on these home visits, the physician is able to determine when the first office or clinic visit will be needed and to address any problems reported by the visiting nurse.

F. **Physical examination**. The physical examination of the well child should be complete, including growth parameters of height and weight at each visit, head circumference at least until age 2, and blood pressure beginning at age 3. The child should be undressed for the examination, with gown covering appropriate to age. In the interest of time, some of the history may be obtained during the examination. Time saved in this way may increase the amount of time for counseling the child and caregivers at the end of the examination. During the physical examination, the child's family can be observed informally to determine the appropriateness of interactive skills by the caregiver and the child's reactions. Evaluation of issues such as nurturing and family's psychological health often are better observed directly by the physician rather than relying solely on information in response to questioning.

G. **Assessment**. At the end of the history and physical examination, an assessment of the child's health can be made and should include an assessment of the child's physical growth, neuromotor development, and family interactions (psychosocial health). The assessment forms the groundwork for subsequent planning for screening tests, immunizations, and anticipatory guidance for the family.

H. **Screening tests**. Routine screening tests are performed in children at different ages according to predetermined standards. These are timed to have the greatest yield of abnormals, determine abnormalities at critical times in a child's life (such as school and puberty), and coincide with immunization visits. Routine blood analysis for hemoglobin and hematocrit and lead, vision, hearing, and tuberculin testing are performed according to standards developed by the American Academy of Pediatrics. Other factors including family history, ethnic background, socioeconomic background, and geographic considerations may suggest the need for additional screening.

I. **Immunizations**. In the United States, children routinely are immunized against diphtheria, tetanus, pertussis, poliomyelitis, *Haemophilus influenzae* type B disease, rubeola, rubella, mumps, hepatitis B, and, most recently, varicella, according to standards set by the American Academy of Pediatrics. Medical records must be maintained to reflect the date of administration, dose, lot number, educational materials given to caregivers, and possible immunization reactions. Government regulations regarding immunizations and routine well-child care visits vary from state to state but may require the parent or legal guardian to sign written consent for immunizations (as part of overall consent to treat or separately). In addition, documentation may be required that information regarding immunizations and side effects has been given to the parent or guardian verbally, in written form, or both.

J. **Anticipatory guidance**. At the end of the patient encounter, the physician should sit down with the parent or guardian and discuss the child's health, progress, and suggestions for care that are appropriate to the child's age, including information pertinent to the period of time until the next well-child examination. Areas to be covered include safety, nutrition, behavior, development, discipline, sexuality, and parenting suggestions that relate to the child's age. Most physicians have age-appropriate written materials that are used in conjunction with these discussions to reinforce key points.

**K. Follow-up**. At the conclusion of the discussion, arrangements for the next well-child examination should be made. Any appropriate referrals also may be arranged at this time with appropriate explanation to parents. Nursing discharge procedure should include reviewing by word or brochure the physician's instructions to the patient, follow-up appointment, and how to reach the physician when necessary.

## Selected Readings

Avery ME, First LR (eds). *Pediatric Medicine*. Baltimore: Williams & Wilkins, 1989.

Committee on Psychosocial Aspects of Child and Family Health 1985–1988. *Guidelines for Health Supervision II*. Elk Grove Village, IL: American Academy of Pediatrics, 1988.

Dodds M, Nicholson L, Muse B et al. Group health supervision visits more effective than individual visits in delivering health care information. *Pediatrics* 91:668–670, 1993.

Marks A, Fisher M. Health assessment and screening during adolescence. *Pediatrics* 80(Suppl):135–158, 1987.

McAnarney ER, Kreipe RD, Orr DP et al. *Textbook of Adolescent Medicine*. Philadelphia: Saunders, 1992.

Osborn LM. Effective well-child care. *Curr Probl Pediatr* 24:306–326, 1994.

Schulman JL, Hanley KK. *Anticipatory Guidance: An Idea Whose Time Has Come*. Baltimore: Williams & Wilkins, 1987.

Sharp L, Pantell RH, Murphy LO et al. Psychosocial problems during child health supervision visits: Eliciting, then what? *Pediatrics* 89:619–623, 1992.

# 2

# History


## Christine L. McHenry


The pediatric history is the foundation on which the future physician-patient/parent relationship is built. It is during the history taking that the physician conveys interest or boredom, concern or annoyance, empathy or lack of understanding. It is also a time when the physician conveys respect for the patient and his or her parent(s), which is demonstrated by how the physician addresses the parent (Mr., Mrs., Ms., Mom, Dad) and patient, how the physician dresses, and how the physician responds to comments and questions from the parent and patient.

The goals of the history are (1) to determine why the parent/patient came to see the physician; (2) to determine what the parent/patient is worried about most and why; and (3) to strengthen the physician-patient/parent relationship by observing, listening, and conveying empathy.

I. **The prenatal interview** has been popularized during the last 15 years and can be the first step in developing a therapeutic physician-parent(s) relationship. Ideally, this interview should take place with both father and mother present. Reasonable goals for the prenatal interview include the following:

   A. **Previous problems.** The physician should identify problems encountered with previous pregnancies and deliveries that might affect the health of the newborn such as preterm labor, jaundice and blood incompatibilities, and diabetes mellitus in the mother.

   B. **Potential health problems.** The physician should identify potential health problems of the newborn such as hereditary diseases (e.g., cystic fibrosis, metabolic disorders).

   C. **Office policy.** The physician should acquaint parents with office policies.

   D. **Hospital procedure.** The physician should discuss the birth hospital's procedures for physician notification, the physician's involvement in the infant's postpartum care, and how complications of newborn care are managed (e.g., availability of consulting neonatologists, transfer to outside facilities, and so forth).

   E. **Well-child care.** The physician should inform parents of the schedule for health maintenance examinations (well-child care).

   F. **Parent concerns.** The prenatal interview gives parents the opportunity to ask questions and voice concerns they may have about being new parents.

   G. **Newborn period issues.** The physician should discuss issues related to the newborn period such as breast-feeding versus formula feeding, choice of formula, circumcision, items needed in a newborn home and nursery.

   H. **Psychosocial issues.** The physician should discuss psychosocial issues that might arise from the pregnancy and delivery as well as family support systems, potential need for social agency involvement, and nursing care.

**II. The comprehensive pediatric interview.** The following is an outline for a comprehensive pediatric interview that occurs as part of the well-child examination during the first office visit to see the physician—whether the first regular postpartum visit or the first visit of an older patient transferring to the physician's care. This is not meant to be an exhaustive list of questions to be asked by the physician but a highlight of areas that should be discussed with the parent and patient. Obviously, the interview can be modified according to the age of the patient and the nature of any problems or concerns the parents might have.

Subsequent well-child interviews of established patients are similar, except that certain unchanging information will not have to be sought again, such as family history, social and environmental history (unless there are changes, such as a move to a new home), immunization history (which will already be recorded on the medical record), and previous hospitalizations and chronic illnesses (which already should be indicated in the previously recorded past medical history and problem list).

**A. History of the present illness—interim history.** A chronological narrative of the symptom(s) or problem(s), if any are voiced, should be recorded as clearly as possible. Important areas to explore include when the symptom began, associated symptoms, location, severity, time of day of the symptom, character of the symptom, and factors that tend to exacerbate or relieve the symptom. Equally important is to ask what the parent thinks is going on, what treatment the parent already may have tried for the symptom, and how the patient's symptom is affecting the family. Similarly, the physician should explore behavior problems raised by the parent, including gathering information about the age of onset, precipitating factors, associated incidents, frequency, how the parent has thus far dealt with them, and what the parent thinks is causing the behavior.

**B. Past medical history**

1. **Prenatal, birth, and neonatal histories** are important during the first 2 years of life and when dealing with the patient who is developmentally delayed or neurologically impaired. Prenatal information should include whether the mother received prenatal care (and, if so, where) and cigarette, alcohol, or drug use (prescription or illegal drugs) during pregnancy. Intrapartum information should include mode of birth (vaginal or C-section) and complications during delivery such as prolonged resuscitation in the delivery suite and low Apgar scores. Information about complications of the newborn period should be sought, including information about respiratory and feeding problems, formula changes, and jaundice. These details often can be found on the nursery discharge papers.
2. **Other past medical history**
   **a.** Recurrent or chronic illnesses such as otitis media or asthma.

b. Childhood illnesses (varicella, measles).
c. Hospitalizations.
d. Surgeries.
e. Previous health care, including location, physician, or clinic; immunizations; and reactions to immunizations.
f. Dental care.

C. **Nutritional history.** In the breast-fed infant, information about adequacy (satisfaction, crying, urine output, leakage, "letdown") and maternal complications (nipple soreness, cracking, bleeding) should be sought. In addition, the physician should discuss supplementation with fluoride, iron, and vitamin D. For the formula-fed infant, it is important to know the formula's brand name and how it is stored and prepared (ready-to-feed, concentrate, or powder) and the fluoride content of the available drinking water. If the water is adequately fluoridated, infant formula (powder or concentrate) prepared with water will not require fluoride supplementation. If the infant eats solid food, the types and amounts should be noted.

D. **Developmental history.** At each visit, information about the four areas of development should be reviewed: gross motor, fine motor, social, and language. Level of skill rather than the age of achievement of that skill is the most important information that has an impact on management.

E. **Allergy history.** Particular attention should be paid to reactions to medications. If a parent or patient says he or she is allergic to a medication, the physician should ask about the type of reaction to differentiate true allergy from medication effects such as nausea (e.g., with erythromycin) or vomiting due to bad taste. Allergy information should be displayed prominently in the medical record and problem list.

F. **Medication history.** A list of the child's current medications, doses, and reasons for use should be recorded. Chronic medications should be recorded on the problem list.

G. **Immunization history.** The child's complete immunization schedule should be recorded in the medical record in a standardized location and updated at each well-child visit. The physician should obtain a careful history of reactions to immunizations with attention to the reaction's severity (degree of fever, degree of warmth, swelling or tenderness at the injection site, timing of the reaction relative to the injection, and treatment received for the reaction). Significant reactions (such as those that preclude further immunization with a particular vaccine) should be recorded on the problem list and displayed prominently in the medical record.

H. **Family history.** The family history includes the age, height, weight, and health status of the child's parents and siblings. Many physicians use this opportunity to obtain and record the names of siblings, including nicknames, for use when talking to the child. Significant familial medical conditions might include diabetes, hypertension, renal disease, arthritis, anemia, endocrine disorders, cancer, migraine headache, inflammatory bowel disease, cystic fibrosis, and tuberculosis. Family history should be sought for both maternal and paternal sides out to two generations.

I. **Social and environmental history.** The purpose of a social and environmental history is to develop a sense of the family support system, the environment the patient lives in, and how they affect health. Social and environmental issues that should be addressed include the type of dwelling, how many people live in the dwelling, fluoridation (city water versus well water), type of heat (gas, electric, hot water), pets, parents' occupations, extended family involvement in care, and religious beliefs. Baby-sitter and day-care information also should be obtained as well as information about the family's support structure. Finally, it is important to obtain some information about family finances and health care coverage to optimally provide affordable health care services. Frequently, this information is obtained at the time of registration by office workers for the clinic or physician. The physician must be aware of the payment mechanisms, as this information may influence certain decisions about timing of immunizations, writing for prescription versus over-the-counter medications, and ordering automated blood counts versus simple office-generated hematocrits.

J. **Review of systems.** The review of systems (ROS) includes age-appropriate questions about all the major organ systems. Much of the ROS will be included in the history of the present illness. "High-yield" areas for questioning include bowel habits (frequency, consistency, history of encopresis), urinary habits (dysuria, enuresis, frequency, nocturia), and sleeping habits (night waking, crying, sleepwalking, sleep talking, nightmares, and night terrors). Behavioral issues that should be addressed include temper tantrums, sibling rivalry, mealtime behavior, homework behavior, and discipline in general. A parent may not volunteer information about these issues, but they are of great importance to the family's overall health. If a concern is uncovered, appropriate counseling and intervention may be initiated before the problem becomes a crisis.

## III. Adolescent interview

A. **Autonomy and confidentiality.** Adolescence is a time of developing autonomy and independence. As a result, the adolescent patient is entitled to a certain degree of confidentiality in his or her interaction with the physician. At the beginning of the physician-patient encounter, parameters for confidentiality should be established between physician and patient and between physician and parent.

B. **The adolescent interview.** The adolescent interview includes certain areas that obviously are not a part of the history of a younger child. Most important, the adolescent interview should include questions regarding the following.

1. **Sexual behavior.** The physician should discuss sexual behavior with the adolescent and include the topics of

dating, age of first intercourse, frequency of intercourse, number of partners, contraception, sexually transmitted diseases, and menstrual history.

2. **School behavior.** The physician should ask the adolescent about homework and future plans.
3. **Extracurricular activities.** The physician should discuss with the adolescent the use of drugs, tobacco, and alcohol; participation in sports; and jobs.
4. **Miscellaneous.** The physician should talk to the adolescent about eating disorders, physical and sexual abuse, moods, thoughts of suicide, and relationships with parents, siblings, and peers.

IV. **The ill visit.** The ill-visit interview focuses on a particular problem and includes the following:

A. A **chief complaint** identifying the symptoms or problem.

B. The **history of present illness** including pertinent ROS in which the illness is explored. It is important to include in the history of the present illness what the parent or patient thinks is going on, what the parent already has tried in terms of management, and what is most worrisome to the parent(s) or patient.

C. **Past medical history** including acute and chronic illnesses, hospitalizations, and surgeries. This is usually necessary only if the physician has not taken care of the patient before or does not have available medical records.

D. **Current medications** the patient may be taking (acute and chronic).

E. An **allergy history** should be obtained at every visit and, when present, prominently recorded in the medical record.

F. **Exposures** including family, school, day-care, and friends.

G. **Immunization history** including whether the patient is up-to-date on routine immunizations and the date of the most recent immunization. This history may have an impact on the process of the evaluation of an acute illness (e.g., a recent diphtheria, tetanus, and pertussis [DTP] vaccine in a febrile infant [vaccine reaction], a recent measles immunization in an infant with a rash [vaccine reaction], and a history of complete pertussis series in a patient presenting with cough). Equally important, however, in the case of a patient with a self-limiting problem, is the opportunity an ill visit may afford the physician to update routine immunizations, especially in the case of a noncompliant patient with a poor track record for routine well-child care.

## Selected Readings

American Academy of Pediatrics. *Guidelines for Health Supervision II*. Elk Grove Village, IL: American Academy of Pediatrics, 1988.

Dimond DA. Let's talk about sex. *Contemp Pediatr* July 1992, Pp 19–29.

Goldenring JM, Cohen E. Getting into adolescent heads. *Contemp Pediatr* July 1988, Pp 75–90.

Green M. 20 interview questions that work. *Contemp Pediatr* November 1992, Pp 47–71.

Hoekelman RA, Blatman S, Friedman SB et al (eds). *Primary Pediatric Care*. St. Louis: Mosby, 1987.

Nowak AJ. What pediatricians can do to promote oral health. *Contemp Pediatr* April 1993, Pp 90–106.

# 3

# Physical Examination

Paul S. Bellet

I. **Approach to the physical examination.** The physical examination of an infant, child, or adolescent must be individualized and have a purpose; there is no routine examination. The assessment begins as soon as the physician sees the child and parents. The physician must quickly assess the acuity and severity of the illness, as this determines the speed of the examination and management of the child. The physician notes the child's degree of illness, mood, cry, respiratory pattern, activity, posture, language, nutrition, and developmental skills. The physician also observes the interaction between the child and parents, including displays of affection, amount of separation tolerance, and response to discipline.

During the interview, the physician should try to form a relationship with the child to instill trust and confidence. This involves talking to the child and sometimes playing together. Children usually respond to a physician who is kind and genuinely likes them. When two or more siblings are to be examined, the older one should be examined prior to examining the others. Usually, the older child will be more cooperative and set a good example for younger siblings. If older children request that parents or younger siblings leave the room during the examination, this wish should be respected. Even when examining young children, the physician should explain in simple terms what he or she is going to do during the examination so that the child will understand or at least be less anxious. A child should have the opportunity to touch and hold some of the instruments, such as the stethoscope, reflex hammer, otoscope, and ophthalmoscope. Holding the instruments gives the child a sense of control and participation rather than a feeling that the physician is doing something against his or her will. (It also can be fun for the child.) The physician should be firm but friendly when instructing the child. The physician should not, however, tell children that potentially painful procedures will not hurt, as doing so deceives the child and compromises any established confidence or trust.

Prior to examining a child, the physician should wash his or her hands in view of the parents. The physician's gentle manner in handling, holding, and talking to an infant or young child presents a model of interaction to the parents. Infants and young children may be examined in the parent's arms or lap, giving them a sense of reassurance. The examination should begin with observation prior to any touching, holding, or manipulation. When a complete examination must be performed, the physician should expose only that part of the body to be examined at that time; thus, the child need not be totally undressed during the entire examination. Modesty should be respected in a child regardless of age.

In infants and young children, the physician should examine the lungs, heart, and abdomen first and then move distally before the child tires or becomes restless. The head, including the tympanic membranes and pharynx, should be examined last because this often requires some holding, and infants often cry. Having the parent hold the child's head against the shoulder with one hand and restraining the child's free arm with the other hand allows the physician to examine the child's ears, eyes, nose, throat, and mouth. If this method is unsuccessful, the child can be placed on the examination table, and the parent can hold the child's forearms while leaning against the child's legs, allowing the physician to control the child's head while performing the examination. Some parents have difficulty holding their children properly, and a nurse's assistance may be necessary. An older child can be examined from head to toe as an adult. Areas of pain should be examined toward the end of the examination. In older girls, the genitalia and anus are examined last. One of the most difficult challenges is completing an examination without producing a physical struggle, a crying child, or an upset parent. Meeting the challenge requires all of a physician's skill in gaining the confidence and trust of the child and parents.

II. **Outline of the physical examination.** The proper method of recording the examination may not be in the order the examination is performed, especially in infants and toddlers. The physical examination includes the following:

A. The **general description** of the patient should include whether the child is well- or ill-appearing and acutely or chronically ill-appearing and the child's degree of distress.

B. **Vital signs** should include pulse rate, respiratory rate, blood pressure, height, weight, and head circumference, including percentiles.

C. **Skin** should be examined for rashes, lesions, color, jaundice, and cyanosis. Abnormalities of hair and nails should be noted.

D. The **lymphatic system** should be examined for size, consistency, mobility, tenderness, and location of lymph nodes.

E. **Head** size and shape, fontanelles, sutures, masses, and tenderness should be noted.

F. **Facial** asymmetry, weakness, tenderness, and edema should be noted.

G. The **eyes** should be examined. Extraocular movements; nystagmus; visual fields and acuity; and the condition of the lids (for ptosis, lid lag, edema), conjunctivae (for color, lesions, discharge), sclerae (for color, pigmentation, lesions), pupils (for size, equality, response to light and accommodation), cornea, and fundi should be noted.

H. The **ears** should be examined, including the external ear, canal (for inflammation, discharge, tenderness), tympanic membranes (for color, architecture, perforation, mobility), middle ear (for effusion), mastoid (for tenderness), and for hearing.

I. The **nose** should be examined for patency, mucous membrane condition (for color, discharge, edema, lesions), septum deviation, masses, and foreign bodies. The sinuses should be examined for tenderness.

J. **Mouth and pharynx.** Lips (for color, lesions); tongue (for size, papillae, movement, lesions); teeth (for caries, staining, plaque); gums (for lesions, inflammation); buccal mucosa, palate, tonsillar area, and pharynx (for color, masses, lesions); and tonsils (for size, color, exudate, peritonsillar tissue) should be examined.

**K.** The **neck** should be examined for mobility, tenderness, masses, condition of thyroid (for size, tenderness, nodules), and torticollis.

**L.** **Breasts** should be given a sexual maturity rating and examined for symmetry, tenderness, masses, and the condition of glandular tissue and nipples (for discharge, retraction, ulceration).

**M.** The **thorax and lungs** should be examined for shape; symmetry; masses; scars; position of the trachea; tenderness of skin, muscle, ribs, and sternum; expansion, retraction, or abnormal movement of the chest; presence and location of wheezes, rhonchi, rales, or rubs; and location of abnormalities by changes in breath sounds, percussion, tactile fremitus, and whispered or spoken sounds.

**N. Cardiovascular system**

1. **Heart.** The physician should ascertain the rate and rhythm, character, and location of the heart's apical pulse; presence of a right ventricular impulse, pulsations, thrills, clicks, rubs, and gallops, intensity and splitting of first and second heart sounds, murmurs (location, timing, intensity [grade 1 to 6], duration, quality, pitch, and radiation).
2. **Peripheral vascular system**
   a. **Jugular veins.** The physician should examine the jugular veins for distention and pulsation, noting the patient's position and distention in centimeters above the clavicle or above the sternal angle.
   b. **Arterial pulses.** The physician should examine the arterial pulses (carotid, radial, femoral, popliteal, posterior tibial, and dorsalis pedis), amplitude and contour of the pulse, and strength of pulses (grade 0 = absent, grade 1 = decreased, grade 2 = normal, grade 3 = increased, and grade 4 = full and bounding).
   c. **Extremities.** The physician should examine the extremities, noting edema, color, temperature, and capillary refill.

**O.** **Abdominal** size, contour, symmetry, scars, distention, visible movements, peristalsis, tenderness, edema, masses (location, size, consistency, tenderness, mobility, pulsations), and hernias should be noted. Palpable organs (liver, spleen, kidneys, bladder, and uterus), and the umbilicus should be examined.

**P. Genital examination**

1. The **male's** penis (for circumcision, prepuce, urethral meatus, discharge, inflammation, lesions), scrotum (testes, epididymis), and perineum should be examined.
2. The **female's** external genitalia (labia, clitoris, introitus, urethral orifice, and perineum) should be examined. Pelvic examination includes examination of the vagina, cervix, fundus, adnexal areas, and cul-de-sac (for inflammation, discharge, tenderness, masses, erosions).

Q. **Anal and rectal** examination includes examination of the perianal area, sphincter (for tone), anal canal, rectum (for masses, tenderness, and blood), and prostate (for size, masses, consistency, and tenderness). Fissures, hemorrhoids, and fistulas should be noted.

R. **Skeletal system**. The physician should examine the back (for scoliosis), hips, upper and lower extremities, bones (for tenderness and deformity), joints (for range of motion, deformity, swelling, redness, warmth, tenderness, and crepitation), ligaments, bursae, and tendons (for swelling, redness, warmth, tenderness, and tendon contracture).

S. **Neurologic examination**

1. The physician should assess the patient's **general status,** including appearance, behavior, speech, language, posture, gait, and gross coordination.
2. The physician should assess function of **cranial nerves I–XII.**
3. The physician should assess the **motor system**, including movement, handedness and muscle mass, strength, tone, coordination, and fasciculation. Contracture, tenderness, tremors, and involuntary movements should be noted.
4. The physician should assess the patient's **sensory system,** including sensitivity to light touch, pain, temperature, position, and vibration; stereognosis; tactile localization; two-point discrimination; and higher cortical function (noting any aphasia, agnosia, and apraxia).
5. **Reflexes** should be assessed, including those of the triceps, biceps, brachioradialis, knee, ankle, sole of the foot (plantar reflex), abdomen, jaw (jaw jerk), cremaster, fingers and toes (grasp reflex), and anus. Strength of reflexes may be described as follows: Grade 0 = absent, grade 1 = decreased, grade 2 = normal, grade 3 = increased, and grade 4 = with clonus. Abnormal reflexes should be noted.
6. **Spinal nerve irritation** should be noted, including meningeal signs and sciatic pain (straight-leg raising).

T. **Mental status examination.** The patient's general behavior and psychological status usually are included in the general description of the patient. When a mental status examination is performed, include the following:

1. **Behavior**. Note unusual or bizarre conduct and mannerisms.
2. **Cognitive function.** Note orientation to time and place, attention, recent and past memory, general information, and judgment.
3. **Thought content**. Note any illogical or bizarre behavior; depersonalized affect; feelings of unreality or persecution; delusions; compulsive, phobic, or obsessive thoughts.
4. **Perception.** Note illusions and hallucinations (auditory, visual, tactile, gustatory, olfactory).
5. **Affect and mood.** Note whether affect and mood are appropriate and whether the patient appears to be anxious, depressed, helpless, hopeless, suicidal, euphoric, manic, guilty, ashamed, panicked, hostile, or irritable.

**III. Newborn**. The physical examination of the newborn should include an initial assessment in the delivery room (including inspection and Apgar scoring) followed by a complete examination in the nursery. The newborn should be examined briefly after birth to determine the general condition of his or her cardiorespiratory, gastrointestinal, and neurologic systems and to detect any gross abnormalities or congenital anomalies. In the nursery, specifics to observe are the following:

**A. General appearance.** Note any dysmorphic features.

**B.** Note **vital signs** and appropriateness of weight for gestational age.

**C. Skin.** Note any jaundice, cyanosis, or rashes.

**D. Head, ears, eyes, nose, and mouth.** Examine the fontanelles, sutures, shape of the ears and position, tongue, and palate. Check for the red reflex, nasal patency, and natal teeth. Look for signs of birth trauma, abnormal eye movements, or cataracts.

**E. Neck**. Note any masses or torticollis.

**F. Breasts.** Note neonatal hypertrophy.

**G. Thorax and lungs.** Note configuration, clavicles, respirations, and breath sounds.

**H. Heart.** Check impulses, heart sounds, murmurs, and peripheral pulses (especially femoral pulses).

**I. Abdomen.** Note distention, hepatosplenomegaly, masses, and bowel sounds. Palpate kidneys, and examine umbilicus.

**J. Genitalia**

1. In the **male**, note phallus length, and examine testes and meatal opening.
2. In the **female**, note clitoral size, examine the introitus, and check for virilization.

**K. Anus and rectum**. Note patency and position of the anus.

**L. Skeletal system.** Examine extremities (for anomalies), the spine (for defects, sinuses), and hips (for dislocation or instability). Note movement and in utero positional deformity versus a fixed deformity.

**M. Neurologic.** Note overall state of alertness, vigor of cry, tone, movement, reflexes (deep tendon and primitive), and response to light and voice.

**N. Behavioral.** Note alertness, response to holding, feeding, voice, and overall degree of activity.

**IV. Subsequent visits**. A complete examination should be performed at each well-child visit with particular attention given to parental concerns or risk (based on the history). Gross and fine motor development, language, and personal social interaction should be assessed at each visit (see Chaps. 9 and 10). Hearing and vision also should be assessed at each well-child visit. The assessment can be done subjectively in a young child and then objectively as the child becomes older. For an illness visit, the nature of the problem dictates the examination.

**A. Two-week visit**. The first regular visit usually occurs at 1–4 weeks of age, depending on infant and parent needs. The physician should be prepared to take the time to listen and answer the parents' questions without hurrying. The examination is generally the same as in the nursery. The physician should pay particular attention to how feeding is progressing and whether any weight gain has occurred, recognizing that due to normal postnatal weight loss, the infant may not regain birth weight until 1 week of age.

B. **Two-month visit**. The hips should be carefully examined for instability or dislocation because congenital dislocation may not be evident at birth. If metatarsus adductus is fixed so that the foot cannot be maneuvered to neutral, the infant should be referred to an orthopedic physician. With flexible metatarsus adductus, the physician should instruct parents in stretching exercises to correct the abnormality.

C. **Four-month visit**. The posterior fontanelle usually is closed by this age. The physician should note the infant's ability to follow an object 180 degrees in the horizontal plane and the presence of penile or labial adhesions.

D. **Six-month visit**. The anterior fontanelle may begin to close (usual range is 9–18 months). The lower central incisors may start to erupt, but this is variable and may be seen normally up to 15 months of age. Any strabismus after 6 months of age is abnormal and may be detected by the central light reflex test or the cover-uncover test. If suspected, the infant should be referred to an ophthalmologist. Hearing should be checked by observing whether the child turns to sound. The tonic neck reflex and Moro's reflex should not be present.

E. **Nine-month visit**. At this age, healthy children may experience slowed weight gain due to decreased milk intake associated with increased intake of solids.

F. **Twelve-month visit**. The Babinski reflex (i.e., upgoing toes) may be normal until 1 year of age.

G. **Fifteen- and 18-month and 2-year visits**. One well-child visit should occur at either 15 or 18 months of age. At these visits, the physician should pay particular attention to growth and developmental parameters.

H. **Three-year visit**. Blood pressure should be measured if it has not been measured previously. Three years is probably the earliest age at which visual acuity can be measured reliably (e.g., Allen picture cards). If vision in either eye is unequal or the gaze is not conjugate, refer the child to an ophthalmologist. If the child's speech is less than 50% understandable or delayed, the physician should consider referral to a speech pathologist.

I. **Four-, 5-, and 6-year-old visits**. At least once between 4 and 6 years of age, objective vision and hearing screening should be performed. A child's development, particularly language and personal social interaction, should be evaluated.

J. **School-age visits**. These examinations may be performed yearly or every other year. Height, weight, and blood pressure should be measured and recorded at each visit. The back should be examined for scoliosis (bend test). School performance should be addressed.

K. **Adolescent visit**. In general, the physical examination of the adolescent should include all aspects of a younger child's examination. Routine visits for well adolescents can be scheduled every 2 years. It is not necessary for the examination to be supervised by either a parent or nurse unless the adolescent wishes the parent to be in the room. When a pelvic or rectal examination is to be performed on a female patient and the physician is a male, a female nurse or nursing assistant must be in the room. The decision about whether to perform a pelvic examination is determined by the patient's complaints and whether she is sexually active.

V. **Other comments.** Breast examination should become a regular part of the physical assessment starting from the time of breast budding, usually between 9 and 12 years of age. It is important to inspect the genitalia and determine the Tanner stage of sexual development. A rectal examination for either a male or female is not part of the routine physical examination but depends on the clinical circumstances.

## Selected Readings

Athreya BH, Silverman BK. *Pediatric Physical Diagnosis*. Norwalk, CT: Appleton-Century-Crofts, 1985.

Avery ME, First LR (eds). *Pediatric Medicine* (2nd ed). Baltimore: Williams & Wilkins, 1994.

Barness LA. *Manual of Pediatric Physical Diagnosis* (6th ed). St Louis: Mosby-Year Book, 1991.

Behrman RE (ed). *Nelson Textbook of Pediatrics* (14th ed). Philadelphia: Saunders, 1992.

American Academy of Pediatrics. *Guidelines for Health Supervision II*. Elk Grove Village, IL: American Academy of Pediatrics, 1988.

Green M. *Green and Richmond Pediatric Diagnosis* (5th ed). Philadelphia: Saunders, 1992.

Hoekelman RA. The Physical Examination in Infants and Children. In B Bates (ed), *A Guide to Physical Examination and History Taking* (6th ed). Philadelphia: Lippincott, 1995.

McAnarney ER, Kreipe RE, Orr DP et al. (eds). *Textbook of Adolescent Medicine*. Philadelphia: Saunders, 1992.

Morgan WL, Engel GL. *The Clinical Approach to the Patient*. Philadelphia: Saunders, 1969.

Rudolph AM (ed). *Rudolph's Pediatrics* (19th ed). Norwalk, CT: Appleton & Lange, 1991.

# 4

# Screening Tests

## Omer G. Berger

Screening tests as a part of health maintenance supervision are performed to identify clinically undetected problems, disorders, or risk factors in childhood. Before deciding to implement a routine screening test, a cost-versus-benefit assessment should be undertaken. *Benefits* include early diagnosis and prevention of disability, retardation, or perhaps even death. *Costs* extend beyond monetary considerations and include psychological trauma and whether effective therapy exists to deal with the identified problem.

I. **Newborn metabolic disorders.** All states require newborn blood sampling for various metabolic and genetic disorders, including phenylketonuria (PKU), congenital hypothyroidism, galactosemia, and homocystinuria. (Early discharge from the hospital may dictate the need for repeat testing to accurately screen for PKU.) In 1987, the National Institutes of Health (NIH) recommended universal screening for hemoglobinopathies, which now has been implemented in many states.

II. **Hypertension.** Routine screening for hypertension should begin at age 3 years. Blood pressure should be taken using an appropriately sized cuff with the child in the sitting position and the arm at the level of the heart. The fourth Korotkoff's sound should be used as the diastolic pressure until children are 12 years of age. Appendix F contains normative values for blood pressure according age, sex, and height. Hypertension is defined as readings from three separate visits that are equal to or greater than the ninety-fifth percentile.

III. **Urinalysis and culture.** Routine urinalysis no longer is recommended as part of routine well-child care, as the yield is very small in the absence of an abnormal history and physical examination. Several historical and clinical aspects of routine care may suggest the need for urinalysis and/or urine culture, however. These include enuresis, dysuria, polyuria, urgency, pollakiuria, family or personal history of hematuria, urinary tract infection, proteinuria, or diabetes mellitus.

IV. **Tuberculosis (TB).** Routine screening for TB is recommended for all children. The frequency and timing of TB testing depend on the prevalence of TB in the geographic area and individual risk factors, including family history or exposure, recent immigration from countries with significant prevalence of tuberculosis, and family or household contact with someone at increased risk (e.g., history of incarceration, human immunodeficiency virus).

A. **For low-risk groups**, TB skin tests traditionally have been performed at 12–15 months, 4–6 years, and early adolescence. Multiple puncture tests no longer are recommended, even for screening, and should be replaced with the intradermal purified protein derivative (of tuberculin) (PPD) test. For children with no high-risk factors based on history and for those who live in areas of the country with a low prevalence of TB, routine testing may be performed less frequently.

**B. For children in high-risk groups** or households with active cases, *annual* intradermal PPD (Mantoux) skin tests are advised.

**V. Anemia and iron deficiency.** The incidence of iron deficiency has decreased but remains the most prevalent deficiency state in children. Because anemia is a late sign of iron deficiency, physicians must be able to use the tests that assist in *early* identification. Red blood cell indices are among the most useful and available. In iron deficiency, the mean corpuscular volume (MCV) is decreased while the red blood cell distribution width (RDW) and protoporphyrins increase. Serum ferritin is the gold standard of iron status determination but tends to be more costly. Most primary care physicians screen with a CBC with red cell indices. If the results suggest iron deficiency, an iron supplementation trial usually is begun without confirmation by serum ferritin. The optimal age of screening is 12–24 months of age, as the toddler diet tends to be low in iron due to the change from iron-fortified formula or breast milk to cow's milk. Infants especially at risk are those older than 12 months of age with prolonged bottle-feeding with cow's milk.

**VI. Cholesterol.** For children older than 2 years of age whose parents or grandparents have a history of coronary disease prior to 55 years of age, the American Academy of Pediatrics recommends a fasting lipid profile. For children whose parents have an elevated total cholesterol level (>240 mg/dl), a total cholesterol level is recommended. In one large study, 38% of all children in whom adequate history was available satisfied criteria for cholesterol testing. Histories, however, are often incomplete or not available. In such instances, the presence of other factors (e.g., obesity or hypertension) may assist in identifying those in need of screening.

**VII. Vision testing.** Subjective vision testing is carried out by history and physical exam at each well-child visit. Objective visual acuity determination using the Snellen charts or Allen cards should be initiated at age 3–4 years. Children with decreased acuity (<20/60) and children with more than two lines of disparity between eyes are indications for referral to an ophthalmologist. One of the goals of screening is to identify children with unilateral refractive errors so that amblyopia can be treated and prevented. Routine vision screening should be carried out every year in school-age children.

**VIII. Hearing testing.** Subjective hearing screening is recommended for each well-child visit. Most parents are aware of their child's auditory acuity and are able to recognize when the infant lateralizes to sound. Children can be objectively screened using pure-tone audiometry by the time the child is approximately 5 years of age. When language delays are identified, audiology referrals may be indicated. Infants with medical problems associated with hearing loss may merit early referral to audiology for field audiometry or auditory brain stem response (ABR). Examples of these entities include anomalies of the external ear, bacterial central nervous system infection, hyperbilirubinemia, family history of hearing loss, marked prematurity, low Apgar scores, and failure of routine neonatal screening tests.

**IX. Lead poisoning.** Risk of lead exposure should be determined in infants by the age of 6 months. High-risk children include those living in dwellings built before 1960, especially those in poor condition, and those with a sibling who has be identified as having an elevated lead level. Children with increased hand-to-mouth behaviors are also at risk. Other factors include a history of home remodeling and certain parental occupations with lead exposure. High-risk children should be screened at age 6 months and every 6 months until the lead has been shown to remain below 10 μg/dl. Children without risk factors may be screened at approximately 12–15 months of age and at 24–30 months of age. Blood lead concentrations greater than 10 μg/dl require follow-up and those above 20 μg/dl should be repeated promptly (venous sample). Blood lead concentrations above 45 μg/dl constitute a medical emergency, and consultation should be obtained.

**X. Development.** An important part of the history and physical examination in routine health maintenance visits is developmental screening, which should be done at every visit. When motor or communication delay is suspected by the physician's screening developmental examination, a follow-up assessment should be made. If a deficit or delay persists, a formal standardized screening test may be indicated.

First published in 1967 and extensively revised in 1992, the Denver Development Screening Test (DDST) is widely used. Administration of the DDST-II requires 20–30 minutes, depending on the child's age and cooperation. This test is standardized and can be administered by nursing and other ancillary personnel following appropriate training. Failure of the DDST indicates referral for evaluation by a pediatric developmentalist.

## Selected Readings

American Academy of Pediatrics, Committee on Nutrition. Statement on cholesterol. *Pediatrics* 90:469–473, 1992.

American Academy of Pediatrics. Tuberculosis. In G Peter (ed), *1994 Red Book: Report of the Committee on Infectious Diseases* (23rd ed). Elk Grove Village, IL: American Academy of Pediatrics, 1994. Pp 480–500.

Centers for Disease Control. *Preventing Lead Poisoning in Young Children*. Atlanta: Centers for Disease Control, October 1991.

Dallman P, Yip R. Changing characteristics of childhood anemia. *J Pediatr* 114:161–164, 1989.

Dennison BA et al. Challenges to implementing the current pediatric cholesterol screening guidelines into practice. *Pediatrics* 94:296–302, 1994.

Frankenburg WK, Dodds J, Archer P et al. The Denver II: A major revision and restandardization of the Denver Developmental Screening Test. *Pediatrics* 89:91–97, 1992.

Romano PE. Vision/eye screening. *Pediatr Ann* June 1990, Pp 359–363.

# 5

# Immunizations

**Robert M. Siegel**

Active immunization by inoculating the host with all or part of a microorganism has been used for centuries. The first attempts at active immunization were pioneered in the Middle East and China by taking the residue of healing smallpox scars and introducing it to a host by intranasal or dermal inoculation. English physician Edward Jenner observed that milkmaids exposed to cowpox were immune to smallpox. Consequently, he developed the first safe, effective vaccine against smallpox using the cowpox virus. With the advent of routine immunization, smallpox has been totally eradicated and several other illnesses significantly reduced in prevalence. Vaccines now have been developed against many infectious agents, and more than 20 vaccines currently are available in the United States (Table 5-1).

I. **Routine childhood immunizations.** Vaccination against childhood illnesses clearly has been one of the most cost-effective responses to illnesses to date. Over the past 50 years, there have been remarkable declines in polio, measles, mumps, rubella, diphtheria, tetanus, and pertussis. Unfortunately, however, immunization rates have fallen in preschool children. Experts estimate that for every $1 spent on immunizations, $10 is saved in treatment costs. In this age of medical reform and cost containment, it is imperative that every effort be made to appropriately immunize every child who comes into contact with the medical system at every opportunity available. The routine immunization schedule of healthy children is shown in Table 5-2.

II. **General principles of childhood vaccination**

A. **Live vaccines**, unless given simultaneously, should not be given within a month of each other. Recent receipt of the oral polio vaccine, however, does not contraindicate receiving the measles, mumps, and rubella vaccine at the appropriate time.

B. In general, vaccines should not be given within 6 months of receiving a **gamma globulin product**, with the exception of hepatitis, rabies, or tetanus prophylaxis vaccines or in the event of international travel.

C. **Premature infants** should be kept on the same vaccination schedule as full-term infants; split doses of vaccine are unnecessary.

D. **Lapsed immunizations** do not require reinstitution of an entire vaccine series; immunizations should be given as though the proper interval has elapsed.

E. **A child whose vaccination status is uncertain** should be considered unimmunized and given appropriate vaccines.

F. A child's **immunization status should be reviewed** at every physician or medical caregiver visit to update immunizations. Even during ill-child visits at the primary care

**Table 5-1. Vaccines licensed in the United States, type of vaccine, and routes of administration**

| Vaccine | Route | Type |
|---|---|---|
| BCG | ID/SC | Live, bacterial |
| Diphtheria | IM | Toxoid |
| Hepatitis A | IM | Inactivated, viral |
| Hepatitis B | IM | Inactivated, viral antigen |
| *Haemophilus influenzae* | IM | Polysaccharide/protein conjugate |
| Measles | SC | Live, viral |
| Meningococcal | SC/IM | Polysaccharide |
| Mumps | SC | Live, viral |
| Pertussis | IM | Inactivated, bacterial |
| Pneumococcal | IM/SC | Polysaccharide |
| Polio IPV | SC | Inactivated, viral |
| Polio OPV | PO | Live, viral |
| Rabies | IM/ID | Inactivated, viral |
| Tetanus | SC | Toxoid |
| Varicella | SC | Live, viral |

BCG = bacille Calmette-Guérin; IPV = inactive polio vaccine; OPV = oral polio vaccine.
Source: Adapted from American Academy of Pediatrics. Active and Passive Immunization. In G Peter (ed), *1994 Red Book: Report of the Committee on Infectious Diseases* (23rd ed). Elk Grove Village, IL: American Academy of Pediatrics, 1994. P 11.

location or emergency facility, immunization status should be considered, as these visits may represent an opportunity to update immunizations (provided the degree of illness does not preclude administration of vaccines). Updating immunization records is especially important for the frequent emergency room visitor for whom medical compliance is unlikely.

**G.** A **pamphlet of patient immunization education materials** listing each vaccine's common adverse reactions should be given to parents, and informed consent should be obtained during each immunization visit.

**H.** There are **no contraindications** to simultaneous administration of multiple vaccines routinely recommended for infants and children.

**III. Immunizations in those who are not up-to-date**

**A.** Tables 5-3 and 5-4 contain guidelines for the immunization of children who are behind in immunizations.

**B.** Whereas most children generally have been fully immunized by school entry, **many American preschool children are behind in immunization status**. Some studies suggest that as many as 50% of inner-city children younger than 2 are underimmunized. Many of these children have missed multiple opportunities by health care workers to immunize them. Common causes of missed opportunities include physicians' misunderstanding of contraindications of vaccination and using only well-child checks for immunization. If a child is behind in immuniza-

**Table 5-2. Recommended vaccine schedule for healthy infants and children**

| Visit | Vaccine | Remarks |
|---|---|---|
| Birth | HBV | Can be initiated at 2 mos and boosted at 4 and 6 mos or initiated at 2 wks and boosted at 4 and 6 mos |
| 1 mo | HBV | — |
| 2 mos | DTP/Hib[a], OPV | 2-mo interval (minimum of 6 wks) |
| 4 mos | DTP/Hib[a], OPV | — |
| 6 mos | DTP/Hib[a], HBV, OPV | OPV and HBV vaccine may be given at 6–18 mos |
| 12–15 mos | MMR[b], DTP/Hib[a], Varc | Tuberculin testing may be done at 12 mos or at this visit<br>DTP booster vaccination should be given a minimum of 6 mos after the third dose of DTP vaccine |
| 4–6 yrs | DTP[d], OPV, MMR[b] | MMR vaccination is recommended at 6 yrs (primary school entry) or 12 yrs (secondary school entry) |
| 14–16 yrs | Td | Repeat every 10 yrs throughout life |

[a]DTP and Hib (conjugate vaccine) vaccines are available combined or separately; acellular pertussis vaccine may be used in those ≥ 15 mos old.
[b]MMR vaccination schedule differs during a measles outbreak.
[c]A single dose of varicella vaccine is recommended between ages 12 and 18 mos and may be given simultaneously with other vaccines recommended at the same age (MMR, OPV, DTP, DTaP, Hib).
[d]DTP vaccine can be given up to 7 yrs of age.
Source: Adapted from American Academy of Pediatrics. Active and Passive Immunization. In G Peter (ed), *1994 Red Book: Report of the Committee on Infectious Diseases* (23rd ed). Elk Grove Village, IL: American Academy of Pediatrics, 1994. P 23.

tions, every effort should be made to vaccinate the child with *every* medical encounter.

IV. **Misconceptions about immunization**. Many misconceptions persist among health care providers about what constitutes contraindications to vaccination. True contraindications are discussed in individual vaccine sections. Table 5-5 lists factors that are *not* contraindications to vaccination but often are erroneously thought to be ("old physicians' tales").

V. **Common side effects and special considerations**

A. **Diphtheria, tetanus, and pertussis (DTP).** The DTP vaccine, because of the pertussis component, is the most

**Table 5-3. Suggested vaccine schedule for children younger than age 7 not immunized during the first year of life**

| Visit | Vaccine | Remarks |
|---|---|---|
| First visit | DTP/Hib, OPV | MMR vaccine if child ≥15 mos; tuberculin, MMR, and HBV[a] testing may be done at the same visit<br>Hib given if child is <60 mos |
| 2 mos after first visit | DTP/Hib, OPV, HBV, Var[b] | Second dose of Hib vaccine is indicated only if first dose was given before 15 mos |
| 4 mos after first visit | DTP, OPV, HBV | Third OPV is optional<br>Alternative HBV vaccination is 0, 1, and 6 mos |
| 10–16 mos after first visit | DTP, OPV | — |
| 4–6 yrs | DTP, OPV, MMR | DTP vaccination is not necessary if fourth dose was given after fourth birthday |
| 11–12 yrs | MMR, HBV series[b] | At entry to secondary school |
| 14 yrs (or 10 yrs after last DTP vaccination) | Td | Repeat every 10 yrs |

[a]HBV vaccine series may be delayed until secondary school entry.
[b]A single dose of varicella vaccine is recommended in children <13 yrs of age without a history of varicella infection. Two doses 4–8 weeks apart are recommended in adolescents age 13 yrs and older without a history of varicella.
Source: Adapted from American Academy of Pediatrics. Active and Passive Immunization. In G Peter (ed), *1994 Red Book: Report of the Committee on Infectious Diseases* (23rd ed). Elk Grove Village, IL: American Academy of Pediatrics, 1994. P 24.

common to cause side effects in children and the vaccine most often involved in litigation. For the two most catastrophic associations of the DTP vaccine—encephalopathy and sudden infant death—no scientific evidence exists suggesting causation, and these complications no longer should be thought to be side effects of the vaccine. The vaccine, however, has many side effects, which are listed in Table 5-6.

Parents should be made aware of all these possible side effects and encouraged to report any adverse events. The pertussis component should be withheld if any of the following adverse events occur after immunization.

1. **Encephalopathy** within 7 days.
2. A **convulsion** with or without fever within 3 days.
3. Persistent, inconsolable **screaming** for 3 or more hours with high-pitched cry within 48 hours.
4. **Collapse or shocklike state** within 48 hours.
5. An immediate **allergic reaction** to the vaccine.

**Table 5-4. Suggested vaccine schedule for children older than age 7 not immunized during the first year of life**

| Visit | Vaccine | Remarks |
|---|---|---|
| First visit | Td, OPV, MMR, HBV | HBV series may be delayed until secondary school entry at 11–12 yrs |
| 2 mos after first visit | Td, OPV, HBV, Var* | — |
| 8–14 mos after first visit | Td, OPV, HBV | — |
| 11–12 yrs old | MMR, HBV series | HBV vaccination if not given earlier Given at this visit, 1 mo, and 5 mos after this visit |
| 10 yrs after last Td | Td | Repeat every 10 yrs throughout life |

*A single dose of varicella vaccine is recommended in children <13 yrs of age without a history of varicella infection. Two doses 4–8 weeks apart are recommended in adolescents age 13 yrs and older without a history of varicella.
Source: Adapted from American Academy of Pediatrics. Active and Passive Immunization. In G Peter (ed), *1994 Red Book: Report of the Committee on Infectious Diseases* (23rd ed). Elk Grove Village, IL: American Academy of Pediatrics, 1994. P 24.

**Table 5-5. False contraindications to DTP immunization**

Reaction to a previous dose of DTP vaccine with only soreness, redness, or swelling in the immediate vicinity of the vaccination or a temperature of <105°F
Mild acute illness with low-grade fever or mild diarrheal illness in an otherwise well child
Current antimicrobial therapy or convalescent phase of illness
Prematurity (vaccines should be given at normal chronological age)
Pregnancy in mother or another household contact
Recent exposure to an infectious disease
Breast-feeding
A history of nonspecific allergies or relatives with allergies
Allergy to penicillin or any other antibiotic agent (except anaphylactic reaction to neomycin or streptomycin)
Duck allergy (no vaccine available in the United States is produced in substrates containing duck antigens)
A family history of convulsions in children who require vaccination against pertussis or measles
A family history of sudden infant death syndrome in children who require DTP vaccination
A family history of an adverse event unrelated to immunosuppression after vaccination

**Table 5-6. Adverse events occurring within 48 hours of whole-cell pertussis immunization**

| Category | Percent |
|---|---|
| Fretfulness | 53.0 |
| Pain at site | 51.0 |
| Fever >100.4°F | 47.0 |
| Swelling at site | 40.4 |
| Redness at site | 37.4 |
| Drowsiness | 32.0 |
| Anorexia | 21.0 |
| Redness >2.5 cm in diameter | 7.2 |
| Vomiting | 6.0 |
| Persistent crying for >3 hrs | 1.0 |
| Fever >104.9°F | 0.3 |
| High-pitched, unusual cry | 0.1 |
| Convulsions | 0.06 |
| Collapse with shocklike state | 0.06 |

Source: Adapted from American Academy of Pediatrics. Pertussis. In G Peter (ed), *1991 Red Book: Report of the Committee on Infectious Diseases* (22nd ed). Elk Grove Village, IL: American Academy of Pediatrics, 1991. P 364.

The only other absolute contraindication to pertussis vaccination is a progressive neurologic disorder. Those with a history of seizures or with a disorder that puts them at risk for seizures should be evaluated on an individual basis.

Recently, the Food and Drug Administration (FDA) approved an acellular pertussis vaccine combined with the DT vaccine (DTaP) for use in children age 15 months–7 years that has a lower incidence of fever and local reaction. This product eventually will be licensed for use in younger children and should be considered in those with a family or personal history of seizures.

B. **Poliomyelitis.** Oral polio vaccine (OPV) (Sabin) has been associated with paralysis on very rare occasions. Immune-compromised individuals are at higher risk for paralysis. The inactive polio vaccine (IPV) has no known serious side effects and should be substituted for OPV in children with the following conditions:
   1. Children with an **immunodeficiency disease or on immunosuppressive therapy**.
   2. Children infected with the **human immunodeficiency virus (HIV)**.
   3. Children who have a household **contact with altered immunity**.

C. **Measles, mumps, and rubella (MMR).** The MMR vaccine is indicated in all healthy children and should be given in 2 doses prior to 12 years of age. Some confusion exists regarding the appropriate age to give the second booster dose. The American Academy of Pediatrics (AAP) chose 12 years of age or secondary school entry for the second dose, and the Centers for Disease Control (CDC) recommended age 6 or primary school entry. The latter recommendation may be more feasible, as most states mandate school sys-

**Table 5-7. Contraindications to the MMR vaccine**

| Condition | Comments |
|---|---|
| Pregnancy | Theoretical risk of fetal damage |
| Anaphylaxis to egg ingestion | Vaccinate after skin testing |
| Anaphylactic allergy to neomycin | Vaccine contains neomycin |
| Immunoglobulin within 3 mos | Blunts immune response |
| Immunocompromised except HIV (includes chronic steroids) | Possibility of severe symptomatic infection |

tems to monitor immunizations and exclude from school those children not appropriately immunized at primary school entry.

The MMR vaccination schedule is altered in areas of increased incidence of measles (first dose at 12 months) or if an outbreak occurs (first dose at 6 months with repeat doses at 15 months and school entry).

The most common adverse reaction to the MMR vaccine is fever in 5–15% of recipients about 1 week after vaccination. Rash is described in 5% receiving the vaccine. Febrile seizures can occur, but there is no evidence of any permanent sequelae. Subacute sclerosing panencephalitis (SSPE), a known, devastating effect of the measles virus, has been described in patients with no history of natural measles infection but with a history of measles vaccination. While SSPE may be a very rare adverse reaction to the MMR vaccine, the incidence of SSPE has declined drastically since the introduction of the vaccine. Table 5-7 lists contraindications to the MMR vaccine.

**D. *Haemophilus influenzae* type B.** Since the introduction of the first *Haemophilus influenzae* type B (Hib) vaccine in 1985 and the conjugate vaccine in 1990, Hib infection has declined dramatically in the United States. Several Hib conjugate vaccines, including one combined with the DTP vaccine (Tetramune by Lederle Laboratories), now exist. Side effects from the vaccines are very rare. All of the available vaccines give immunity with one dose when given to a child who is 15 months or older. Most of the conjugate Hib vaccines except Connaught's vaccine (Prohibit) are given routinely at 2, 4, and 6 months of age simultaneously with the DTP vaccine primary series to achieve immunity at a younger age. There should be 2 months between vaccinations when given before 15 months of age. A booster dose is recommended between 12 and 15 months of age. One of the conjugate Hib vaccines (Tetramune) has been combined with the DTP vaccine for easier administration at these ages. Table 5-8 summarizes the Hib immunization schedule.

**E. Hepatitis B virus (HBV).** In 1992, the AAP recommended the HBV vaccine be administered to all infants and high-risk children and adolescents. Immunization of healthy adolescents was recommended when feasible. The standard regimen of vaccination at 0, 1, and 6 months of age or at 2, 4, and 6 months of age is acceptable. All infants

**Table 5-8. *Haemophilus influenzae* conjugate vaccine recommendations**

| Age at first dose | Required no. of doses |
|---|---|
| 2–6 mos | 4* |
| 7–11 mos | 3 |
| 12–14 mos | 2 |
| 15–59 mos | 1 |

*If PRP-OMP from Merck is used, only three doses are required at 2, 4, and 12 mos of age.

Source: Adapted from American Academy of Pediatrics. *Haemophilus influenzae* Infections. In G Peter (ed), *1994 Red Book: Report of the Committee on Infectious Diseases* (23rd ed). Elk Grove Village, IL: American Academy of Pediatrics, 1994. Pp 211–212.

**Table 5-9. Recommended doses of hepatitis B vaccines**

| Group | Recombivax HB[a] | Enerix-B[b] |
|---|---|---|
| Infants of HbsAg-positive mothers (Hepatitis B immunoglobulin, 0.5 ml, is given at the same time as the first dose of vaccine) | 5 μg | 10 μg |
| Age <11 yrs | 2.5 μg | 10 μg |
| Age 11–19 yrs | 5 μg | 20 μg |
| Age >19 yrs | 10 μg | 20 μg |
| Dialysis patients and immunosuppressed adults | 40 μg | 40 μg |

[a]10 μg/ml (adult formulation); 5 μg/ml (pediatric formulation).
[b]20 μg/ml.

Source: Adapted from American Academy of Pediatrics. Hepatitis B. In G Peter (ed), *1994 Red Book: Report of the Committee on Infectious Diseases* (23rd ed). Elk Grove Village, IL: American Academy of Pediatrics, 1994. P 229.

born after April 1, 1992, should be given an HBV vaccine along with their other childhood immunizations. Those born prior to this date should receive their HBV vaccination series as young adolescents. There are no recommendations for HBV vaccine booster doses at this time.

Dosing of the HBV vaccine depends on the patient's age and the type of vaccine used. Dosages are summarized in Table 5-9.

F. **Varicella.** In 1995, the varicella vaccine was licensed for routine use, and the AAP recommended this vaccine be administered routinely to all children between the ages of 12 and 18 months of age in a single dose. Older children (18 months to 13 years of age) should be immunized similarly if they lack a reliable history of varicella infection. Adolescents past their thirteenth birthdays who have not been immunized previously and do not have a history of varicella infection should receive 2 doses of the varicella vaccine 4–8 weeks apart. The vaccine may be given simultaneously with other routine vaccines (MMR, Hib, DTP, and DTaP vaccines; OPV or IPV).

Side effects include a mild maculopapular or varicelliform rash with a median of two to five lesions at the vaccine site or elsewhere within 1 month of the vaccine in 7-8% of children and adolescents and pain, tenderness, or redness at the injection site in about 25% of recipients.

The varicella vaccine is contraindicated in children with immunosuppression (e.g., congenital immunodeficiency, HIV infection, and immunosuppressant therapy); chronic, high-dose (>2 mg/kg/day of prednisone) steroid use of greater than 1 month's duration; malignancies; pregnancy; or neomycin allergy (history of anaphylactoid reaction). The vaccine should be considered, however, in children with acute lymphocytic leukemia in remission (see recommendations of the AAP Committee on Infectious Diseases referenced below). Varicella vaccine should not be administered to children who have received immunoglobulin within at least 5 months. Furthermore, the vaccine manufacturer recommends that salicylates be withheld from children for 6 weeks after varicella vaccine administration, although a connection with Reye's syndrome is unknown.

## Selected Readings

American Academy of Pediatrics. Active and Passive Immunization. In G Peter (ed), *1994 Red Book: Report of the Committee on Infectious Diseases* (23rd ed). Elk Grove Village, IL: American Academy of Pediatrics, 1994.

American Academy of Pediatrics Committee on Infectious Diseases. Recommendations for the use of live attenuated varicella vaccine. *Pediatrics* 95:791–796, 1995.

Edwards KM. Pediatric immunizations. *Curr Probl Pediatr* 23:186–216, 1993.

Garber MR, Mortimer EA. Immunizations: beyond the basics. *Pediatr Rev* 13:98–106, 1992.

Peters G. Childhood immunizations. *N Engl J Med* 327:1794–1800, 1992.

6

# Nutrition

## Anita Cavallo and Mary Pat Alfaro

Appropriate intake of the various nutritional components in balanced proportions is essential for optimal physical growth and cognitive development.

I. **Recommended dietary allowances (RDAs)** are the levels of daily intake of essential nutrients recommended for the average healthy, moderately active population to ensure physiologic needs will be met. These levels do not necessarily constitute the minimum or optimal requirements; adjustments may be needed for individuals based on size, activity, and health status (see the revised RDA chart in Appendix D).

II. **Nutritional assessment**. Each well-child visit should include a nutritional history and nutritional anticipatory guidance. A review of the child's diet and formulation of plans for the dietary management for the next interim period between well visits are important even when growth is adequate.

A. **History** should include types and amount of nutrients, feeding patterns, and nutritional supplements such as vitamins, iron, and fluoride.

B. **Growth.** Length (or height) and weight are plotted on appropriate growth charts at each well-child visit. Variations in the rate of linear growth or weight gain should be analyzed carefully along with the data obtained by history.

C. **Head circumference.** In the first 2 years of life, it is essential to review the growth of the child's head circumference along with nutritional data. Brain growth velocity is highest in the first 9 months of life, and infant malnutrition has been linked to lower intelligence.

III. **Nutritional requirements**

A. **The first year.** The average daily caloric requirement (kcal/kg/day) is highest during the first year of life and decreases from 120 at birth to 115 at 1 month, 105 at 2 months, 95 from 3 to 5 months, and 90 from 6 to 12 months of age.

1. **Breast milk or infant formula** is the main source of nutrition in the first year of life. Breast-feeding is preferable and should be encouraged over formula feeding. Breast milk provides the appropriate balance of nutrients required in the first 6 months of life in an easily digestible form. Additionally, breast milk provides protection against some infections and appears to reduce the risk of development of certain illnesses, such as diabetes mellitus, Crohn's disease, and atopic disease.

   Feeding options should be discussed during the prenatal visit, and plans to provide appropriate support for the mother who chooses to breast-feed should be made prior to her expected date of delivery. Appropriate teaching and support for the mother are extremely important for successful breast-feeding. Special attention should be given to individual plans such as the mother's return to work away from home, pumping breast milk, part-time jobs, and so forth.

The lactating mother has special dietary needs (see Appendix D), and successful breast-feeding also requires time, dedication, and a supportive family. Stressful environments and preoccupations with job, finances, and family often impair successful breast-feeding. When adequate support is available, breast-feeding has a high success rate. Mothers should be encouraged to breast-feed but should not feel guilty if social conditions do not permit or if breast-feeding is unsuccessful.

When breast-feeding is not available, the nutritional needs of the infant in the first year of life can be met using infant formulas based on cow's milk or soy and fortified with iron. The source and amount of nutrients vary among the different commercial preparations (see Appendix B).

It is not well-established at what age exclusive breast-feeding or formula feeding becomes insufficient as a source of nutrients. Generally, it is recommended to begin solid foods (see sec. **III.A.2**) around 6 months of age to provide adequate nutrition, introduce nutrients that have different textures and flavors, promote the development of swallowing independently from sucking (between 4 and 6 months of age), and promote chewing (between 8 and 12 months of age). The recommended nutritional intake for the normal infant during the first year of life is summarized in Table 6-1.

2. **Solid foods**. In the normally developing child, solid foods may be introduced between 4 and 6 months of age. The decision about when to initiate solid foods depends on the infant's feeding frequency and amount of feedings. Attention should be given to distinguish hunger from other causes of crying in infants.
   a. **Cereal** is generally the first solid food introduced in the infant diet. Cereal should be offered from a spoon from the start rather than mixed with formula in the bottle; the infant needs to learn to swallow food presented with a spoon.
   b. **Vegetables and fruits** may be introduced at 6–8 months of age. Commercially prepared or homemade strained foods are adequate but should be cooked without added salt. Foods should be introduced one at a time, allowing a 1-week interval between to ascertain tolerance.
   c. **Meats and other sources of protein.** Commercially prepared or home-cooked strained beef, chicken, veal, lamb, beans, tofu, split peas, yogurt (plain), cottage cheese, and egg yolk can be introduced gradually between 7 and 9 months of age. Note: Egg

**Table 6-1. Feeding guidelines for the first 12 months of life**

| Age | Formula: Amount at each feeding (no. of feedings) | Formula: Total per 24 hours | Juices (per day) | Cereal[a] (per day) | Fruits[b] (per day) | Vegetables (per day) | Meats (per day) | Egg yolk[c] (per day) | Starch[d] (per day) |
|---|---|---|---|---|---|---|---|---|---|
| 1–2 wks | 2–3 oz (6–8) | 22 oz | — | — | — | — | — | — | — |
| 2–8 wks | 3–5 oz (5–6) | 28 oz | 1 oz (1/2 strength) | — | — | — | — | — | — |
| 2–4 mos | 4–6 oz (4–5) | 30 oz | 3–4 oz (full strength) | — | — | — | — | — | — |
| 4–6 mos | 5–7 oz (4–5) | 32 oz | 3–4 oz | 2 tbsp × 2 | — | — | — | — | — |
| 6–8 mos[e] | 7–8 oz (3–4) | 28 oz | 4 oz | 1/3 cup × 1 | 2–4 tbsp × 2 | 2–4 tbsp × 2 | 1 tbsp × 2 | 1 tbsp | — |
| 8–12 mos[f] | 8 oz (3–4) | 24 oz | 4 oz | 1/2 cup × 1 | 4 tbsp × 3 | 2–4 tbsp × 2 | 2–4 tbsp × 2 | 1 tbsp | 2 tbsp |

[a]For breast-fed infants, cereal is prepared with infant formula.
[b]Infant may start as early as 4 months. Use strained fruits, no mixtures.
[c]Egg yolk (from medium egg) may be given 2–3 times per week.
[d]For example, use mashed potatoes and pasta.
[e]Infant begins to use cup. Use strained solid foods, one new food per week.
[f]Infant learns to chew. Use mashed or chopped solid foods; avoid hot dogs, grapes, and nuts.

white is not recommended before 1 year of age because of possible allergic reactions.

3. **Water.** Breast milk and infant formulas provide normal water requirements during the first 4–6 months of life. Care must be taken to avoid excess water intake; up to 4 oz of water (without added substances) may be offered per day during the first few months of life and more liberal amounts thereafter. Juices may be introduced by 2 months of age but initially should be diluted.
4. **Supplements.** Although supplementation with vitamins is controversial (see sec. **III.D**), it is a common pediatric practice to supplement the breast-fed infant in the first year of life with vitamin D and iron (e.g., Tri-Vi-Sol with iron infant drops). Fluoride supplementation, if needed, should be started at 6 months of age.

**B. The toddler and child**. The average caloric requirement by body weight declines during childhood and differs significantly between males and females during and after puberty as indicated in Table 6-2.

Caloric requirements are considerably lower in the second year than in the first 6 months of life, and often parents worry unnecessarily about the child's seemingly decreased appetite, frequently describing their toddler as being a "picky eater."

In the second year of life, a wide assortment of table foods provides the necessary nutrients, and the child usually receives three meals and three snacks per day. The source of protein now is more varied than in early infancy and includes milk, meats, eggs, and vegetables. The child should consume 2–3 cups of homogenized milk enriched with vitamin D. Yogurt and cheese may substitute for milk. Excessive milk intake often is accompanied by reduced intake of the wider variety of foods required to meet the nutritional needs of the toddler, and iron deficiency anemia may develop.

Eating patterns, good or bad, will be established during the toddler and early childhood years. It is important to remind the parent that the child's appetite may fluctuate from day to day; therefore, sweet snacks and other high-calorie snacks without nutritional value should be avoided. Anticipatory guidance should emphasize prevention of nutritional deficiencies and obesity.

By school age, the number of meals and snacks usually is reduced to four or five on school days. Food likes and dislikes, as well as cultural patterns, are established at this time. Activity level is an important determinant of the child's nutritional requirements.

**C. The adolescent**. Physical growth and pubertal maturation are accompanied by greater nutritional requirements, particularly of protein, calcium, iron, zinc, and vitamins (see Appendix D for the daily allowances of these nutrients). Eating disorders and obesity are a common concern with adolescents.

**Table 6-2. Average caloric intake requirements by age, body weight, and sex**

| | Kcal/kg/day | |
|---|---|---|
| Age (years) | Females | Males |
| 1–3 | 100 | 100 |
| 4–6 | 90 | 90 |
| 7–10 | 70 | 70 |
| 11–14 | 47 | 55 |
| 15–18 | 40 | 45 |
| 19–24 | 38 | 40 |

Source: Adapted from Subcommittee on the Tenth Edition of the RDAs. Energy. In National Academy of Science National Research Council (ed), *Recommended Dietary Allowances* (10th ed). Washington, DC: National Academy Press, P 33, 1989.

**D. Supplements**

1. **Iron.** Breast milk and iron-fortified formula provide adequate iron for infants, with the possible exception of the premature infant being fed exclusively breast milk; supplementation is needed only if the infant is receiving a formula without iron, which is not recommended. Beyond infancy, a well-balanced diet also provides sufficient iron.
2. **Fluoride.** Supplemental fluoride (250 μg/day for infants 6 months to 2 years old) should be given if the infant receives ready-to-use formula or if the drinking water or the water used to prepare the formula contains less than 0.3 ppm of fluoride. Note that although the local water source may be fluoridated, the family may be using bottled water for drinking or preparation of the formula.
3. **Vitamin D.** No supplementation is needed for the formula-fed infant; whether the breast-fed infant needs supplementation is controversial. The current recommendation is to give vitamin D, 400 IU/day, to breast-fed infants with limited sun exposure. Children on a milk-free diet may receive insufficient vitamin D and calcium, so supplementation then may be necessary.
4. **Other vitamins and trace elements.** Although the requirements have not been established with certainty, it is believed that both the breast-fed and the formula-fed infant receive appropriate amounts of these nutrients. Nutritional deficiencies may be seen in children with inadequate diets.

**IV. Special dietary concerns**

**A. Cholesterol.** Prevention of atherosclerosis in adults should begin in childhood. Dietary recommendations are applicable only for children older than 2 years because the high growth rate in infancy requires an energy-dense diet.

After the child's second birthday, the recommended intake is as follows:

1. Saturated fatty acids: less than 10% of total calories.
2. Total fat: up to 30% of total calories.
3. Cholesterol: less than 300 mg/day.

Such recommendations are for the healthy population, and the goals can be reached by adhering to the following guidelines:

Use lean meats and low-fat dairy products.
Limit the amount of fried foods, prepared snacks, and desserts.
Limit "fast food" meals.

Cholesterol screening and special dietary adjustments need to be considered in select cases. Children who have a parent with a cholesterol level of 240 mg/dl or greater should be screened. Screening also should be considered for children whose parent or grandparent had one of the following at younger than 55 years of age: documented atherosclerosis, myocardial infarction, angina pectoris, cerebrovascular disease, peripheral vascular disease, or sudden cardiac death.

**B. Dietary fiber** intake appears to have a protective role in adults against diseases of the colon, obesity, and coronary heart disease. Excess fiber, however, may impair absorption of nutrients. The infant in the first year of life needs little dietary fiber. After the first year, diet should include whole grain cereals, breads, fruits, and vegetables. The physician should be aware, however, of excessive emphasis on fiber and low-calorie foods, which may affect adequate provision of energy, protein, and other nutrients necessary for normal growth.

**C. Obesity** is the most prevalent nutritional problem in the United States. When excess caloric intake relative to energy needs is the cause of obesity, the child is generally taller for age and genetic potential. On the other hand, obesity associated with congenital or acquired syndromes usually is associated with decreased linear growth rate. The diet history often is inconclusive because of the tendency to underreport food intake and overestimate physical activity. To date, limited success has been achieved with weight-loss programs for children.

In pediatric practice, great emphasis should be placed on prevention of obesity (e.g., encouraging avoidance of overfeeding in infancy and the use of food treats for behavioral management and offering advice about appropriate exercise).

**D. Food allergies.** Adverse reactions (food sensitivities) are categorized as food hypersensitivity (an immune mechanism is operative) and food intolerance. The reported incidence of food allergies varies from 0.3% to 20.0% in infants and declines with age. Genetic predisposition and early introduction of certain foods in the infant diet are the main factors in the development of food allergies; breast-feeding reduces this risk. It is possible, however, for an offending food allergen to be passed to the infant through breast milk.

The dominant food allergies in infants are eggs, cow's milk, peanuts, and soy, and in children, tree nuts, fish and other seafood, and wheat and other cereal grains. Most children outgrow cow's milk allergy and egg allergy by age 3 or 4 years, but other food allergies tend to persist longer and sometimes are lifelong.

Food allergies must be treated by strict avoidance of the allergen. When multiple food allergies are suspect or present, their avoidance may have a significant deleterious impact on the child's nutrition, and referral to a registered dietitian should be made for adequate nutritional planning and education.

E. **Vegetarian diet.** Vegetarianism has become more popular in the United States in recent years. Vegetarian diets are classified as lacto-ovo-vegetarian, lacto-vegetarian, or pure vegetarian. Plant-based diets supplemented with milk or milk and eggs are nutritionally similar to diets that contain meat. The pure vegetarian diet also can be nutritionally adequate but requires more careful planning to provide adequate amounts of amino acids, calcium, riboflavin, iron, vitamin A, vitamin D, and vitamin $B_{12}$. Cereal grains combined with legumes, nuts and seeds, and fortified soy or nut beverages should be included. In general, a dietitian should be consulted to help the parent formulate an adequate vegetarian diet for a child.

Health advantages of vegetarianism include decreased cholesterol levels and lower rates of obesity, hypertension, and gallstones. The main concerns about vegetarian diets in children are sufficient caloric intake and inclusion of all essential nutrients.

F. **Sports.** The caloric demands of sports activities are above those needed for optimal growth. Because the average diet in the United States is already high in protein, an overall increase in food consumption without significant alterations in the proportions of the dietary constituents generally suffices despite the known increased protein use during exercise. There is no evidence supporting the need for additional vitamin supplementation of the athlete, but an iron supplement may be necessary to cover for iron loss related to exercise. Fluid and electrolyte balance must be maintained. Beverages with glucose, chloride, sodium, and potassium may be beneficial, particularly in hot climates, but they must always be hypotonic. Water intake should be encouraged during and after exercise.

## Selected Readings

American Academy of Pediatrics. *Pediatric Nutrition Handbook* (2nd ed). Elk Grove Village, IL: American Academy of Pediatrics, 1985.

Pipes PL. *Nutrition in Infancy and Childhood.* St. Louis: Times Mirror/Mosby College Publishing, 1989.

Subcommittee on the Tenth Edition of the RDAs. *Recommended Dietary Allowances* (10th ed). Washington, DC: National Academy Press, 1989.

Suskind RM, Lewinter-Suskind L. *Textbook of Pediatric Nutrition*. New York: Raven, 1993.

# 7

# Anticipatory Guidance

Julie Jaskiewicz

Every health supervision visit gives the primary care physician an opportunity to share information and suggestions for parenting that enhance good parent-child interactions and facilitate health promotion. This process is called *anticipatory guidance*, and it allows the physician to anticipate for parents the child's development, behavior, and issues that arise at various ages. Parents are made aware of the changes that occur in their children over time and are offered suggestions for adapting to those changes. Every physician will develop his or her own style for guiding individual families. The primary goal is to help parents relate positively to their children and enjoy them.

**I. Principles**

**A. Partnership.** Ideally, physicians and parents work as partners to provide the best possible nurturing environment for the child. Parents should be encouraged to see themselves as the best caregivers and teachers of their children, with the physician as a guide and support. When parents view themselves as competent caregivers, their self-esteem and self-confidence are enhanced, which may in turn improve compliance with preventive health maintenance.

**B. Parents' agenda**. The physician should ask parents about their specific concerns, questions, or problems with the child rather than present them with a laundry list of predetermined topics. It often is not possible to discuss all issues at each health maintenance visit. Carefully listening to parents' concerns enables the physician to determine the information that needs to be shared at that visit and what can wait until a later time. A few minutes of specific advice for a parent's most pressing concern is better than a long discussion of issues that may seem insignificant at that moment to an overwhelmed parent. The physician should try to avoid a judgmental or dogmatic approach. When there is a problem with the child, the physician should ask parents what they already have tried in order to avoid suggesting something the parents already have done that has failed.

**C. Anticipate normal development.** A key principle of anticipatory guidance is to enlighten parents ahead of time about normal development and expected changes in routine (e.g., starting solid foods) or potential problems (e.g., nighttime awakening). It is preferable to discuss potential problems with parents before they occur. If parents are made aware that certain behaviors can be expected and are normal (e.g., temper tantrums in toddlers), they will be more equipped to handle them and less likely to develop the misconception that their child's behavior is bad or a result of their failure as parents.

**D. Timing.** The timing of anticipatory guidance within the health maintenance visit varies among physicians and from one visit to another. Issues may be discussed at the end of the visit, or some issues may be raised as the physical examination proceeds. Many physicians provide written materials about these issues to supplement office discussion. The smart physician takes advantage of unique opportunities, too. For example, if an infant is left unattended on the examination table by a parent who is across the room, the physician can use that opportunity to discuss with the parent safety issues for infants and can model in the office more appropriate care.

## II. Components

**A. Development.** Most anticipatory guidance issues are related directly to a child's developmental stage and projected development over time. At each visit, the parents should be given an update on the child's developmental progress (cognitive, somatic, motor, and sexual milestones) and advised about what the child should be capable of doing by the time of the next health maintenance visit. The appropriate time to begin discussing the concept of sexuality as a normal, lifelong developmental process (much like sleeping, feeding, or elimination) is early in infancy with parents first, and then with the child. Adolescence is too late to bring up sexuality issues for the first time; a teen-ager may be uncomfortable talking about these issues with a physician who has never mentioned the subject before. By starting these discussions in infancy and continuing throughout childhood, parents will feel more knowledgeable and comfortable as sexuality educators of their children.

**B. Nutrition.** The physician should discuss with parents diet and caloric requirements at different ages, the variability in appetite among individual children, and the normal development of feeding skills. Parents often are concerned more about the feeding behaviors of their child than the nutritional aspects of food. Some parents use their child's feeding success as proof of their success or failure as a caregiver. Some children learn quickly that they exert tremendous control over the family by their behavior at mealtime. The physician should anticipate for parents the different psychosocial-developmental issues that relate to a child's feeding behavior, such as the usual decrease in appetite during the toddler years and the need for self-feeding in spite of the mess it creates. By discussing these issues with parents before the child is developmentally capable of the behaviors, parents will feel more in control, less anxious, and less responsible for their child's normal, though often challenging, feeding behavior.

**C. Safety.** The dangerous situations children get into are directly related to their developmental capabilities. Parents often do not anticipate these dangers because they are unaware of their child's abilities. Parents should be prepared early about what to expect and how to ready themselves and the child's environment by relating their child's developmental stage to potential common hazards. Specific hazards in a child's environment, such as living next to a busy, four-lane highway, merit specific discussion. The physician should be sure to emphasize seasonal safety (discuss water safety beginning in the spring) and stress the need for appropriate supervision.

D. **Behavior and discipline.** Some of the most challenging behaviors exhibited by children, such as temper tantrums, are actually the result of the child's developmentally appropriate expression of normal feelings. When parents understand that these new feelings and expressions are normal and necessary for their child's successful maturation, they may be more able to tolerate the behavior and set age-appropriate limits. The physician should talk to parents about the normal, yet challenging, behavior their children are likely to demonstrate before they actually do; thus, parents will feel empowered to manage their child before he or she gets out of control. Setting consistent limits, complimenting good behavior, and ignoring unappreciated behavior are the hallmarks of good discipline. When discussing a child's difficult behavior with parents, it is worthwhile for the physician to take a moment to explore with them their own feelings of frustration and anger. A little understanding of the parents may be a tremendous support for them. Occasionally, a group meeting between parents with children of similar ages can be helpful for sharing ideas and helping parents realize their experience is not unique. A mnemonic for remembering how to discuss discipline with parents is "*r*earing *c*hildren *h*as *a* *r*eward": *r*emove temptation, *c*onsistency, *h*ouse rules (and consequences of breaking them), *a*void physical punishment (replace with time-out and behavior modification), and *r*eward the positive and ignore the negative (within limits).

E. **Parenting.** This component of anticipatory guidance includes the central theme of good parenting—namely, the mutual enjoyment of parent and child. Physicians can help parents view child rearing as rewarding and enjoyable by remaining sensitive to the extreme challenges some parents may experience, especially single or medically or emotionally limited parents. The physician should give parents practical and age-appropriate tips to enhance interaction with their children and compliment their good parenting skills. They should be encouraged to keep a sense of humor too. It is easy for many parents to get so bogged down in the drudgery of day-to-day child care that the joy is overlooked, and the environment may then become a potential for neglect or even abuse. Each health maintenance visit is an opportunity for the physician to continually reassess the parent-child interaction, identify potential problems, and intervene as necessary.

III. **Anticipatory guidance by age**

A. **The prenatal visit.** The purpose of the prenatal visit is to become acquainted with the parents and explain the philosophy and structure of the physician's practice (e.g., office hours, how to reach the physician in an emergency, and fee schedule). Ideally, the prenatal visit should take place during the last trimester with both parents present. The physician should allow the parents the opportunity to ask questions and be particularly sensitive to the concerns of first-time parents. Issues that should be covered include what to expect at the time of delivery (heel stick, eye drops, separation from infant after delivery), who will examine the infant in the hospital (the physician, the physician's partner, staff physician), rooming in, circumcision, and clothes for going home. The prenatal visit is also the opportunity to take a detailed family history, including household composition, health issues in family members (especially congenital or genetic conditions), and attitude of the parents about the pregnancy (excited, depressed, unwanted). The physician should discuss the following issues at the prenatal visit:

*Nutrition*
Breast- versus bottle-feeding
Feeding schedule in the hospital, at home
Father's involvement in feeding
Vitamin and mineral supplementation if indicated

*Safety*
Smoke detector
Stroller
Car safety restraint before leaving hospital
Water thermostat set <120°F
Safe furniture, crib with slats less than 2⅜" apart, tight-fitting mattress

*Parenting*
Prenatal classes
Potential changes in the relationship
Maternal health and emotional issues between parents
Sibling needs
Schedule of health maintenance visits
Discouragement of smoking and alcohol
Social supports
Printed literature about the office and general newborn care

**B. Newborn.** The newborn visit usually takes place in the hospital within the first 24 hours after delivery. Whenever possible, the physician should examine the infant with both parents present so the normal features of the baby can be explained. The physician should discuss the following with parents at the newborn visit:

*Development*
Normal infant reflexes
Crying pattern (2–3 hours per day)
Distinguishing hunger from other cries
Stooling patterns
Hiccups and sneezing normal
Sleep pattern (2–4 hours at a time, 15–20 hours per day total)
Vaginal discharge, breast engorgement, erections normal

*Nutrition*
Postnatal weight loss
Breast- versus bottle-feedings

Bottle preparation
Supplementing breast-feedings
Burping and spitting
Bottle propping discouraged
Vitamins and fluoride supplements if necessary
Schedule, frequency of feedings, demand versus regular schedule, volume of feeding (2–4 oz per feeding)

*Safety*
Leaving the infant unattended
Leaving alone with siblings or pets
Use of car restraint
Adequate heat in home
Sibling aggression

*Behavior and Discipline*
Emphasis on infant individuality
Infantile colic
Temperament (easy and cuddly versus difficult to console)
Need for holding, close contact with parents

*Parenting*
Bathing (skin and umbilical cord care)
Diaper changes, dressing advice
Pacifier for non-nutritive sucking
Thermometer instructions
Review finances if necessary; discuss availability of funds from Women, Infants, and Children (WIC) program
Emphasis on enjoyment of infant
When and how to call physician for problems
Management of siblings' negative reactions (spending time alone with older siblings while someone else watches the infant so siblings continue to feel important and loved)
Maternal postpartum issues (time for mother; adequate rest; involvement of family supports, especially father)
Plans for first regular office or clinic visit

**C. 2 weeks.** The physician should discuss the following at the infant's 2-week visit:

*Development*
Emphasis on infant's abilities (focuses on face, responds to mother's voice)
Review of development during next 2 months (lifting head up, response to tactile and visual stimuli)
Need for holding, cuddling, and talking to infant while bathing, feeding, and diapering
Most still awaken at night, nap for parent during day while infant sleeps
Normal variations in stool frequency, color, and consistency
Crying increases during first 8 weeks and may have no identifiable cause; fussiness is infant's temperament, not parental inadequacy
Strong urine stream in boys, no dribbling
Variable timing of milestones

*Nutrition*
Problems with breast- or bottle-feeding
Discourage bottle propping
No solids until 4–6 months
Fluoride and vitamin supplements if necessary
Review of usual feeding interval and amount (3 oz/lb/day)

*Safety*
Car restraint
Bath safety
Never leave unattended
Avoid shaking
Never leave alone with siblings, pets
Avoid excessive sun exposure
Crib safety (avoid loose cradle gyms and small objects in crib)

*Behavior and Discipline*
Review of temperament, individuality
Counseling if colicky behavior present

*Parenting*
Encourage cuddling, talking to infant
Time alone for parents together
Sibling attention
Choosing a baby-sitter
Day-care plans if mother returns to work
When to call the doctor
Review immunization schedule
Plans for next visit

**D. 2 months.** The physician should discuss the following at the infant's 2-month visit:

*Development*
Review skills and anticipate new accomplishments during next 2 months (increased smiling, head control, vocalization, rolling)
Reinforce need for cuddling, talking to infant, stimulation
Stooling patterns
Review of crying and feeding behavior

*Nutrition*
Feeding intervals every 3–4 hours, longer at night
Vitamins and fluoride supplements as needed
Iron supplementation for premature infants, 2 mg/kg/day elemental iron, 15 mg/day maximum
No solids until 4–6 months
No solids in bottle

*Safety*
Car restraint
Never leave unattended
Discourage walker
Can use playpen for safe space
Unbreakable toys, no detachable parts or sharp edges
Avoid holding infant while drinking hot liquids

*Parenting*
Upper respiratory infection, fever management
Child care arrangements, baby-sitter
Enjoyment of infant
Time set aside for siblings
Review when to call the doctor
Plans for next visit

**E. 4 months.** The physician should discuss the following at the infant's 4-month visit:

*Development*
Review skills, anticipate new developments during next 2 months (rolling, reaching, laughing, increased vocalizing, response to vocalizing, sitting with support)
May have predictable sleep pattern but developmental variability
Drooling starts now, teething starts by 6 months; suggest teething ring, acetaminophen
Review crying and stooling patterns

*Nutrition*
Introduce solid foods at 4–6 months beginning with iron-fortified cereal (by spoon), followed by fruits, vegetables; one new food at a time
Continue breast milk or formula to 12 months
Vitamin and fluoride supplements if necessary
Iron supplements (iron-fortified formula, cereal, or iron drops)
No bottle in bed

*Safety*
Review previous guidance
Car restraint
Never leave unattended
Infant reaching, keeping small objects out of reach
Discourage use of walker
Safe toys without removable parts
Avoid baby powder (risk of aspiration)

*Behavior and Discipline*
Stranger anxiety between 6 and 8 months
Thumb-sucking normal
Review temperament
Discourage physical punishment

*Parenting*
Emphasis on stimulation, talking with infant as a way to encourage speech development
Encourage play; interaction of infant, parents, and siblings
Enjoyment of infant
Parental relationship, stress
When to call the doctor
Plans for next visit

**F. 6 months.** The physician should discuss the following at the infant's 6-month visit:

*Development*
Review skills; anticipate new developments by 9 months (pincer grasp, sitting well alone, pulling to stand, cruising, babbling)
May resist sleep due to separation anxiety (use favorite toy as transitional object)
Nighttime waking common
Stooling patterns
Teething not associated with high fever
Dental care

*Nutrition*
Breast- or bottle-feeding until 12 months
Solid foods, 2–3 meals per day
Finger foods between 7 and 9 months
Discourage milk or juice as pacifier
No bottle in bed
Begin to offer cup
Vitamin and fluoride supplementation if necessary

*Safety*
Increased mobility between 6–9 months means injury prevention crucial
Child-proof home: gates on stairs, electrical outlets covered
Car restraint
Never leave unattended
Syrup of ipecac
Bathtub safety
Discourage walker

*Behavior and Discipline*
Stranger anxiety, separation anxiety (not deliberately trying to annoy parents)
Discourage hand slapping
Sharp "*no*" by 9 months

*Parenting*
Encourage age-appropriate, safe toys
Enhance parent-child interaction by playing
Enjoyment of infant games together
Stimulate speech with frequent talking
Shoes unnecessary except for protection
Review when to call the doctor
Plans for next visit

**G. 9 months.** The physician should discuss the following at the child's 9-month visit:

*Development*
Review skills; anticipate new developments by 12 months (walking alone, speaking 2–3 words, imitation, improving hand-eye coordination)
Sleep patterns, bedtime routine, nighttime waking, allowing infant to soothe self back to sleep
Stooling patterns
Teething, dental care

*Nutrition*
Finger and table foods
Four meals per day with family at the table
Self-feeding
Weaning from bottle, encourage cup
Decreased food intake by 12 months
Introduce cow's milk at 12 months
No bottle in bed
Vitamins and fluoride supplementation as needed

*Safety*
Avoid access to sharp objects
Syrup of ipecac
Change to toddler car restraint when >20 lb
Child more mobile; secure against potential falls
No small foods that can be aspirated such as peanuts, hot dogs, popcorn, raisins, and grapes
Provide The Injury Prevention Program (TIPP) and American Academy of Pediatrics sheets

*Behavior and Discipline*
Stranger anxiety, separation anxiety (related to object permanence, not spoiling)
Discourage physical punishment; physically remove from potential dangers
Anticipate autonomy issues of toddlerhood
Consistent limit setting

*Parenting*
Encourage exploration
Discuss developing autonomy as normal
Assess family functioning
Plans for next visit
Explain difference between setting limits and punishment
Encourage social games between parents and child to promote interaction and imitation

**H. 12 months.** The physician should discuss the following at the child's 12-month visit:

*Development*
Review skills; anticipate new developments by 15 months (walking well, taking stairs, three- to six-word vocabulary, understands simple commands)
Understands praise
Likes to give and get hugs
Teething and dental care
Sleep usually consistent pattern

*Nutrition*
Review self-feeding
Eat only sitting at the table
Decreased appetite in second year
Cow's milk by 12 months
No bottle in bed
Wean from bottle
Table foods, minimal sweets

Vitamins and fluoride supplements as needed
Discourage food as a reward or removal of food for punishment

*Safety*
No small foods that can be aspirated such as peanuts, popcorn, M&Ms, hot dogs
Poison-proof home
Syrup of ipecac
Never leave unattended
Reinforce tap water temperature <120°F
Review water, car, and stair safety; burn risks
Provide TIPP sheets

*Behavior and Discipline*
Discourage physical punishment
Consistent limits
Firm "*no*" for unwanted behaviors
Physically remove from dangers
Praise for desired behavior
Developing autonomy
Unable to remember prohibitions, will need reminding, not scolding

*Parenting*
Encourage speech development with frequent talking
Point out body parts and objects by name and encourage imitation
Picture books with one picture/one word on a page
Emphasize developing independent behaviors as normal, not just in opposition
Play alone and with others
Reinforce concept of discipline
Enjoyment of child
Plans for next visit

**I. 15 months.** The physician should discuss the following at the child's 15-month visit:

*Development*
Review skills; anticipate new developments by 18 months (understands simple commands, enhanced motor skills making climbing and running possible)
Discuss toilet training; some children developmentally ready by 18–24 months; buy a potty seat; let the child take the lead; do not force
Dental care
Regular bedtime routine; one to two naps per day

*Nutrition*
Self-feeding
Eating with family
Begin to encourage spoon
Phase out bottle
No bottle in bed
Usually three meals, two to three nutritious snacks
Vitamins not usually needed
Good table manners not expected
Appetite low, slower weight gain normal

*Safety*
Toddler car restraint
Secure gates, doors of stairwells
Lower crib mattress
Poison-proof home if not already
Hot water thermostat <120°F
Syrup of ipecac
Protect against falls, electrical dangers
Plastic bags and balloons unsafe; discuss injury and burns
Never leave unsupervised
TIPP sheets
Water safety
No small foods that can be aspirated
No chewing gum

*Behavior and Discipline*
Discourage physical punishment
Discuss temper tantrums
Autonomy and curiosity are normal and necessary for sense of competence
Appropriate limit-setting and removal from dangerous situation if necessary
Build self-esteem by lots of praise for good behavior; ignore unwanted behavior
Consistency by all caregivers, including grandparents
Self-comforting behaviors, thumb-sucking normal

*Parenting*
Appropriate toys such as dolls, books, pull toys, musical toys, and pots and pans; riding toys
Encourage interactive games and supervised exploration
Stimulate language development by reading, singing, talking
Encourage imitative behaviors
Show affection
Sibling rivalry
Plans for next visit

**J. 18 months.** The physician should discuss the following at the child's 18-month visit:

*Development*
Review skills; anticipate new developments by 2 years
Toilet training readiness between 18 and 24 months
Masturbation is age-appropriate way to self-comfort and handle stress
Nightmares
Night awakenings
Variable need for naps
Bedtime ritual

*Nutrition*
Self-feeding well
Use of spoon and cup
No bottle
Eat meals as a family
Discourage snacks
Pickiness normal

Prevention of mealtime as a battle
Modest food requirement
Respect of child's autonomy, no forced feeding

*Safety*
Car restraint
Stair, window, water safety
Supervised play
Never leave unattended
TIPP sheets
Syrup of ipecac
Protect from falls, electrical injury, burns

*Behavior and Discipline*
Respect need for autonomy and independence; allow reasonable choices
Responds well to praise for accomplishments and is pleased by parental approval
Praise for positive behavior; ignore negative behavior
Discourage food as reward for good behavior
Consistent verbal limits
Discourage physical punishment
Occasional clinging behavior normal
Sharing toys not likely at this age

*Parenting*
Encourage parents to play games; pretend play enjoyed
Durable toys, toys that can be taken apart and put together
Read simple stories and bedtime stories
Enjoyment of child
Assign simple chores
Encourage show of affection
Parental relationship, stress
Plans for next visit

**K. 2 years.** The physician should discuss the following at the child's 2-year visit:

*Development*
Review skills; anticipate new developments during the second year: climbing and jumping well, beginning to form gender identity
Speech should be intelligible to parents but some dysfluency normal, vocabulary of 50 single words
Variable need for naps
May be ready to move to regular bed
Toilet training readiness
Imitates use of toothbrush
Genital curiosity normal
Develops imaginary friends

*Nutrition*
Encourage self-feeding
May be "picky eater"
Avoid control struggles around feeding
Discourage non-nutritious snacks
Encourage family being together at mealtimes
Eat sitting at the table

*Safety*
Car restraint
Stair, water, window safety
Be alert to ingestion potential
Syrup of ipecac
Growing autonomy makes wandering more common; never leave unattended
TIPP sheets

*Behavior and Discipline*
Autonomy leads to enhanced exploration
Clinging behavior at times is age-appropriate
Firm "*no*" understood but not easily remembered
Play with one or two others better than group
Review temper tantrum management
Pleased with parental approval
Sharing still unlikely
Consistent, age-appropriate limits

*Parenting*
Encourage play with peers, physical activity
Simple chores
Limit television
Read frequently
Encourage praise of good behavior
Parent relationship issues
Plans for next visit

**L. 3 years.** The physician should discuss the following at the child's 3-year visit:

*Development*
Excellent motor skills
Brushes teeth
70% continent at night
Masturbation normal
50% of speech intelligible to everyone, some dysfluency normal
Curiosity about babies and differences between boys and girls; use correct terms for genitalia
Regular bedtime ritual and time, napping variable

*Nutrition*
Encourage balanced diet
Avoid junk foods
Entirely self-feeding

*Safety*
Seat belt in car at 4 years or 40 lb
Close supervision for outside play
Strangers, strange dogs or animals
Inappropriate touching
Water and street safety
TIPP sheets

*Behavior and Discipline*
Encourage independence, self-discipline, positive sibling relationship
Explain consequences of unacceptable behavior

Discourage physical punishment
Enjoys pretend play
Begins to take turns, share
Provide choices
Consistent limits

*Parenting*
Encourage exploration, communication, initiative, pretend play
Assign chores and give praise for accomplishments
Out of home experiences
Limit television, watch television with child
Sitter, day-care, preschool readiness
Plans for next visit

**M. 4 years.** The physician should discuss the following at the child's 4-year visit:

*Development*
Bedtime ritual
Toilet training
75% dry at night
Masturbation normal
School readiness in terms of cognitive, emotional skills (ability to separate from parent, can follow commands, listen, verbally communicate)
Encourage privacy for bathing, dressing, undressing
Sexuality education, use proper terms, child's level of understanding, interest in same sex common

*Nutrition*
Balanced diet
Small portions with seconds available
Social atmosphere of mealtime
Avoid conflict between family members at mealtime

*Safety*
Emphasize car seat belt
Continued close supervision
Water, street, fire safety
Strangers, stray animals
Inappropriate touching
Teach name and address
Helmet if riding bicycle
TIPP sheets

*Behavior and Discipline*
Enjoys interacting with peers
Can understand, keep agreement
Likes chores
Growing independence with need for limits
Reprimand privately (away from friends)
Explain consequences for breaking house rules

*Parenting*
Encourage interaction with peers, pretend play, simple board games
Go with child on outings, trips
Assign chores and praise accomplishments

Show interest in child's activities
Limit television
Plans for next visit

**N. 5 years.** The physician should discuss the following at the child's 5-year visit:

*Development*
School readiness in terms of cognitive and emotional skills (see 4-year visit)
Referral for educational evaluation if question of intellectual readiness
Avoid promoting sense of failure if child not ready
Dresses self, bedtime ritual, story reading or storytelling
Continue sexuality education, facilitate parents' knowledge if necessary
Dental care
Enuresis

*Nutrition*
Balanced diet
Pleasant mealtime atmosphere

*Safety*
Emphasize car seat belt
Constant supervision around water
Bicycle safety, helmet use
Strangers
Memorize name, address, phone number
TIPP sheets

*Behavior and Discipline*
Review balance between independence and need for limits
Able to play by the rules
Offer choices
Discipline in private

*Parenting*
Promote interaction with peers
Assign chores, praise for accomplishments
Show affection, pride in school progress
Communication with school, teachers
Parental pleasure in child and family life
Plans for next visit

**O. 6–10 years.** The physician should discuss the following issues that are appropriate for a child between the ages of 6 and 10 years old:

*Development*
School progress in terms of cognitive development
Physical activity related to motor skills
Child responsible for own dental care, brushing, and flossing
Sexuality, same sex-peers, interest in reproduction, "dirty" jokes, anticipate pubertal changes by 8–10 years of age
Enuresis
Rules for bedtime

*Nutrition*
Self-balanced diet
Three meals daily including breakfast
Avoid "junk" foods
Mealtime with family

*Safety*
Car seat belt
Bicycle helmet
Learn to swim
Adult supervision when parents away
Strangers

*Behavior and Discipline*
Growing independence and self-responsibility
House rules and consequences for breaking house rules
Enjoys hobbies
Discipline in private
Avoid physical punishment
Offer choices

*Parenting*
Encourage promotion of good health habits and self-care
Reinforce age-appropriate independence and self-responsibility
Rules for chores, homework, outside activities
Parents as role models
Allowance
Show affection
Praise child's accomplishments
Do hobbies with child
Encourage reading, library card
Limit television
Plans for next visit

P. **Adolescence.** The social and emotional aspects of an adolescent's life have a great impact on physical health, and these concerns are stressed in adolescent anticipatory guidance. Whereas in the child's early years parents are the focus of the physician's suggestions and guidance, in adolescence, the teen-ager becomes more involved with his or her own care at each visit. Psychological and physical development more than chronologic age determine issues to be discussed at each visit. The content of anticipatory guidance during the adolescent years is guided by an understanding of the developmental tasks that occur during adolescence, including (1) acceptance of the physical changes that result in an adult body and reproductive capability, (2) attainment of independence from the family, (3) emergence of a stable identity, and (4) development of adult thinking patterns.

1. **Early adolescence (11–14 years)** is a period of rapid physical and sexual development. The primary question of the early adolescent is "Am I normal?" The early adolescent is commonly egocentric and primarily concrete operational, has an undifferentiated concept of sexuality, and identifies primarily with same-sex peers. The hallmarks of this stage are ambivalence and insecurity,

leading to the "hot and cold" attitude some parents will recognize. The physician should discuss the following with the early adolescent:

*Health Habits*
Self-responsibility
Balanced diet
Maintenance of appropriate weight
Physical exercise
Limit television
Weight training guidelines
Dental care
Breast and testes self-examination
Illicit drugs, alcohol, smoking

*Sexuality*
Physical changes of puberty, emphasizing "normal" is variable
Body image
Sexual orientation
Nocturnal emissions and masturbation
Dating responsibility
Right to say "*no*" to illicit drugs, alcohol, sexual behavior
Delaying sexual activity
Contraception
Sexually transmitted diseases
Gynecomastia in boys
Menstruation in girls

*Safety*
Seat belt at all times
No drinking and driving
Bicycle helmet
Anticipate risk-taking behaviors
Protection from physical or sexual assault

*School*
Review progress
Pride in own performance
Self-responsibility
Future goals in concrete terms

*Social*
Peer group and peer pressures
Extracurricular activities
Communication with peers, parents, physician

*Parenting*
Chores, allowance, work outside the home
Allow age-appropriate decision-making
Promote self-responsibility, independence
Encourage communication, listening skills
Ambivalence to be expected
Respect for privacy with appropriate supervision
Show interest in activities, friends, praise for accomplishments
Promote self-esteem
Show appropriate affection

Spend time with adolescent
Help parents understand egocentrism is normal
Parents as role models
Fair house rules
Plans for next visit

2. **Middle adolescence (15–16 years).** By this stage, most physical growth and development has occurred. The primary question of middle adolescence is "Who am I?" Middle adolescents often demonstrate formal operational thinking with an increasing ability to understand feelings with insight into the future. Sexuality usually is directed toward opposite-sex partners. The hallmark of middle adolescence is a striving for independence, with issues of autonomy, conflict with authority, testing of limits, and experimentation at their peaks. The physician should discuss the following with the middle adolescent.

*Health Habits*
Self-responsibility
Balanced diet
Avoid junk foods
Maintenance of appropriate weight
Regular physical activity
Dental care
Breast and testes self-examination
Need for sufficient sleep
Illicit drugs, alcohol, smoking

*Sexuality*
Review physical changes of puberty and assure adolescent of normalcy
Feelings about sexuality, sexual activity; delay of sexual activity; right to say *"no"*
Dating responsibility, contraception
Sexually transmitted diseases

*Safety*
Stress self-responsibility
Discuss risk-taking behaviors
Seat belt at all times
No drinking and driving; designated driver
Bicycle, motorcycle helmet
Hitchhiking

*School*
Review progress
Pride in own performance
Self-responsibility
Encourage staying in school
Future goals, college, work

*Social*
Peer group and peer pressure
Extracurricular activities
Communication with peers, parents, physician

*Parenting*
Parents as role models
Stress communication
Show affection, praise
Build self-esteem
Respect for privacy, decision-making, appropriate supervision, reasonable rules
Emphasize limit testing; conflict with authority is developmentally normal
Plans for next visit

3. **Late adolescence (17–20 years).** The primary question of the late adolescent is "Who am I in relation to others and to the future?" Late adolescents may demonstrate separation anxiety as they contemplate moving away from home. The hallmark of late adolescence is concern about the future, with issues of education, vocation, sexuality, and individuation from the family most important. The physician should discuss the following with the late adolescent.

*Health Habits*
Maintenance of appropriate weight
Regular physical activity
Dental care
Need for sufficient sleep
Breast and testes self-examination
Illicit drugs, alcohol, smoking
Balanced diet, avoid junk foods, salt, cholesterol
Need for continued routine health maintenance once separated from family
Self-responsibility

*Sexuality*
Feelings about sexuality, sexual activity
Self-responsibility
Right to say "*no*"
Dating, partner responsibility
Contraception, sexually transmitted diseases

*Safety*
Review seat belt use
No drinking and driving
Responsibility for behaviors
Designated driver

*School*
Review progress
Future plans, goals, values

*Social*
Separation from family, friends for college, work
Communication with peers, parents, partner, and physician
Changing peer group
Marriage, child rearing

*Parenting*
Parents as role models
Parental difficulty with separation and letting go
Allow independence
Support decisions
Emphasize separation anxiety for parents and adolescent is developmentally normal
Plans for future health care, referral to internist, family practitioner

## Selected Readings

American Academy of Pediatrics. *Guidelines for Health Supervision II*. Elk Grove Village, IL: American Academy of Pediatrics, 1988.

Schulman JL, Hanley KK. *Anticipatory Guidance: An Idea Whose Time Has Come*. Baltimore: Williams & Wilkins, 1987.

Rudolph AM. Counseling and Anticipatory Guidance. In AM Rudolph (ed), *Rudolph's Pediatrics*. Norwalk, CT: Appleton & Lange, 1991.

Schmitt B. *Your Child's Health* (rev ed). New York: Bantam Books, 1991.

Kreipe RE, McAnarney ER. Psychosocial aspects of adolescent medicine. *Semin Adol Med* 1:33–45, 1985.

# 8

# Infant Dental Care

James F. Steiner

The American Academy of Pediatric Dentistry recommends a visit to the pediatric dentist when the first primary tooth erupts but no later than age 12 months. Prior to that visit, oral health recommendations should be provided by the primary care physician. This chapter gives the health care provider the tools needed to recognize high-decay risk behaviors by providing a list of targeted historical questions, keys to recognizing early physical findings caused by high-decay risk behaviors, and, finally, anticipatory guidance recommendations that ensure continued oral health.

**I. History**. The well-baby dental history should identify oral health risk factors as follows:

- **A. Feeding practices**. Does the infant sleep with the nursing bottle or, if breast-feeding, with mother? If the child is eating table food, is the meal schedule regular or is the child's eating and drinking unsupervised? Are multiple caretakers involved in feeding, such as child care centers or grandparents?
- **B. Oral hygiene routines.** Who cleans the child's teeth? How are they cleaned? What is the frequency of cleaning? Is fluoride toothpaste used and how much?
- **C. Fluoride use.** Is the family's drinking water optimally fluoridated? If not optimally fluoridated, have fluoride supplements been prescribed?
- **D. Non-nutritive sucking.** Does the child suck a digit or a pacifier? What is the frequency and intensity of sucking? Is the pacifier worn on a cord around the neck? Prior to use, is the pacifier dipped in a sweetened liquid?

**II. Oral examination**. The physician should perform this part of the physical examination with the infant supine on the examination table. A bright light, tongue blade, and gloves are needed.

- **A. Number of teeth present.** The mandibular primary incisor is the first primary tooth to erupt at around 6 months of age. The 20-tooth primary dentition is completed by 36 months of age.
- **B. Plaque** is a soft, white material that collects on teeth. Cariogenic bacteria reside in plaque and convert dietary carbohydrates to acid. The acid demineralizes enamel, beginning the decay process. Plaque should be cleaned from the teeth daily with a toothbrush.
- **C. Demineralized enamel.** If plaque is observed, it is removed with gauze and the underlying enamel inspected. Demineralized areas, whiter than the surrounding normal enamel, are the initial clinical signs of dental caries. Daily tooth cleaning stops the demineralization and prevents progression to a cavity.
- **D. Dental caries.** If plaque is not removed regularly, demineralization continues and caries develops. Caries is a

**Table 8-1. Recommended daily fluoride intake (mg/day) relative to the fluoride concentration in the local water supply**

| Patient age | <0.3 ppm* | 0.3–0.6 ppm* | >0.6 ppm* |
|---|---|---|---|
| 6 mos–3 yrs | 0.25 | 0 | 0 |
| 3–6 yrs | 0.50 | 0.25 | 0 |
| 6–16 yrs at least | 1.00 | 0.50 | 0 |

*Fluoride concentration in drinking water in parts per million (ppm).

break in the enamel that will continue to slowly enlarge. Dental treatment is indicated.

**III. Anticipatory guidance.** Providing oral health information for families during the first year of life can establish healthy routines. The physician should offer advice regarding the following:

**A. Feeding practices.** Bottle-fed children should be held when feeding and should not sleep with the bottle, which puts them at high risk for nursing bottle caries. The upper front teeth develop decay as early as age 12 months, and if the practice continues, decay affects other newly erupted teeth.

Infants who sleep with their mothers and breast-feed unsupervised while their mothers sleep are at similar risk for nursing caries. The physician should remind caretakers at each well-baby visit that unsupervised sleep-time bottle- or breast-feeding is a high-risk behavior for dental decay. When weaning is introduced and table foods enter the diet, caretakers should be advised that children with unrestricted access to food and drink increase their risk for decay. The physician should recommend a feeding pattern of regular meal times and two or three snacks daily.

**B. Oral hygiene.** Cleaning the gum pads once daily using a clean, moist cloth or gauze but with no toothpaste should begin in early infancy. As teeth erupt, parents should change to an infant toothbrush and brush the teeth at least once daily to remove plaque. At 24 months, a very small smear of fluoride toothpaste on the brush is introduced. Adults should supervise and assist with brushing until children develop the fine motor skills necessary to brush effectively, which usually coincides with the ability to tie shoes.

**C. Fluoride.** Water fluoridation reduces the incidence of dental caries 40–50%. If drinking water is not optimally fluoridated, the physician should prescribe fluoride supplements as indicated in Table 8-1. Supplements are available as liquids, chewables, tablets, and vitamin fluoride combinations in 0.25-, 0.50-, and 1.0-mg concentrations. The local water department can be contacted for fluoride levels in the community water supply. If the family has well water, health departments and commercial laboratories can analyze well water for fluoride concentration. Fluoride toothpaste also prevents caries. Parents should be advised to select a toothpaste that has the American Dental Association seal on the packaging. Fluoride products must be stored out of children's reach.

D. **Non-nutritive sucking.** If an infant begins to suck a thumb or finger, parents should try to interest the infant in a pacifier, which is easier to discontinue. Pacifiers never should be hung on a cord around the baby's neck (due to risk of strangulation), nor should the pacifier be coated with honey or other sugary substance. The physician should encourage pacifier weaning at about age 3 years and thumb- or finger-sucking intervention begins at 5–6 years. A very gentle technique to help children stop the sucking habit is described in the book *David Decides about Thumbsucking* by S.M. Heitler.

E. **The first dental visit.** Refer infants to the pediatric dentist when the first primary tooth erupts or no later than age 12 months.

## Selected Readings

American Academy of Pediatric Dentistry. *Reference Manual: Pediatric Dentistry Special Issue* 15(7), 1993–94.

Heitler SM. *David Decides about Thumbsucking*. Denver: Reading Matters, 1985.

Nowak AJ. What pediatricians can do to promote oral health. *Contemp Pediatr* 4:90, 1993.

# 9

# Normal Speech and Language Development

Ann W. Kummer

The ability to communicate affects all activities of daily living, including the ability to learn and develop social relationships. The pediatrician or primary care practitioner should be knowledgeable about the normal stages of communication development in order to be able to answer questions from parents and identify children at risk for a speech or language disorder. Since a communication disorder can have a significant adverse effect on the developing child, early identification and intervention are important. In addition, early treatment often results in faster progress and a more favorable prognosis.

**I. Definitions**

**A. Speech**, or articulation, can be defined as the physical production of individual sounds. It involves movement of the articulators (i.e., the lips, tongue, jaw, and velum) in coordination with respiration and phonation to form speech sounds known as phonemes. These movements, and thus sounds, are produced in sequence to form spoken words.

**B. Language.** Whereas speech is the physical component of verbal communication, language is the cognitive component. Language can be defined as the meaning or message conveyed between individuals, which can be accomplished through speech and written or gestural modes. In assessing a child's language development, it is important to look at both receptive and expressive language.

1. **Receptive language** is the child's ability to understand the language of others. This is demonstrated by appropriate responses to questions or requests and the ability to follow directions.
2. **Expressive language** refers to the child's ability to choose appropriate words in conveying a message (semantics), use the appropriate word forms (morphology), and put the words together in an appropriate order (syntax). Expressive language also includes the ability to use language in an appropriate way following the social rules of conversation (pragmatics).

   Both articulation and language skills begin to develop at birth. Although these skills develop concurrently, each component is discussed separately in this chapter for the sake of clarity. Table 9-1 summarizes the basic speech and language milestones of normal development.

**II. Articulation development**

**A. Birth–6 months**

1. **Birth cries.** Articulation development actually begins with the birth cry. With early cries, the infant must coordinate respiration, phonation, and oral movements to produce sound.

**Table 9-1. Milestones for speech and language development**

| | |
|---|---|
| 0–6 mos | Coos |
| | Responds to speakers with eye contact |
| | Cries for communication |
| 6–12 mos | Babbles |
| | Jargons |
| | Responds to simple commands with gestures |
| | Uses vocalizations and gestures for communication |
| 12–18 mos | Articulates with plosives and nasals |
| | Listens to conversations |
| | Responds to verbal requests and commands |
| | Uses single words and gestures for communication |
| 18–24 mos | Begins articulating with fricatives and affricates |
| | Understands concepts and many compound or complex commands |
| | Begins using 2–3 word combinations |
| 2–3 yrs | Shows interest in explanations |
| | Uses phrases and short sentences |
| | Tells about experiences |
| 3–6 yrs | Speech is intelligible most of the time |
| | Uses complete sentences although errors in syntax are common |

2. **Cooing.** Purposeful sound making begins at around 2 months of age when the infant begins to coo, which consists of sighs and various vowel sounds produced as a form of vocal play. Cooing is an important stage of articulation development because during this stage, the child learns to manipulate the oral mechanism to produce sounds in a purposeful manner. The child also learns to associate tactile-kinesthetic sensations with an acoustic result, thus developing an important oral-auditory feedback loop. Cooing becomes more intonated by 4–6 months of age as the child learns to produce contrasts in pitch, amplitude, and resonance.

**B. 6–12 months**

1. **Babbling** begins at around 6 months and is characterized by the production of consonant sounds in a repetitive manner (e.g., ma ma ma, ba ba ba). Like cooing, babbling provides the child with an opportunity to practice sound production and develop the oral-auditory feedback loop to produce sounds purposefully. During the babbling stage, the child learns to produce many of the early developmental phonemes, or speech consonants. When classified by place of production, these include the bilabial sounds (p, b, m), lingual-alveolar sounds (t, d, n), and velar sounds (k, g).

   The babbling sounds are developed early because the place of production is easy to access and the manner of production is relatively easy. For some of the babbling sounds, the oral cavity is completely closed by either the tongue or the lips. Air pressure builds in the oral cavity and is released suddenly. Since the sudden release of air pressure is explosive in nature, these sounds are called *plosives*. Examples of plosives include /p/, /b/, /t/, /d/, /k/, and /g/. Other early sounds, called *nasals,* also require the oral cavity to be closed by the lips or the tongue. With these sounds, only the velum remains down during production, as in humming, resulting in nasal resonance. Nasal sounds include /m/, /n/, and, later, /ng/.

2. **Jargon.** At 9–10 months, the child begins to use early developmental sounds in a variety of combinations rather than in a repetitive manner. Since various intonational patterns are used with the sound combinations, it may seem as if the child is actually speaking, but in a foreign language. In fact, many parents report that their child is talking in sentences but just cannot be understood. Of course, jargon is merely sound practice and not meaningful speech.

C. **12 months–3 years.** The next stage of articulation development involves the acquisition of sounds produced by forcing the air stream through a narrow opening, causing a high-frequency friction sound. These sounds appropriately are called *fricatives* and include /f/, /s/, /z/, and /sh/. Not only are these sounds more difficult to produce than the early developmental sounds, they require the assistance of teeth. Most of the fricative sounds develop between 12 months and 3 years of age. Once fricative phonemes are acquired, the child begins to produce affricate phonemes such as /ch/ and /j/. Affricates may be difficult to produce because they combine a plosive sound with a fricative—for example, /ch/ is produced by combining /t/ plus /sh/, and /j/ is produced by combining /d/ and /zh/. The child must be able to produce both plosive and fricative sounds individually before these phonemes can be combined to produce the affricate sound.

D. **3–6 years.** The last sounds to be developed are usually /l/, /r/, /th/, and occasionally /v/. These sounds require more fine motor control than early developmental phonemes; therefore, many children have difficulty with one or more of these speech sounds until the age of 6.

E. **Referral guidelines.** During the first year of life, most of the early developmental sounds should be well established because they lay the groundwork for the development of the other sounds. If the infant is not cooing by 4 months or babbling by 8 months, the physician should monitor the child's developmental progress closely and consider a referral to a speech-language pathologist. Evidence of oral-motor dysfunction, such as difficulty with feeding or swallowing, should prompt a referral. Not producing a variety of sounds in different combinations by the age of 12 months also may indicate reason for concern. By age 3, the child should have acquired the use of most speech sounds so that his or her speech is intelligible most of the time. If speech is very difficult to understand at this age, a referral should be considered. By age 6, the child should have essentially "perfect" speech with no errors in articulation. If articulation errors persist after this age, a referral to a speech-language pathologist is indicated.

**III. Language development.** Because we cannot actually hear or see the process, the development of receptive language is inferred. More is known about the process children go through in the development of expressive language, however, because it is more easily observed and documented.

**A. Newborns.** At birth, the infant is aware of sounds in the environment and startles or cries in response to loud or sudden noises. Studies suggest that infants are aware of even the differences between similar speech sounds (e.g., /p/ and /b/). Awareness and discrimination form the basis of later understanding. Expressive language development begins with early cries, which are reflexive and stimulated by physical or environmental conditions, such as hunger or pain. The infant soon learns, however, that these cries bring about a caregiver response, such as feeding or attention. As a result, the infant begins to use crying and various vocalizations to bring about a response. Within the first few months, most parents are able to distinguish their infant's cries of hunger, pain, and needing attention.

**B. 2–6 months.** By 2 months of age, the infant achieves and maintains eye contact with others as they speak. By 4 months, the infant begins to vocalize directly to others with cooing and learns to imitate and take turns in sound production. In the first 6 months, the infant is taking in all that he or she hears in the environment and may be beginning to understand that speech has meaning. The infant does not demonstrate much understanding at this point, however.

Caregivers and other speakers in the environment unknowingly assist the infant in learning to listen to and understand language by using a unique speaking style characterized by the use of short utterances and very simple syntax. A small core vocabulary is used, and topics are limited to the here and now. The same utterance often is repeated, and verbal rituals or games, such as "so big" or "patty cake" are used frequently. The speaker also alters his or her tone of voice when speaking to an infant, tending to use a high pitch with great pitch variation and intonation. Facial expressions and gestures are exaggerated during speech to capture the infant's attention.

**C. 6–12 months.** At 6–8 months of age, the child begins to display an association of meaning to the sound combinations heard in speech. The child looks up in response to his or her name, may respond to "no," and responds to simple commands such as "Come here." Gestures accompanied by vocalizations are used as a form of expressive language at this developmental stage.

By 7–8 months, most babies have begun to use a pointing or reaching gesture that may mean one of two things: "I want that" or "Look at that." This gestural form of communication is very effective at this age and communicates all the child's needs at that time.

By 10–12 months of age, the child is able to point to body parts, common objects, and simple pictures following a request. The child demonstrates understanding by responding to many simple, one-part commands. The child also babbles and jargons to others and occasionally uses single words with gestures for communication.

**D. 12–18 months.** After the first birthday, the child follows many simple commands and seems to understand much of what is said to him or her. Since comprehension precedes production, the child is able to understand far more than he or she is able to say.

First words begin to emerge at 9–18 months of age; most children use at least one or two words by their first birthday. Many first words sound much like babbling (e.g., mama, dada, bye bye). They become true words when these sound combinations are used in an appropriate and meaningful way.

The child's first words are typically holophrastic in nature. In other words, "milk" may mean "I want the milk," "I don't want the milk," or "I spilled the milk." Most first words are substantive words, such as nouns or verbs. Some functional words, such as "all gone," " no," "more," or "that," also emerge as first words. A few social words are acquired early in development as well, such as "hi" and "bye bye."

The development of vocabulary skills is a very complex process that involves much more than mere memorization of labels. For children to learn a simple word such as "chair," they must first develop a mental prototype of this word based on perceptual features, functional features, or both. For example, a chair has the perceptual features of four legs and a flat surface. These features also apply to a table or a sofa, however. A chair has the functional features of something to sit in, but this is also true of a sofa. The child needs to determine which perceptual and functional features most clearly define the word "chair" for understanding and appropriate use to occur.

Children often make mistakes while learning the meaning of words. They commonly overgeneralize words—for example, a child initially may assume that all animals with a snout, four legs, and a tail are dogs. A less common error is one of exclusion—for example, a child may assume a Chihuahua cannot be a dog because it is too small. The process of learning to code and categorize words appropriately is obviously very complex, yet it must take place for the development of much of the entire lexicon.

**E. 18–24 months.** At 18–24 months, the child understands more complex language, showing an understanding of some concepts such as adjectives, possessive pronouns, and plural forms. The child can follow many compound and complex commands and begins to combine words together for short utterances. At first, words are combined without regard to syntactical order. Each word usually has a downward intonational contour, suggesting that the word represents a complete sentence—for example, the child may say "dish," "broke," and "Michael" as three separate sentences. The child then learns to combine words in an appropriate syntactic order for two- and three-word utterances. The child may later say, for example, "Broke dish" or "Michael broke dish."

Although much is written about the two-word stage of language development, most children begin combining two, three, and even four words around the same time. By the age of 2 years, the child should be combining at least two words together for short utterances.

F. **2–3 years.** At 2–3 years, the child demonstrates an understanding of long and complex sentences and shows an interest in verbal explanations of why and how. The child understands most forms of syntax and follows everyday conversation easily. From this point on, receptive language continues to develop, but primarily in the area of vocabulary and understanding idioms or subtle meanings. At this stage, the child's expressive language consists of phrases and short sentences. The child uses different syntactical forms, such as pronouns, plurals, past tense, questions forms, and negation. The child first learns the rules of syntax and then the exceptions to those rules. Therefore, syntactical errors are very common in the normal developmental process, such as the following: "I talk gooder than you," "I runned outside," "I got stang by a bee," "I have two feets." These errors actually show that the child has learned the rule and how to apply it; however, learning all the exceptions takes time. Therefore, these errors of regularizing irregular syntactic forms may persist even past school age.

G. **3–6 years.** By the age of 3, the normally developing child communicates with long and structurally complex sentences and begins to develop the pragmatic skills that relate to the social rules of conversation. For instance, the child learns to initiate a conversation appropriately, usually by saying "hi" followed by the listener's name. The child becomes aware that, in a conversation, the speaker needs to reference pronouns before using them. The speaker also needs to consider what the listener knows about the topic so that the conversation can be geared appropriately. The child learns that it is not appropriate to end a conversation on the telephone without saying "good-bye." At this stage, the child begins to understand that the meaning of what is said often has to be inferred. For example, "Could you please pass the salt?" is actually a command and does not require an affirmative answer, and the idiom "Two heads are better than one" should not be interpreted literally.

H. **Referral guidelines.** If the child does not use any single words by 16–18 months of age and cannot follow simple commands, a speech-language pathology assessment should be considered. If the child does not combine words for short utterances by the age of 2 or use complete sentences by the age of 3, an evaluation is indicated. Finally, if the child's sentence structures are noticeably defective or the child has difficulty communicating ideas effectively at age 4, a referral should be made for a speech and language evaluation.

## IV. Key points

A. Although speech and language development are very individual and minor variations occur in the rate and sequence of development, the primary care physician should be knowledgeable about the stages of normal development and proactive in screening for communication difficulties.

**B.** Whenever there is a suspicion that the child is not developing speech or language skills normally, the child should be referred to a speech-language pathologist for a professional evaluation.

**C.** The pediatrician always should listen to parents' concerns because parents are usually good observers of their own children. If parents are worried about the child's speech and language development, a referral for evaluation is appropriate. Even if therapy is not recommended at that time, the speech-language pathologist can provide the parents with developmentally appropriate activities to stimulate speech and language development in the home.

**D.** Early intervention is very important and ultimately can affect the long-term prognosis for normal communication skills. Ideally, intervention should occur in the preschool years to take advantage of the brain's plasticity for developing speech and language skills. If the communication disorder persists into the school-age years, not only does the child have more difficulty acquiring language skills, but habit strength makes the disorder more difficult to correct. An investment in early intervention can pay off in the future in regards to treatment and educational costs.

## Selected Readings

Bloom L, Lahey M. *Language Development and Language Disorders*. New York: Wiley, 1978.

Coplan J. *The Early Language Milestone Scale* (ELM-2). Austin, TX: Pro-Ed, 1993.

Coplan J. Normal speech and language development: An overview. *Pediatr Rev* 16:91, 1995.

Foster S. *The Communicative Competence of Young Children: A Modular Approach*. London: Longmans, 1990.

Lindfors JW. *Children's Language and Learning*. Englewood Cliffs, NJ: Prentice-Hall, 1980.

Owens RE. *Language Development: An Introduction* (3rd ed). New York: Merrill, 1992.

Reed V. *An Introduction to Children with Language Disorders*. New York: Macmillan, 1986.

Skinner PH, Shelton RL. *Speech, Language and Hearing* (2nd ed). New York: Wiley, 1985.

# 10

# Normal Motor and Cognitive Development

**Rosemary E. Schmidt and Sonya Oppenheimer**

Developmental assessment of the young child is a key function of all physicians who provide primary care to infants and children. Development is a dynamic process that must be monitored throughout the child's growing years. Acquisition of normal motor milestones does not necessarily equate with normal cognition; children who become autistic may have normal motor milestones just as children with delayed motor milestones due to cerebral palsy may have normal cognition.

I. **Normal developmental milestones** traditionally are divided into four areas: major motor, minor motor, social adaptive, and language. The average ages and age ranges at which accomplishments in each of these areas occur in the normal infant have been quantitated and are the basis of the Denver Developmental Screening Test (DDST), which is commonly used to assess development as part of well-child care. The Revised DDST-II (see Appendix J) contains the standard milestones in chronological order. The authors of the DDST suggest it be administered in the standardized manner with specific tools. It is also useful, however, as a reference for the primary care physician because it shows the age range for acquisition of developmental milestones.

Ideally, the DDST would be administered to all infants and children at all well-child visits. More practically, however, most practitioners incorporate some of these milestones into the developmental history and physical examination to estimate the infant's or child's functional age. When the developmental age seems delayed, more quantitative testing is performed using a tool such as the DDST, or referral for developmental evaluation is made.

Early identification of the child with developmental delays is desirable so that an intervention program can be planned. Public Law 1029–119, in place since 1986, mandates an appropriate education in the least restrictive environment for all children with developmental problems. Children from birth to 3 years of age are entitled to intervention services that may include an early childhood developmentalist, an occupational therapist, a physical therapist, and a speech therapist. The services required are determined by the developmental assessment and the family wishes. Every state has its own laws that, in general, require local availability of resources. The primary care physician must be aware of these resources in order to provide appropriate referrals as necessary.

II. **Cognitive development.** A number of methods can be used to determine cognitive development and intelligence. When testing these functions in children, the physician must realize that cognitive development and intelligence are affected by many factors in addition to genetics, many of which may not be readily apparent at the time of testing. These factors include environmental stimulation, motor function and development, and sensory function and development. Formal tests of cognitive development and intelligence include the following:

A. **Bayley Scales of Infant Development** (0–2½ years)
B. **Gesell Developmental Schedule** (0–5 years)
C. **Stanford-Binet IV** (2 years to adult)
D. **Wechsler Preschool Primary Scale of Intelligence** (4–6 years)
E. **Wechsler Intelligence Scale of Children** (5–15 years)

III. **Motor development.** During early childhood development, primitive reflexes are replaced by voluntary motor control regulated by higher cortical centers. Motor development generally proceeds in a cephalocaudad direction characterized by the acquisition of oculomotor control at birth (by 16 weeks), head and arm control (16–28 weeks), trunk and hand control (28–40 weeks), walking and running (second year), and mature motor control by 5 years. It is important to observe symmetry of motor movements as well as the regular acquisition of developmental milestones. Delays in motor skills may indicate global developmental delay (mental retardation), primary motor delays (such as that seen in cerebral palsy), or environmental deprivation. Physicians should look for the following developmental milestones:

A. **2–3 months.** The infant gains head control using the neck muscles against gravity.
B. **3–4 months.** The infant demonstrates progressive shoulder and upper-trunk control and lifts his or her chest off flat surfaces.
C. **4 months.** The infant's ability to roll over prone to supine is demonstrated.
D. **6–7 months.** Trunk control is gained and leads to sitting.
E. **9–17 months.** Locomotion begins with rolling and is followed by the "commando crawl," creeping in the quadruped position, bear-walking on hands and knees, standing, "cruising," and eventually free walking (average 12 months). Subsequently, there is ongoing improvement in balance and coordination.
F. **22 months.** The child can throw a ball overhand.
G. **30 months.** The child can pedal a tricycle.
H. **36 months.** The child balances on one foot for 1 second.
I. **48 months.** The child can hop on one foot.
J. **4–4½ years.** The child demonstrates the heel-to-toe maneuver.
K. **4½ years.** The child can catch a bouncing ball.
L. **5–7 years.** The child begins riding a two-wheel bicycle.

IV. **Primitive reflexes in the infant**. Normal motor development depends on intact peripheral and central nervous systems, normal muscle tone, the presence and later integration of primitive reflexes, and the development of postural and righting reflexes. Persistence of primitive reflexes can interfere with normal motor development.

In addition to the routine developmental milestones suggested by the DDST (which are ascertained routinely as part

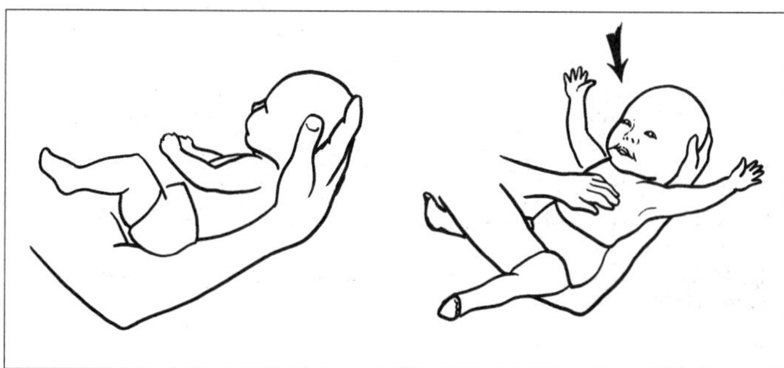

**Fig. 10-1. Moro's reflex. Left, infant held by examiner; right, movement of infant elicited by downward motion.**

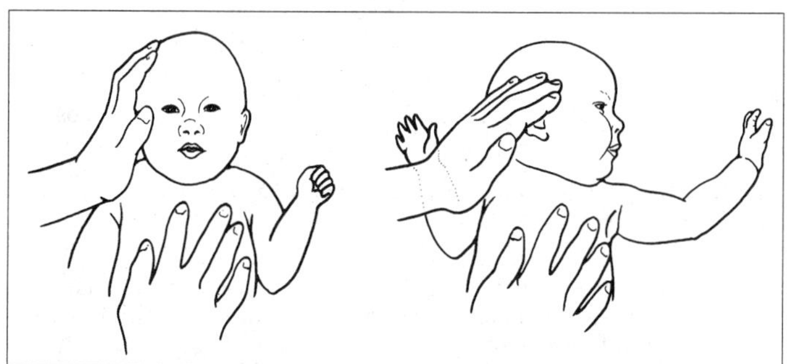

**Fig. 10-2. Asymmetric tonic neck reflex. Left, infant with head in neutral position; right, position of arms after head turned to left.**

of the well-child examination), the neurologic examination of the infant should include an evaluation of several primitive reflexes, which, while normal in the first 3–4 months of age, should disappear at certain ages. Persistence should alert the physician to neurodevelopmental abnormalities such as cerebral palsy. At the same time, certain postural reflexes develop as neurodevelopmental maturation occurs. These primitive and postural reflexes are described below.

**A. Moro's reflex** (Fig. 10-1). The infant is cradled in a semi-reclined position of about 45 degrees with his or her head supported by the examiner's hand. With the examiner's hand and forearm under the infant's head and trunk, the examiner drops the infant's body downward and back. The sudden loss of support without letting the baby's head fall back unsupported should produce Moro's reflex—that is, the infant extends his or her arms, quickly opening the hands and fingers. This movement is good for early detection of asymmetry in the upper extremities. The response should disappear at approximately 4 months of age.

**B. Asymmetric tonic neck reflex** (Fig. 10-2). The infant is placed on his or her back. Keeping the infant's neck and body aligned and stabilizing the trunk with one hand, the

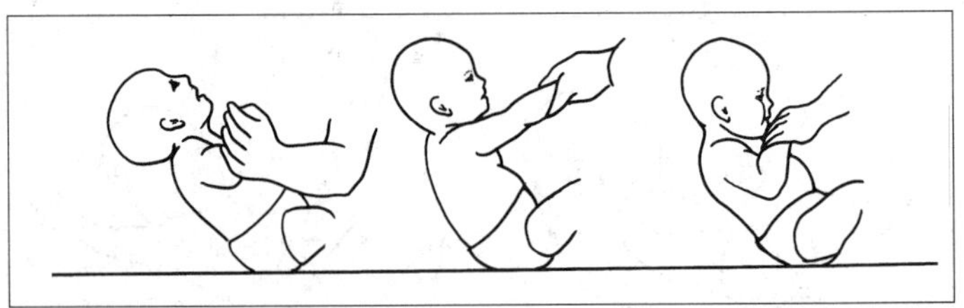

**Fig. 10-3. Pull to sit. Left, less than 4 months of age; middle, 4–5 months of age; right, more than 5 months of age.**

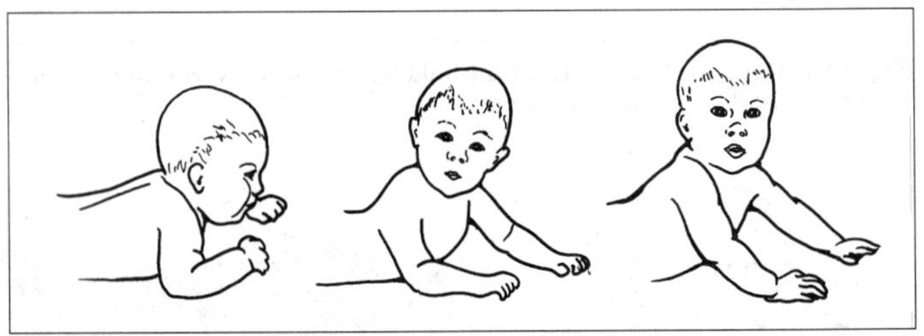

**Fig. 10-4. Body lying prone. Left, 0–2 months of age; middle, 2–4 months of age; right, 6 months of age.**

examiner gently turns the infant's head to one side and holds it for about 10 seconds, watching the child's arms. An infant responds positively (e.g., when his or her head is turned to the left) by flexing the right elbow and straightening the left arm. The asymmetric tonic neck reflex normally is present in infants 1–4 months old.

C. **Pull to sit** (Fig. 10-3)
   1. **Younger than 4 months.** The infant's head lags behind the body.
   2. **4–5 months.** The infant keeps the head in line with the body.
   3. **Older than 5 months.** The infant's head leads the body.

D. **Body lying prone** (Fig. 10-4)
   1. **0–2 months.** The infant's head is in line with the body.
   2. **2–4 months.** The infant can elevate his or her head about 45 degrees.
   3. **6 months.** The infant can elevate his or her head 90 degrees.

E. **Sitting posture**. With the child in the sitting position, the observer notes the spine's curvature. Normal responses are the following:
   1. **Younger than 4 months.** The infant's spine is completely rounded.
   2. **4 months.** The infant's spine extends, or straightens, to the level of the third lumbar segment.
   3. **6–7 months.** The infant extends, or straightens, the upper and lower back and props forward with the hands.
   4. **8 months**. The infant sits erect with no difficulty.

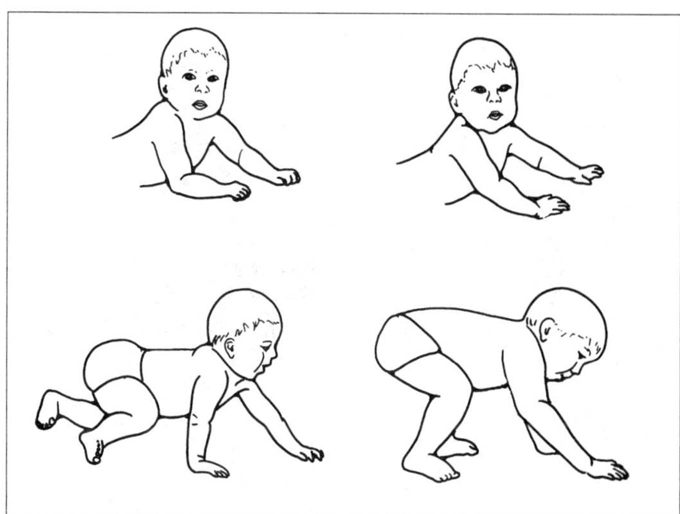

**Fig. 10-5. All fours. Top left, 3½ months of age; top right, 5 months of age; bottom left, 7–9 months of age; bottom right, 10–12 months of age.**

F. **All fours** (Fig. 10-5) refers to the child's ability to assume the all-fours position. The physician should note the following progression of this ability:
   1. **3½ months.** The infant props on the forearms and hands.
   2. **5 months.** The infant supports himself or herself on the hands.
   3. **7–9 months.** The infant can get on the hands and knees.
   4. **10–12 months.** The child can assume the plantigrade position on hands and feet.

G. **Head in space.** The infant is held in vertical suspension and tilted slowly—first sideways each way and then forward and backward. In an infant with poor head control or in a premature newborn, the examiner should be careful not to hyperextend the neck when tilting the child backward. When tilted, the infant should try to adjust his or her head so that it remains upright regardless of body position, with the eyes and mouth horizontal and the nose vertical. This reaction normally begins to appear at about 1-1/2 months of age and is complete by 4 months.

H. **Downward parachute** (Fig. 10-6). The test for the downward parachute response should be attempted only after the child has demonstrated head control. The child is lifted vertically some distance from the examination table. Once the infant's legs are somewhat flexed, the examiner rapidly lowers the child 2–3 feet to produce the sensation of falling. If no response is elicited by lowering the child to the table top, lower the child to the floor. The normal infant at about 4 months of age reacts by straightening and spreading the legs and turning the feet outward.

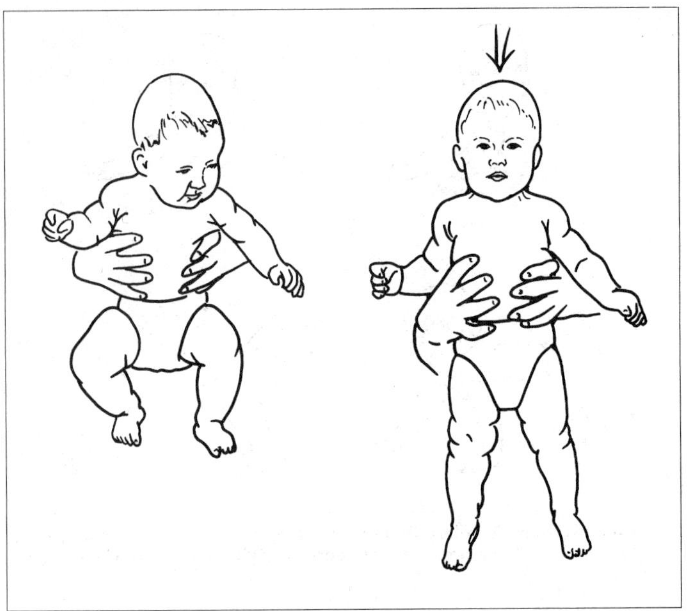

**Fig. 10-6. Downward parachute. Left, infant in position; right, protective movement (straightening of lower extremities) with downward motion.**

I. **Standing ability**. To test the infant's ability to stand, hold the infant upright above the examining table. Note whether the child can support his or her weight well. Normal development of this ability is the following:
   1. **5 months.** The infant is able to support his or her own weight; legs are semiflexed.
   2. **8 months.** The infant is able to stand with support with trunk slightly forward and hips flexed.
   3. **10 months.** The child is able to stand erect with support.
   4. **12 months.** The child is able to stand independently.

   Primitive supporting reactions are tested by holding at least part of the infant's weight. An infant younger than 2 1/2 months immediately stiffens the legs in extension ("positive supporting"); if the child is between 2 1/2 and 5 months of age, the legs should collapse as you lower him or her toward the table ("astasia").

J. **Sideways parachute** (Fig. 10-7). After the age of 6 months, a normal infant tries to protect himself or herself from falling by extending an arm and open hand.

K. **Forward parachute** (Fig. 10-8). Like the other parachute reactions, this reaction should not be tested until the child has demonstrated head control. The infant is held firmly at midtrunk level with his or her back to the examiner. Suspended vertically above the table, the infant is then tilted forward suddenly. A normal infant reacts by

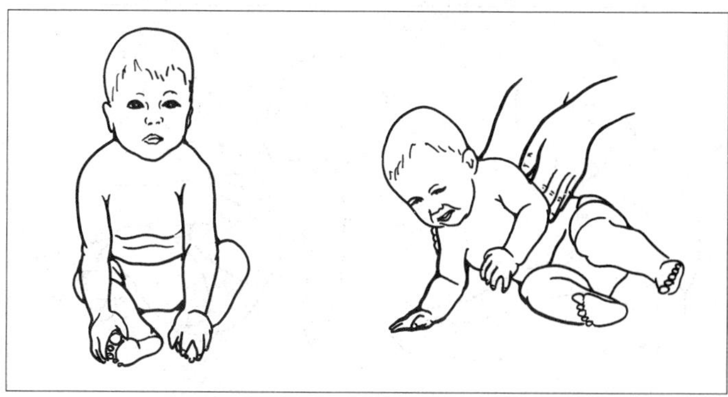

**Fig. 10-7. Sideways parachute. Left, infant in position; right, protective movement (abduction of upper extremity) with push.**

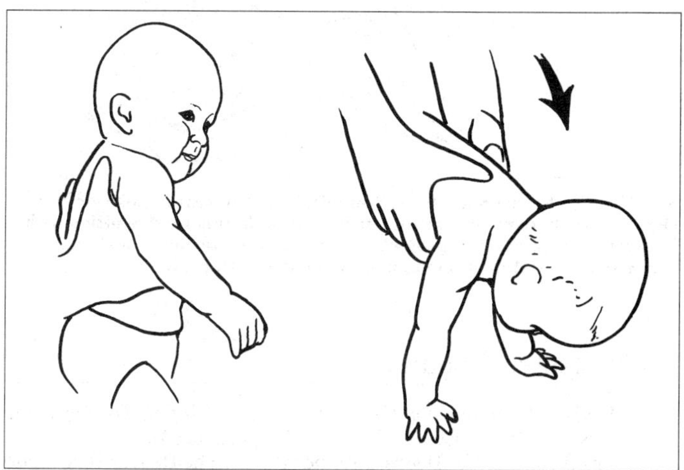

**Fig. 10-8. Forward parachute. Left, infant in position; right, protective movement (straightening of upper extremities toward table or floor) with forward motion.**

straightening the arms forward and extending the fingers. This reaction may be seen in infants as young as 7 months. Asymmetry in the upper extremities can be detected using this maneuver.

L. **Backward parachute** (Fig. 10-9). Holding the child in the sitting position, the examiner gently tips him or her backward. Usually, a child age 9 months or older reacts to the sudden imbalance by either extending both hands behind or rotating to one side to catch himself or herself with a hand. This should not be tested in a child who does not demonstrate good head control to avoid rapid flexing and extension of the neck.

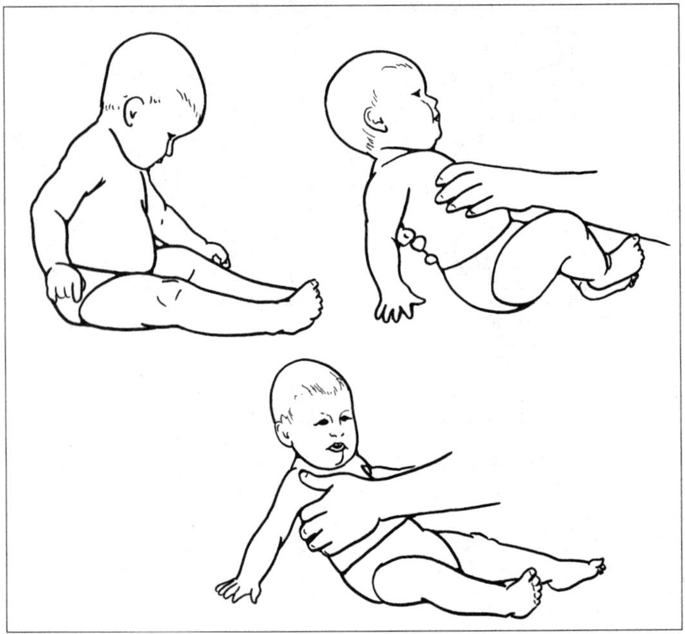

**Fig. 10-9. Backward parachute. Top left, infant in sitting position; top right, protective movement (extension) of both upper extremities with backward push; bottom, protective movement (rotation of body and extension/abduction of one upper extremity) with push.**

## Selected Readings

Bayley N. *Manual for the Bayley Scales of Infant Development.* San Antonio, TX: Psychological Corporation, 1969.

Frankenberg WK, Dodds J, Archer P et al. The Denver II: a major revision and restandardization of the Denver Developmental Screening Test. *Pediatrics* 89:91, 1992.

Frankenberg WK, Thornton SM, Cohrs ME. *Pediatric Developmental Diagnosis*. New York: Thieme-Stratton, 1981.

Gesell A, Amatruda CS. *Developmental Diagnosis*. New York: Harper & Row, 1967.

Thorndike RL, Hagen EP, Sattler JM. *The Stanford-Binet Intelligence Scale: Guide for Administering and Scoring* (4th ed). Chicago: Riverside, 1986.

Wechsler D. *The Wechsler Pre-School and Primary Scale of Intelligence (WPPSI)*. New York: Psychological Corporation, 1967.

Wechsler D. *Wechsler Intelligence Scale for Children—Revised Manual (WICS-R)*. New York: Psychological Corporation, 1974.

# II

# The Problem Visit—Medical

# A

# Dermatologic Disorders

11

# Atopic Dermatitis (Eczema)

Raymond C. Baker

Atopic dermatitis, or eczema, is an inherited, chronic skin condition related to the other atopic diseases, asthma, and allergic rhinitis and conjunctivitis (hay fever). It usually is associated with a positive family history, personal history of other atopic diseases, elevated serum IgE, dry skin, and eosinophilia.

I. **Description.** Eczema begins in the first few months of life as a red, pruritic dermatitis primarily of the cheeks, trunk, and extensor surfaces. As the child grows older, it commonly concentrates on the flexured areas of the body (e.g., antecubital fossae, popliteal fossae, nape of neck, hands, feet).

Associated skin conditions include dry skin (almost always), keratosis pilaris, pityriasis alba, and ichthyosis vulgaris. The skin typically shows erythema, papules, crusting, and oozing (especially with superinfection) with secondary excoriations, lichenification, and hyperpigmentation. Prominent features at all times are dry skin, itch (which waxes and wanes), and hypersensitivity of the skin to external contacts (e.g., harsh soaps, irritating cloth) resulting in itch, scratch, and skin lesions—the "vicious cycle" of atopic dermatitis.

II. The **treatment** of atopic dermatitis consists of attention to the four "*I's*" of eczema: *i*tch, *i*nflammation, *i*nfection, and *i*mmersion in water.

A. **Itch** is a constant feature of eczema. In the young infant, evidence of itch is the parent's complaint about the infant's difficult or restless sleeping. At all ages, excoriations and lichenification (from rubbing pruritic skin) are evidence of itch. Treatment of itch may require antihistamines to control until other interventions take effect. Diphenhydramine (1.5–2.0 mg/kg PO q4h) or hydroxyzine (0.5 mg/kg PO q4h) especially at bedtime is usually effective.

B. **Inflammation** typically is controlled with topical steroids (1.0% and 2.5% hydrocortisone), applied thinly and rubbed into the skin bid–tid. The higher-strength preparation usually is given initially if the inflammation is severe for 3–4 days. The weaker preparation then can be used for maintenance. More potent, fluorinated steroid creams should be avoided whenever possible in children, especially in naturally occluded areas (groin, axilla) and on the face due to the increased possibility of local side effects (cutaneous atrophy, steroid rosacea, striae, and telangiectasia).

C. **Infection** should be sought any time an exacerbation occurs or typical crusting and oozing develop. Superinfection with skin organisms, especially *Staphylococcus aureus*, is common and requires systemic antibiotics such as erythromycin.

D. **Immersion in water (hydration).** Perhaps the most important aspect of care is skin rehydration. Dry skin tends to produce itch and subsequent exacerbation of the dermatitis; therefore, skin should be kept hydrated at all times. This is best accomplished by frequent bathing or soaking in the bathtub (qd routinely, bid to bring an exacerbation under control) with limited use of soaps. Soaking is followed immediately by applying a topical cream or ointment (lotion is not as effective for this purpose; ointment is most effective) to trap the water in the skin to keep it hydrated. Specific instructions to the parent are to allow the child to play or soak in the water until the skin is thoroughly hydrated. Then, before drying, apply topical preparations (topical steroids first, then creams or ointments to maintain hydration of the skin). Sometimes the two can be combined into one if the vehicle of the steroid is appropriate, but this tends to be more expensive. In general, younger children better tolerate ointments (e.g., Vaseline, Aquaphor), which are more occlusive to prevent water loss from the skin and less expensive, whereas older children object to the greasy feel of ointments and better tolerate creams (e.g., Eucerin, Nivea).

## Selected Readings

Cohen B. Atopic dermatitis: breaking the itch-scratch cycle. *Contemp Pediatr* August 1992, Pp 64–81.

Hurwitz S. *Clinical Pediatric Dermatology* (2nd ed). Philadelphia: Saunders, 1992.

Weston WL, Lane AT. *Color Textbook of Pediatric Dermatology*. St. Louis: Mosby-Year Book, 1991.

12

# Diaper Dermatitis

**Raymond C. Baker**

I. **Diaper dermatitis** occurs in up to 35% of infants, peaking at 7–9 months of age. The majority of such rashes are due to prolonged skin contact with moisture (urine), which results in overhydration and maceration of the skin. Rubber pants over cloth diapers and paper diapers with plastic outer layers and fitted legs exacerbate the diaper's humid environment by preventing ventilation, thereby increasing maceration and epidermal breakdown. This commonly is followed by further damage from diaper chafing, irritants in the stool, and superinfection with *Candida albicans*. Other common etiologies of diaper dermatitis that must be distinguished clinically are atopic dermatitis, seborrheic dermatitis, and bullous impetigo.

II. **Treatment** of diaper dermatitis depends on the etiology, severity, and the period of time it has been present. The following recommendations are in order of both increasing severity and length of time present.

A. **Routine care** of the diaper area in the infant without dermatitis consists of frequent diaper changes as feasible and cleansing with tepid water or prepackaged diaper wipes with each change. Mild soap, such as Dove or Johnson's Baby Soap, or prepackaged wipes may be used after defecation. Talcum powder is unnecessary except as a deodorant.

B. **Chafing diaper dermatitis** (mild erythema sparing the folds of skin; shiny, glazed surface) may be relieved simply by applying corn starch or talcum powder to decrease friction produced by the skin's rubbing against the diaper, which caused the rash. The physician should caution parents about leaving containers of talcum powder within reach of the infant, who may mistake a container for a bottle and ingest or inhale some of the powder.

C. **Moderate irritant dermatitis** (mild erythema, epidermis intact, indistinct border) may be treated by increasing the frequency of diaper changes and gently cleaning the diaper area at diaper changes with tepid water. It is also important that the diaper area be adequately ventilated, which may be achieved by (1) using cloth diapers without rubber pants, (2) cutting or tearing the fitted legs of paper diapers to allow air entry, or (3) exposing the diaper area to air for 5–10 minutes at each diaper change. In addition, Vaseline, petrolatum, A&D, Desitin, or other ointment may be applied at bedtime to protect skin from contact with urine overnight. Ointment should be removed gently with the morning bath.

D. **Severe irritant dermatitis (erythema, superficial ulceration) with *C. albicans* superinfection (intense erythema, satellite lesions)** may require an antifungal agent (nystatin, clotrimazole) tid and an ointment or paste containing zinc oxide (Balmex, Desitin, Caldesene) at night. Overnight ointments should be removed in the morning with gentle soap-and-water cleansing (or baby oil for ointments and pastes such as Desitin, which may be difficult to remove with just soap and water) followed by antifungal cream. Occasionally, topical **nonfluorinated** steroids such as 0.5–1.0% hydrocortisone used sparingly and for a limited period of time (2–4 days) may reduce the rash's inflammatory component and improve patient comfort more rapidly.

**E. Bullous impetigo** of the diaper area is characterized by large, flaccid vesicles and blisters (bullae) of varying size that may be filled with cloudy fluid or pus. Bullous impetigo is treated with oral systemic antibiotics (semisynthetic, beta-lactamase–resistant penicillins, erythromycin, or cephalosporins with activity against *Staphylococcus aureus*) and topical skin care.

## Selected Readings

Hurwitz S. Skin lesions in the first year of life. *Contemp Pediatr* January 1993, Pp 110–128.

Lane AT. Resolving controversies in diaper dermatitis. *Contemp Pediatr* April 1986, Pp 45–54.

Rasmussen JE. Diaper dermatitis. *Pediatr Rev* 6:77, 1984.

Weston WL, Lane AT, Weston JA. Diaper dermatitis: current concepts. *Pediatrics* 66:532, 1980.

# 13

# Impetigo

## Raymond C. Baker

Impetigo contagiosa is the most common childhood bacterial skin dermatitis. There are two classic forms of impetigo: nonbullous impetigo and bullous impetigo.

I. **Nonbullous impetigo** is the more common type of impetigo in children. The typical lesion begins as an erythematous papule, commonly resulting from skin trauma as a result of scratching, insect bites, viral exanthema, and so forth. This lesion spreads rapidly to become an amber-colored crust on an erythematous base, ranging in size from several millimeters to 1–2 cm. The lesions occur most commonly on the extremities and around the nose and mouth. Nonbullous impetigo is seen more commonly during the summer months in preschool and early school-age children. The diagnosis is made by the clinical appearance of the lesions; bacterial culture usually is unnecessary.

The **etiology** of nonbullous impetigo is *Streptococcus pyogenes*, *Staphylococcus aureus*, or both. **Treatment** should be selected to cover both organisms. Oral antibiotic choices are erythromycin, cloxacillin, dicloxacillin, cephalexin, amoxicillin-clavulanate, cefpodoxime, cefprozil, cefaclor, or loracarbef for 10 days. Topical therapy with mupirocin (Bactroban) applied tid has been shown to be as effective as oral erythromycin. The choice of treating orally (systemically) versus topically is influenced by the area of skin to be covered and the local prevalence of erythromycin-resistant *S. aureus,* which is significant in some communities. Treatment of impetigo caused by *S. pyogenes* does not prevent the complication of acute poststreptococcal glomerulonephritis.

II. **Bullous impetigo** is less common and exclusively due to *S. aureus*. The organism produces epidemolytic toxin, which acts locally to cause separation within the layers of the epidermis, encouraging bulla formation. The bullae are flaccid, may be filled with cloudy fluid, and arise from normal-appearing skin. Lesions are 0.5–3.0 cm in diameter. After they rupture, a thin, clear varnish-like coating appears over the denuded area. The lesions may enlarge even after the bulla has ruptured; they often are found in small groups of three to six bullae confined to a single area. In the newborn, lesions often are found in the perineal, periumbilical, and axillary areas. In older children, they usually occur on the extremities. The diagnosis usually can be made clinically, although a bacterial culture is confirmatory. Systemic antistaphylococcal antibiotics such as those listed above should be given for a 10-day course. There are insufficient data on topical mupirocin treatment in bullous impetigo to suggest its use.

## Selected Readings

Barton LL, Friedman AD, Sharkey AM et al. Impetigo contagiosa III. Comparative efficacy of oral erythromycin and topical mupirocin. *Pediatr Dermatol* 6:134, 1989.

Dagan R. Impetigo in childhood: changing epidemiology and new treatments. *Pediatr Ann* 22:235, 1993.

Demidovich CW, Wittler RR, Ruff ME et al. Impetigo: current etiology and comparison of penicillin, erythromycin, and cephalexin therapies. *Am J Dis Child* 144:1313, 1990.

Goldfarb J, Crenshaw D, O'Horo J et al. Randomized clinical trial of topical mupirocin versus oral erythromycin for impetigo. *Antimicrob Agents Chemother* 32:1780, 1988.

McLinn S. Topical mupirocin versus systemic erythromycin treatment for pyoderma. *Pediatr Infect Dis J* 7:785, 1988.

Rasmussen JE. Impetigo: changing bacteria, changing therapies. *Contemp Pediatr* 9:14, 1992.

14

# Lice and Scabies

## Raymond C. Baker

I. **Head lice (pediculosis capitis)**

A. **Life cycle**. The egg of the *Pediculus humanus capitis* incubates for 8–9 days, and the offspring mature in 10–15 days. The adult feeds about five times per day, and the female lays about six eggs a day for a 2- to 3-month period. The eggs are laid close to the scalp for warmth, requiring a temperature of about 87°F for optimal growth; they are cemented firmly to the hair shaft and not easily removed. Eggs can survive for about 30 days off the host; the adult can survive only a few days off the host.

B. **Epidemiology**. Females are infested more frequently by head lice than males, children more frequently than adults, and whites much more frequently than blacks, in whom lice infestation is rare. The greatest incidence of head lice is in the fall and winter. Spread is by the direct hair-to-hair or fomite-to-hair (e.g., hats, brushes) transfer of adult lice, not eggs.

C. **Diagnosis** of head lice is made by a history of itch, exposure, and presence of nits in the hair (the greatest concentration of nits is usually at the occiput). Nits appear as white to gray, smooth, oval particles firmly attached to the hair shaft close to scalp. They fluoresce weakly with a Wood's lamp, which is useful in screening large numbers of children, as in school. Excoriations, especially at the back of the neck, may be present. Particles of dandruff, which may resemble nits, are distinguished easily by their easy removal from hair, whereas nits are firmly attached to the hair shaft. If in doubt about lice infestation, microscopic examination of a hair with a nit provides an unmistakable diagnosis. Adult lice are seen sometimes, especially with heavy infestations, but less often than nits.

D. **Treatment.** Several effective treatments are available for head lice. Kwell Shampoo (lindane) is applied to dry hair in a quantity large enough to wet the hair, left on 5–10 minutes, then lathered with water and removed; this procedure should be repeated in 1 week. Nits must be removed mechanically with a fine-toothed comb. Pyrethrins (e.g., RID, A-200) are used similarly to Kwell Shampoo. Nix Cream Rinse (permethrin) has the advantage of being more ovicidal. This product is applied to the hair after washing and towel drying, left on 5–10 minutes, and rinsed off with water; repeat application is usually unnecessary. Since this product is ovicidal, removal of nits is not as important; however, most schools and day-care facilities will not accept a child with nits in the hair.

Fomites should be washed in hot water and dried in a hot dryer, dry cleaned, or stored in a sealed plastic bag 2–3 weeks, by which time the parasites will have died without a food source.

**II. Pubic lice infestation (pediculosis pubis)**

**A.** The **life cycle** of the causative organism *Phthirus pubis* is similar to that of the head louse.

**B. Epidemiology.** The peak age of infestation is 15–40 years. Blacks and whites are affected equally, females more commonly under age 19, males more commonly over age 18. The adult louse usually is transmitted during sexual intercourse; thus, pubic lice should be considered a sexually transmitted disease.

**C. Diagnosis** is made by a history of itch and exposure. Nits and adult lice are visible in the pubic hair on examination. Excoriations may be present, including characteristic sky-blue spots (maculae ceruleae) in the pubic area.

**D. Treatment** is similar to that for head lice. Kwell lotion may be used but must be left on overnight. Sexual partners should be treated also, and evaluation and testing for other sexually transmitted diseases should be considered.

**E. Phthiriasis palpebrum**. Infestation of the eyelashes and lids with pubic lice is seen in children with infected parents. Treatment is petrolatum applied 4–5 times a day followed by the mechanical removal of nits with forceps.

**III. Scabies**

**A. Life cycle**. The impregnated female *Sarcoptes scabiei* burrows superficially into the epidermis, forming a burrow at a rate of 1–5 mm per day and laying eggs at a rate of about 2–3 a day. The adult life span is about 30 days. Eggs hatch in 3–5 days, and offspring mature in 8–17 days, ready for impregnation. Males do not burrow and die shortly after copulation.

**B. Epidemiology**. Men are affected more than women, girls more than boys. The most common age of infection is age 15–40 years, although scabies is seen fairly commonly in children. Spread is by skin-to-skin contact as during sexual intercourse or mother-to-child contact. Fomites have little involvement in the organism's transmission.

**C. Pathogenesis**. The symptoms in scabies are most likely the result of allergic sensitization to the mite and its products. Evidence of an allergic pathogenesis includes (1) the observation that symptoms are delayed until 30 days after first infestation yet develop within 24 hours after reinfestation; (2) reinfestation is uncommon, suggesting that the allergic inflammatory response kills or attenuates the organism; (3) the patient has a positive intracutaneous skin test with crude extract (immediate reaction); and (4) the patient has a positive Prausnitz-Kustner passive transfer test.

**D. History.** The characteristic history in scabies is itch, itch, itch! The itch of scabies typically has a gradual onset, is progressive, and is usually worse at night. The scratching it evokes is severe enough to cause bleeding. There is almost always someone else in the family infested with whom the affected child sleeps (siblings or parents).

**E. Physical examination** reveals a characteristic distribution that includes the flexured areas of the body (wrists, ankles, elbows, axillae, umbilicus, interdigital web spaces, penis, nipples). In young children, palms and soles commonly are affected. Primary lesions are burrows, papules, vesicles, and pustules; secondary lesions are excoriations, impetiginization, urticaria, and nodules.

F. **Diagnosis** is made using the combination of a characteristic history, characteristic distribution and appearance of the lesions, identification of burrows, and demonstration of the mite on skin scraping. The latter is unnecessary if burrows are identified. Skin scrapings are performed by placing a drop of mineral oil or immersion oil on the suspicious lesion, gently scraping back and forth with a scalpel blade held at 90 degrees from the skin, then placing the scraped material onto a microscope slide for viewing under low, dry power. A scraping is positive if any of the following are seen in the scraping: scabies mite, eggs, egg casings, or fecal pellets (scybala).

G. **Treatment.** The preferred treatment of scabies is topical permethrin (Elimite) cream applied and left on overnight (adults and children). Alternatively, Kwell (lindane) lotion can be applied and left on overnight in adults, 6 hours in children. Adjunctive therapy sometimes includes oral antihistamines for itch, topical steroids for inflammation, and oral antibiotics (to cover *Staphylococcus* and *Streptococcus*) for superinfection (e.g., erythromycin, cephalexin, Augmentin).

## Selected Readings

Colven RM, Prose NS. Parasitic infestations of the skin. *Pediatr Ann* 23:436, 1994.

Gurevitch AW. Scabies and lice. *Pediatr Clin North Am* 32:987, 1985.

Honig PJ. Bites and parasites. *Pediatr Clin North Am* 30:563, 1983.

Hurwitz S. *Clinical Pediatric Dermatology* (2nd ed). Philadelphia: Saunders, 1993.

Weston WL, Lane AT. *Color Textbook of Pediatric Dermatology*. St. Louis: Mosby-Year Book, 1991.

# 15

# Tinea Capitis


## Christine L. McHenry


Tinea capitis is a fungal scalp infection seen most frequently in toddlers and young school-age children. Three organisms are primarily responsible for the disease in the United States: *Trichophyton tonsurans* (>90% of cases), *Microsporum audouinii*, and *Microsporum canis*.

**I. Clinical presentation and differential diagnosis**

**A. Clinical presentation.** *T. tonsurans* is transmitted between humans and is more common in African-American children. It can cause several different types of infection: (1) seborrheic, with diffuse scaling and pruritis; (2) "black dot," with alopecia and hair remnants within the follicular orifice giving the appearance of black dots on the scalp; (3) kerion, which represents an immune response to the dermatophyte that presents as an erythematous, boggy, tender mass that may be accompanied by systemic symptoms such as fever and lymphadenopathy; and (4) pustules or scabbed areas without scaling or significant alopecia. Major complications of tinea capitis include tinea corporis, secondary bacterial infection (usually with *Staphylococcus aureus* [uncommon]), permanent alopecia, and trichophytid reactions ("id" reactions).

**B. Differential diagnosis.** The differential diagnosis for a child with a scaling scalp, alopecia, or both includes psoriasis, seborrheic or atopic dermatitis, alopecia areata, bacterial folliculitis, trichotillomania, and traction folliculitis.

**II. Diagnosis.** Because many children with tinea capitis do not have areas of alopecia and broken hairs, they frequently are not diagnosed initially. A definitive diagnosis can be made by fungal culture, which is usually positive within 1–2 weeks. Two other tests can be performed at the time of presentation: a Wood's lamp examination and a KOH preparation. A Wood's lamp examination may be helpful if the infection is secondary to an ectothrix organism, such as *Microsporum* species, in which the hyphae and spores are on the surface of the hair shaft. This causes a characteristic fluorescence under the Wood's lamp. *T. tonsurans*, however, causes an endothrix infection, with hyphae and spores within the hair shaft; therefore, it does not fluoresce. A KOH preparation of either the involved hairs or scales may reveal the characteristic hyphal and spore appearance.

**III. Management.** Treatment consists of oral microcrystalline griseofulvin at 10–15 mg/kg PO qd given with a meal (fatty food in the meal enhances absorption). If ultramicrocrystalline griseofulvin is used, the dosage is cut in half. Grifulvin V (125 mg/5 ml) is the only form of griseofulvin available as an oral suspension. A short course of oral prednisone may be considered if a kerion is present. The child should be seen at 3-week intervals to evaluate progress, to encourage compliance, and for reculture. Treatment with griseofulvin should be continued until a negative culture is obtained (usually 6–8 weeks) and clinical infection has resolved. Reported side effects of griseofulvin include leukopenia, aplastic anemia, hypersensitivity, photosensitivity, gastrointestinal disturbance, and paresthesias. It probably is not necessary to monitor blood counts while the child is on a 6- to 8-week course of griseofulvin. Shampooing twice weekly with selenium sulfide (Selsun) will decrease spore shedding and help prevent spread of the infection. Combs, brushes, ribbons, and hair accessories should not be shared. Children can go back to school once griseofulvin therapy is started. If the physician suspects tinea capitis but elects not to begin griseofulvin until culture results are back, the child should still shampoo twice weekly with selenium sulfide so spore dissemination will not occur in the school setting.

## Selected Readings

Frieden I. Diagnosis and management of tinea capitis. *Pediatr Ann* 16:39, 1987.

Hurwitz S. *Clinical Pediatric Dermatology* (2nd ed). Philadelphia: Saunders, 1993.

Krawchuk D, Lucky A, Primmer S et al. Current status of the identification and management of tinea capitis. *Pediatrics* 72:625, 1983.

Rasmussen JE. Cutaneous fungus infections in children. *Pediatr Rev* 13:152, 1992.

Sheretz EF. Are laboratory studies necessary for griseofulvin therapy? *J Am Acad Dermatol* 22:1103, 1990.

B

# HEENT Disorders

16

# Acute Otitis Media

Raymond C. Baker

Acute otitis media (AOM) is the most common bacterial infection in pediatrics, accounting for as many as one-third of all illness visits to the primary care physician. At least two-thirds of children experience one or more episodes of AOM during the first year of life, and half have had at least three episodes by age 3 years.

I. **Epidemiology.** The highest incidence of AOM is in the first 2 years of life due largely to three factors: (1) Infants have increased susceptibility to upper respiratory tract infections; (2) infants have relatively larger nasopharyngeal lymphoid tissue at the opening of the auditory tube, which results in obstruction; and (3) the auditory tube is less competent in infants than in older children. Other factors associated with an increased incidence of AOM during infancy and early childhood are the following:

   A. **Bottle propping** (with reflux of milk through the auditory tube)
   B. **Siblings** in the home
   C. **Family history** of recurrent AOM
   D. **Cow's milk formula** (immunologic factors found in breast milk are absent)
   E. **Day-care attendance**
   F. **Smoking** in the home
   G. **Cold weather** months of the year, resulting in increased incidence of viral respiratory tract infections
   H. **American Indian or Eskimo ethnic background**
   I. **Presence of cleft palate** (virtually 100% incidence of recurrent AOM)
   J. **Down's syndrome**

II. **Pathogenesis.** The normal functions of the auditory tube are (1) ventilation of the middle ear space, (2) protection from the nasopharynx, and (3) clearance of secretions from the middle ear space. The primary cause of AOM is interference with these normal functions, resulting in blockage of the exit of middle ear fluid through the auditory tube, stasis of fluid in the middle ear space, and superinfection with bacteria from the nasopharynx. While the most common cause of obstruction is swelling due to viral infection, other causes are hypertrophied lymphoid tissue (adenoids) or tumor, allergic inflammatory edema, impairment of the opening mechanism from muscular dysfunction (tensor veli palatini muscle), and excessive tubal wall compliance.

III. **Diagnosis**. In the very young infant, symptoms of AOM are nonspecific, as in most other illnesses at this age, and may include irritability, rhinorrhea, poor feeding, diarrhea, cough, and fever. In the older child, symptoms are otalgia, fever, rubbing or pulling at the ears (in the preverbal infant), otorrhea, and decreased hearing.

The diagnosis is made most accurately with the pneumatic otoscope, which may reveal a bulging tympanic membrane (TM) secondary to pus under pressure in the middle ear canal; immobility or decreased mobility of the TM; opacity, thickness, or erythema (due to tympanitis) of the TM; pus visible through the TM; or perforation of the TM with pus exuding. Sometimes, especially in early AOM, before the development of pus in the middle ear space, erythema due to tympanitis may be the only sign of AOM. Since crying also may cause TM erythema, this finding must be associated with other symptoms or signs suggestive of AOM to make a diagnosis.

IV. **Microbiology of AOM**

A. **The etiology of AOM** in otherwise healthy infants and children is the same regardless of age as follows (based on 4,157 tympanocenteses—Giebink):

1. ***Streptococcus pneumoniae*** (30%)
2. **No growth** (presumably includes viral—see sec. **IV.C** below) (28%)
3. ***Haemophilus influenzae***, nontypeable (20%)
4. **Miscellaneous** and mixed (12%; all <2% of total)
5. ***Moraxella catarrhalis*** (higher in some regions of the country) (6%)
6. ***Staphylococcus aureus*** (2%)
7. ***Streptococcus pyogenes*** (2%)

B. **Amoxicillin resistance** (based on the combined data from two studies—Kovatch and Shurin)

1. ***H. influenzae***, nontypeable (20%)
2. ***M. catarrhalis*** (80%)
3. **Total organisms causing AOM resistant to amoxicillin** (25%)

C. Up to 10% of AOM may have a **viral etiology** (based on 1,221 tympanocenteses—Ruuskanen) including the following:

1. **Respiratory syncytial virus** (5.5%)
2. **Rhinoviruses** (1.4%)
3. **Influenza viruses** (1.1%)
4. **Adenovirus** (0.9%)
5. **Enteroviruses** (0.5%)
6. **Parainfluenza viruses** (0.4%)
7. ***Rotavirus*** (0.1%)

V. **Treatment.** The choice of antibiotic should be based on sensitivities of the organisms likely to cause AOM and concentrations of antibiotic that can be obtained in the middle ear. Antibiotics may be divided into first-line (new-onset AOM), second-line (first treatment failure), and third-line (subsequent treatment failures). In general, third-line antibiotics are more expensive but have a broader spectrum, especially against beta-lactamase–producing organisms.

A. **First-line. Amoxicillin** (e.g., Amoxil), 15–20 mg/kg PO tid. Not effective against beta-lactamase–positive *Haemophilus* (25–30%) and most *Moraxella.*

B. **Second-line**

1. **Trimethoprim-sulfamethoxazole** (Septra, Bactrim), 0.5 ml/kg PO bid
2. **Pediazole** (erythromycin plus sulfisoxazole), 0.25 ml/kg PO qid

C. **Third-line**
   1. **Cefprozil** (Cefzil), 15 mg/kg PO bid.
   2. **Amoxicillin-clavulanate** (Augmentin), 10 mg/kg PO tid. Augmentin has a significant incidence of diarrhea.
   3. **Cefixime** (Suprax), 8 mg/kg PO qd.
   4. **Cefaclor** (Ceclor), 13–15 mg/kg PO tid; Ceclor has a significant incidence of serum sickness-like rash.
   5. **Loracarbef** (Lorabid), 15 mg/kg PO bid.
   6. **Cefpodoxime** (Vantin), 5 mg/kg PO bid.
   7. **Ceftriaxone** (Rocephin), 50 mg/kg (maximum dose 1,000 mg) IM one time. This regimen is useful in an emergency department setting where medication compliance and follow-up are in question.

   The treatment period is traditionally 10 days, although several studies have suggested a shorter course in uncomplicated AOM (5–7 days for oral antibiotics; single injection of ceftriaxone).

D. **Adjunctive treatment** for AOM includes acetaminophen for fever, acetaminophen or ibuprofen for pain, and topical antibiotics (if TM is perforated). Decongestants or combinations of decongestant and antihistamine have not proved effective in preventing complications of AOM.

E. **Treatment failures** may be due to noncompliance with the antibiotic regimen, a resistant organism, or an adverse (real or imagined) reaction to the antibiotic that prompts the caregiver to discontinue it. Comparing second infections or treatment failures following treatment for AOM, *S. aureus* and beta-lactamase–positive *H. influenzae* are found more commonly. The majority of organisms isolated, however, are sensitive to the original antibiotic.

VI. **Resolution of tympanic membrane abnormalities**. Follow-up of AOM is most appropriate at 4–6 weeks postinfection, as the purpose of follow-up is to document **resolution**. If seen at 2 weeks, one-third to one-half of children still will have an abnormal exam; 90–95%, however, are normal at 1 month. Early follow-up by telephone to determine response to antibiotic may be appropriate at 48–72 hours. One would expect defervescence and some pain resolution by this time.

## Selected Readings

Baker RC. Pitfalls in diagnosing otitis media. *Pediatr Ann* 20:591, 1992.

Giebink GS. The microbiology of otitis media. *Pediatr Infect Dis J* 8:S18, 1989.

Green SM, Rothrock SG. Single-dose intramuscular ceftriaxone for acute otitis media in children. *Pediatr Infect Dis J* 91:23, 1993.

Harrison CJ, Belhorn TH. Antibiotic treatment failures in acute otitis media. *Pediatr Ann* 20:600, 1992.

Harrison CJ, Marks MI, Welch DF. Microbiology of recently treated otitis media compared with previously untreated acute otitis media. *Pediatr Infect Dis J* 4:641, 1985.

Hendrickse WA, Kusmiesz H, Shelton S et al. Five versus 10 days of therapy for acute otitis media. *Pediatr Infect Dis J* 7:14, 1988.

Kovatch AL, Wald ER, Michaels RH. Beta-lactamase–producing *Branhamella catarrhalis* causing otitis media in children. *J Pediatr* 102:261, 1983.

Ruuskanen O, Arola M, Putto-Laurila A et al. Acute otitis media and respiratory virus infections. *Pediatr Infect Dis J* 8:94, 1989.

Schwartz RH, Rodriguez WJ, Brook I et al. The febrile response in acute otitis media. *JAMA* 245:2057, 1981.

Shurin PA, Marchant CD, Kim CH et al. Emergence of beta-lactamase–producing strains of *Branhamella catarrhalis* as important agents of acute otitis media. *Pediatr Infect Dis J* 2:34, 1983.

# 17

# Acute, Subacute, and Chronic Sinusitis

Christine L. McHenry

Sinusitis is an inflammation of the mucosal lining of one or more of the paranasal sinuses. It can be classified according to duration of symptoms as acute (<30 days), subacute (30–120 days), and chronic (>120 days). Obstruction of sinus ostia, impaired ciliary function, and overproduction of or increased viscosity of secretion lead to the retention of secretions in the paranasal sinuses. Upper respiratory tract infections (URIs) and allergies are the most common predisposing factors. Clinically, most cases of sinusitis in children involve the maxillary and ethmoid sinuses. After age 10 years, the frontal sinuses take on a greater clinical importance. Isolated sphenoid sinusitis is rare.

## I. Acute sinusitis

**A. Clinical presentation.** Common symptoms of acute sinusitis in adolescents and adults include headache, fever, and facial pain; however, children may have fairly nonspecific complaints. Sinusitis should be suspected if (1) URI symptoms persist beyond 10 days without improvement, especially with persistent cough; (2) the child with an URI seems sicker than usual with high fever and has purulent nasal drainage and periorbital swelling; or (3) the allergic child has an acute exacerbation of respiratory symptoms, the respiratory symptoms are difficult to control with usual management, or both. Findings on the physical examination that suggest sinusitis include mucopurulent discharge from the nose, erythematous nasal mucosa, facial tenderness, periorbital edema, and malodorous breath.

**B. Infectious agents.** Acute sinusitis may be a viral, bacterial, or mixed infection. The most common bacterial pathogens isolated are nontypeable *Haemophilus influenzae* (20%), *Streptococcus pneumoniae* (30–40%), *Moraxella catarrhalis* (20%), *Streptococcus pyogenes*, and alpha-hemolytic streptococcus. Anaerobes are recovered about 10% of the time. Viral pathogens include rhinovirus, influenza, and parainfluenza.

**C. Management.** Given that up to 50% of children with acute sinusitis have a spontaneous clinical cure and that approximately 80% of bacterial agents in acute sinusitis do not produce beta-lactamase, amoxicillin, 10–20 mg/kg/dose PO tid, is an appropriate initial antibiotic. If the patient does not improve or worsens during the first 48 hours of antibiotics, changing antibiotics to a beta-lactamase–resistant drug, such as trimethoprim-sulfamethoxazole (Bactrim, Septra), 0.5 ml/kg PO bid; erythromycin-sulfisoxazole (Pediazole), 0.25 ml/kg PO qid; amoxicillin-clavulanate (Augmentin), 10 mg/kg PO tid; or cefuroxime axetil (Ceftin), 250 mg or 500 mg bid, may be beneficial. In addition, sinus aspiration should be considered if an air-fluid level is present on x-ray. Therapy is continued 14–21 days depending on clinical response. The effectiveness of either topical or systemic decongestants or antihistamines on the clinical recovery of sinusitis has not been studied adequately; topical decongestants may provide some symptomatic relief.

**D. Complications** of sinusitis include orbital cellulitis or abscess, osteomyelitis, epidural or subdural abscess, cavernous sinus thrombosis, meningitis, and brain abscess. Obviously, such complications require hospitalization with IV antibiotics and appropriate subspecialty consultation. Because of a higher incidence of intracranial complications with frontal and sphenoid sinusitis, initial management of these patients requires hospitalization.

**II. Subacute and chronic sinusitis**

**A. Clinical presentation.** Children with subacute and chronic sinusitis may present with mucopurulent nasal discharge, nasal congestion (obstruction), cough (especially at night), sore throat, snoring, and sleep disturbance. Headache, fever, and facial pain are less common than in acute sinusitis. Findings on physical examination may include mucopurulent nasal discharge, erythematous nasal mucosa, injected pharynx, acute or serous otitis media, and malodorous breath.

**B. Infectious agents.** Nontypeable *H. influenzae, S. pneumoniae*, and *M. catarrhalis* are the most common bacterial agents recovered. Anaerobes appear to play a minor role in subacute and chronic sinusitis in childhood.

**C. Management** of subacute and chronic sinusitis is similar to the management of acute sinusitis. If a patient has not had a recent course of antibiotics, amoxicillin is a reasonable first choice. If the patient does not respond clinically to amoxicillin or has had a recent course of antibiotics, an antibiotic that covers beta-lactamase–producing organisms should be started. In most instances, treatment should be continued for 21 days.

## Selected Readings

Goldenhersh MJ, Rachelefsky GS. Sinusitis: Early recognition, aggressive treatment. *Contemp Pediatr* 6:22, 1989.

Richards W, Roth RM, Church JA. Underdiagnosis and undertreatment of chronic sinusitis in children. *Clin Pediatr* 30:88, 1991.

Tinkelman DG, Silk HJ. Clinical and bacteriologic features of chronic sinusitis in children. *Am J Dis Child* 143:938, 1989.

Wald E. Diagnosis and management of acute sinusitis. *Pediatr Ann* 17:629, 1988.

Wald E. Sinusitis in children. *N Engl J Med* 326:319, 1992.

Wald E. Sinusitis. *Pediatr Rev* 14:345, 1993.

# 18

# Pharyngitis and Tonsillitis

Paul S. Bellet

Pharyngitis, an inflammation of the mucous membranes and underlying structures of the throat, may be divided into two categories: illness with nasal involvement (nasopharyngitis) and illness without nasal involvement (pharyngitis, tonsillitis, or tonsillopharyngitis).

I. **Nasopharyngitis.** Viruses nearly always cause nasopharyngitis (adenoviruses, parainfluenza viruses, influenza viruses, and less commonly, rhinoviruses and respiratory syncytial virus). Nasopharyngitis also may occur in children with rotavirus gastroenteritis. The clinical findings include rhinorrhea, coryza, usually fever, and mild pharyngeal erythema. This is an acute, self-limited illness lasting 4–10 days. The treatment of rhinorrhea and coryza is the same as that for the common cold (see Chap. 19). Symptomatic treatment for sore throat is discussed below.

II. **Pharyngitis** without nasal involvement usually is due to viruses (adenoviruses, parainfluenza viruses, influenza viruses, Ebstein-Barr virus, enteroviruses) and bacteria (*Streptococcus pyogenes*). Less common causes include herpes simplex virus, *Mycoplasma pneumoniae*, other streptococci (B, C, and G), mixed anaerobic infections (*Bacteroides* spp., *Peptostreptococcus*, *Fusobacterium* spp.), and *Neisseria gonorrhoeae* (sexually active adolescents or exposed children and adolescents). The onset of illness is usually acute with sore throat and fever. The pharynx, tonsils, or both are inflamed with erythema, exudate, ulceration, or vesicles. The cervical lymph nodes may be enlarged and tender. Exudate on the pharynx and petechiae on the soft palate are seen most frequently with *Streptococcus pyogenes* (group A *Streptococcus*) and infectious mononucleosis. Ulcerative and vesicular lesions are seen most frequently with enteroviral infections (herpangina) and herpes simplex virus.

III. **Diagnosis.** Children with nasopharyngitis, herpangina, pharyngoconjunctival fever, or pharyngeal vesicles have a viral disease and do not require culture or antibiotic therapy. The child with acute pharyngitis and exudate suggests group A streptococcal infection, which is confirmed with a rapid streptococcal antigen test (with culture back-up if negative). Many children, however, fall between these extremes, and a throat swab for a rapid streptococcal antigen test, throat culture, or both should be performed, especially if there is a positive exposure history.

IV. **Treatment.** Effective treatment for group A streptococcal infection includes several options:

   A. **Single IM injection of benzathine penicillin G** (600,000 U for children less than 60 lb; 1,200,000 U for those more than 60 lb).

   B. **Penicillin V**, 250 mg tid for 10 days. With good compliance, penicillin V, 250 mg PO bid, also is effective.

C. **In patients allergic to penicillin, erythromycin estolate,** 20–40 mg/kg/day PO divided bid–qid for 10 days (maximum dose 1,000 mg/day).

D. **Symptomatic treatment** of sore throat includes acetaminophen or ibuprofen PO plus cold liquids, Popsicles, and ice cream in younger children. Older children and adolescents may find some relief from gargling with warm saline solution or drinking warm liquids (e.g., hot chocolate, tea, soup).

## Selected Readings

American Academy of Pediatrics. Group A Streptococcal Infections. In G Peter (ed), *1994 Red Book: Report of the Committee on Infectious Diseases* (23rd ed). Elk Grove Village, IL: American Academy of Pediatrics, 1994.

Bass JW. Antibiotic management of group A streptococcal pharyngotonsillitis. *Pediatr Infect Dis J* 10:S43, 1991.

Cherry JD. Pharyngitis (Pharyngitis, Tonsillitis, Tonsillopharyngitis, and Nasopharyngitis). In RD Feigin, JD Cherry (eds), *Textbook of Pediatric Infectious Diseases* (3rd ed). Philadelphia: Saunders, 1992.

Gerber MA, Spadaccini LJ, Wright LC et al. Twice daily penicillin in the treatment of streptococcal pharyngitis. *Am J Dis Child* 139:1145, 1985.

Klein JO. Management of streptococcal pharyngitis. *Pediatr Infect Dis J* 13:572, 1994.

Shulman ST. Complications of streptococcal pharyngitis. *Pediatr Infect Dis J* 13:S70, 1994.

Shulman ST. Streptococcal pharyngitis: Diagnostic considerations. *Pediatr Infect Dis J* 13:567, 1994.

19

# Upper Respiratory Tract Infection (The Common Cold)

Paul S. Bellet

An upper respiratory tract infection (the common cold) is an acute, communicable viral infection. Viruses that usually cause upper respiratory tract infections include rhinoviruses, parainfluenza viruses, respiratory syncytial virus, and coronaviruses. Other agents that occasionally cause upper respiratory tract infections include adenoviruses, enteroviruses, influenza viruses, reoviruses, and *Mycoplasma pneumoniae*. Children usually average three to eight colds per year.

I. **Diagnosis.** Upper respiratory tract infections are characterized by nasal stuffiness, rhinorrhea, sneezing, coryza, throat irritation, and low-grade or no fever. Other manifestations include cough, malaise, headache, muscle ache, vomiting, and diarrhea. The duration of illness is usually about a week, but cough and nasal discharge may persist for 2 weeks or more. The physical examination reveals inflamed, swollen turbinates with clear or mucopurulent discharge. The diagnosis is clinical, but a specific diagnosis can be made by virus isolation from nasal secretions (nasal wash technique). The primary disorder to consider in the differential diagnosis is allergic rhinitis (seasonal or perennial). The most common complications of upper respiratory tract infection are otitis media, sinusitis, and pneumonia.

II. **Treatment.** No therapy is necessary in most cases of upper respiratory tract infection in children. Symptomatic care can be considered in the individual case when needed. Relief of nasal obstruction is most important in infants so they can feed and sleep more comfortably; isotonic saline drops and gentle aspiration usually are effective. In children and infants older than 6 months, oral decongestants such as pseudoephedrine (Sudafed) may be used. Topical decongestant nose drops and sprays can be useful, but persistent use for more than 3–5 days may lead to rebound obstruction. In children 6–24 months of age, phenylephrine (Neo-Synephrine) ⅛% nose drops may be used q4h. In children 2–6 years of age, oxymetazoline (Afrin) pediatric nose drops or spray 0.025% may be used q8–12h. In children older than 6 years, Afrin adult nose drops or spray 0.05% may be used q8–12h. Antihistamines have no place in the routine therapy of the common cold, although they are included in many over-the-counter cold medicines. If allergic rhinitis is possible, a combination of oral decongestant and antihistamine can be used; examples of over-the-counter decongestant and antihistamine combinations are Novahistine, Triaminic, and Actifed.

## Selected Readings

Cherry JD. The Common Cold. In RD Feigin, JD Cherry (eds), *Textbook of Pediatric Infectious Diseases* (3rd ed). Philadelphia: Saunders, 1992.

Schmitt BD. Ambulatory Pediatric Drugs. In M Green, RJ Haggerty (eds), *Ambulatory Pediatrics IV*. Philadelphia: Saunders, 1990.

# 20

# Conjunctivitis

## Raymond C. Baker

The conjunctiva becomes colonized by a number of saprophytic organisms soon after birth, such as *Staphylococcus, Corynebacterium xerosis, Proteus, Pseudomonas,* and, occasionally, fungi. A variety of organisms have been isolated in conjunctivitis; the most common ones are shown in Table 20-1.

Most ocular infections are benign, self-limiting diseases that present with itch, foreign body sensation, and acute inflammation of the conjunctiva, usually with mucopurulent or mucous discharge. Nonpurulent conjunctivitis is seen in Kawasaki disease and toxic shock syndrome. Treatment differs by age groups.

I. **Ophthalmia neonatorum**, or neonatal conjunctivitis, usually is related to pathogens acquired during the infant's passage through the birth canal. The most common organisms are *Neisseria gonorrhoeae, Chlamydia trachomatis,* and herpes simplex virus. Other pathogens that may be acquired soon after birth are *Haemophilus* and *S. aureus.*

Conjunctivitis occurring in the first 3 weeks of life should be evaluated with a Gram stain and culture with Thayer-Martin medium for gonococci, tissue culture for viruses and chlamydia, and routine bacterial culture. When culturing for chlamydia, the lower palpebral conjunctiva is swabbed and the swab placed into transport medium. The nasopharynx also should be swabbed and the swab placed in the same transport medium as the conjunctival swab, saving the cost of one tissue culture. From a treatment perspective, it is not important whether the organism grows from the conjunctiva or nasopharynx, as both should be treated systemically.

A. **Gonococcal conjunctivitis.** Gram stain evidence of gram-negative intracellular diplococci requires hospitalization and treatment for presumptive *N. gonorrhoeae* infection. Isolated conjunctivitis should be treated for 7 days with ceftriaxone, 50 mg/kg/day IV or IM as a single daily dose, or cefotaxime, 25 mg/kg IV or IM q12h. If the isolate is sensitive to penicillin, aqueous penicillin G, 100,000 units/kg/day IV divided q6h for 7 days is effective. Frequent saline irrigations are needed for the accompanying copious discharge.

B. ***C. trachomatis* conjunctivitis** also requires systemic treatment. Erythromycin estolate, 30–40 mg/kg/day PO in 3–4 divided doses, should be given for 14 days to eliminate the organism from the upper and lower respiratory tract.

It should be assumed the organism came from a nontreated or inadequately treated mother; therefore, parents should be screened for gonococcal and chlamydial infection and treated if positive.

C. **Chemical conjunctivitis** manifests with hyperemia, watery discharge, and chemosis within hours of silver nitrate instillation in the neonate. It resolves spontaneously within 24–48 hours.

**Table 20-1. Common bacteria and viruses isolated in conjunctivitis**

| Bacteria | Viruses |
|---|---|
| *Haemophilus* spp. | Adenovirus |
| *Streptococcus pneumoniae* | Enterovirus |
| *Staphylococcus aureus* | Coxsackievirus |
| *Neisseria gonorrhoeae* | Herpes simplex |
| *Neisseria meningitidis* | Varicella-zoster |
| *Moraxella* spp. | Epstein-Barr virus |
| *Escherichia coli* | Molluscum contagiosum |
| *Pseudomonas aeruginosa* | Measles virus |
| *Chlamydia trachomatis* | |

D. **Herpes simplex conjunctivitis.** Referral to ophthalmology is necessary.

E. **Other organisms in the newborn.** When appropriate tests do not identify any of the above specific pathogens, broad-spectrum topical antibiotics may be applied, pending more specific information from the culture. Effective topical antibiotics include polymyxin (Polysporin), erythromycin, gentamicin, tobramycin, and sulfacetamide.

II. **Infancy and childhood**

A. **Nasolacrimal duct obstruction** causes a persistently wet eye and intermittent mucopurulent discharge of varying degrees in infants from birth to 12 months of age. Intermittent mucopurulent discharge (recurrent superimposed conjunctivitis) should be treated with topical antibiotics as above. If the condition has not resolved spontaneously by 1 year of age, referral to ophthalmology is necessary for possible probing.

B. **Infectious.** Most conjunctivitis beyond the neonatal period is self-limiting, whether viral or bacterial. Examination of the child should include the ears, as otitis media frequently is associated with nontypeable *Haemophilus influenzae* conjunctivitis. Recovery of the ocular infection appears to be more rapid with the use of topical therapy, applied qid until the infection has resolved. The choice of drug is empirical; sulfacetamide, Polysporin, gentamicin, tobramycin, or erythromycin can be used. Topical steroids are not indicated in acute conjunctivitis. Ointments have the advantage of lasting longer and being easier to apply in most circumstances.

In the young, uncooperative patient, who typically resists by squeezing shut the eyes, the following technique can be used with ophthalmic drops: The parent sits on the floor with legs slightly abducted and extended. The infant is positioned supine on the floor with his or her upper extremities trapped beneath the parent's legs and the child's head held by the parent's upper legs at the crotch. The drops are placed at the inner canthus of the eye (which is usually tightly closed). The parent then sets the eye drop bottle down and with the thumbs of both hands pulls the lids apart gently, allowing the drops to enter the eye.

C. **Allergic conjunctivitis.** The typical presentation of allergic conjunctivitis is watery discharge, itchy eyes (and often itchy nose), tearing, and edema of the conjunctiva (chemosis) and lids. Effective treatment consists of topical decongestants with or without antihistamine (e.g., Vasocon or Naphcon ophthalmic solution). Cromolyn sodium 4% solution (Opticrom) also may be used prophylactically. Oral antihistamines may be used alone or in conjunction with topical therapy as well. Topical steroids are effective for allergic conjunctivitis, but their use should be with ophthalmologic consultation (due to potential exacerbation of unrecognized herpetic conjunctivitis).

III. **Control measures.** Hand washing is the most important control measure to prevent the spread of infectious conjunctivitis. Some school systems require a physician's note before the child is allowed back in school, even though isolated conjunctivitis is not a medical reason for exclusion from school. In day-care facilities, the concern of spread is greater, and some day-care centers allow the child to return only after being seen by a physician.

## Selected Readings

Gigliotti R. Acute conjunctivitis of childhood. *Pediatr Ann* 22:353, 1993.

Hammerschlag MR. Chlamydia trachomatis in children. *Pediatr Ann* 23:349, 1994.

Hammerschlag MR. Neonatal conjunctivitis. *Pediatr Ann* 22:346, 1993.

Lohr JA. Treatment of conjunctivitis in infants and children. *Pediatr Ann* 22:359, 1993.

Weiss AH. Acute conjunctivitis in childhood. *Curr Prob Pediatr* 24:4, 1994.

Weiss AH. Chronic conjunctivitis in infants and children. *Pediatr Ann* 22:366, 1993.

21

# Common Oral Conditions in Infants and Children

James F. Steiner

Parents commonly bring their infants and children to the physician with problems and concerns about the mouth and teeth. The primary care physician needs to have a working knowledge of common oral conditions to recognize and manage the problem, reassure the parents if the condition is benign and self-limiting, or make a dental referral. The following are examples of typical oral problems the physician might see as part of routine primary care. They are predominantly clinical conditions that present during the child's first 24 months or situations that appear later but begin in this period.

I. **Epstein's pearls.** Found in more than half of newborns, Epstein's pearls are white, raised, circular, 1-mm epithelial inclusion cysts in the midline of the hard palate. These resolve without treatment.

II. **Tongue tie.** The lingual frenum, a band of tissue that courses from the ventral surface of the tongue to the floor of the mouth, occasionally may limit lingual movement when the tongue is protruded. Treatment rarely is indicated because this condition alone usually does not affect speech. Before referring for frenectomy (also known as tongue clipping), a speech pathologist should be consulted.

III. **Eruption conditions.** The first primary tooth erupts at about 6 months, and all 20 primary teeth are usually in place by 36 months.

A. **Natal and neonatal teeth.** Teeth present at birth are natal teeth; those erupting during the first month are neonatal teeth. Eighty-five percent of both natal and neonatal teeth are the normal primary incisors and not supernumerary teeth. If they are quite loose, consideration should be given to their removal. An associated, rare condition, Riga-Fede disease, is a traumatic ulcer on the ventral surface of the infant's tongue caused by a sharp spot on the natal or neonatal tooth. Pain from the ulcer may prevent nursing. When the sharp spot is smoothed, however, the ulcer will heal and feeding will resume.

B. **Teething.** Many symptoms are attributed to teething. Those that probably *are* associated with teething are drooling, irritability, and occasionally low-grade fever. A fever of more than 101°F never should be considered secondary to teething, however, and a source of fever should be sought. Many folk remedies for teething pain have inconsistent results; a cool, water-filled teething ring and oral acetaminophen may offer relief.

C. **Eruption hematoma.** As teeth move toward eruption, a blue, blood-filled swelling may surround the emerging tooth. This so-called eruption hematoma usually requires no treatment, as it ruptures and resolves when the tooth penetrates the gingiva.

D. **Delayed eruption.** When no teeth have erupted by 12–14 months in a well baby, the physician should rule out missing teeth. If radiographs reveal teeth, continued watchful waiting is appropriate. Two conditions that may delay eruption are hypothyroidism and fibromatosis gingivae (in which dense gingivae prevent eruption).

E. **Ectopic tooth eruption** commonly is seen when permanent teeth begin replacing primary teeth at around 6 years of age. They present most frequently as a double row of teeth in the mandibular anterior area in which the permanent incisors erupt behind the primary incisors. If the primary incisor is loose, parents should encourage the child to manually manipulate the loose tooth to encourage exfoliation. If the primary tooth is not loose, extraction is indicated.

IV. **Discoloration** presents as extrinsic, easily removed surface stains or intrinsic subsurface discoloration incorporated within the enamel and dentin of the tooth crown.

A. **Iron stain.** A gray to black, easily removed extrinsic stain may be seen in infants taking iron drops. Switching to chewables or tablets will prevent the stain.

B. **Trauma.** When primary teeth are concussed, the dental nerve (known as the pulp) may hemorrhage into the dentin, resulting in light to dark gray discoloration of the crown. A stronger force may sever the neurovascular bundle supplying the pulp, resulting in eventual pulp necrosis and a similar crown discoloration. Watchful waiting is appropriate. If pain, swelling, or a draining fistula through the gingiva develops, dental referral is indicated.

C. **Fluorosis.** Mild fluorosis is a lacy, white intrinsic color change observed in the enamel of permanent teeth resulting from ingestion of greater-than-optimal amounts of fluoride during enamel formation. Young children who drink optimally fluoridated water or, in nonfluoridated areas, are on systemic fluoride supplements are at risk for fluorosis if they swallow toothpaste while brushing. To reduce the risk of fluorosis, toothbrushing should be supervised by an adult until age 5–6 years, and only a smear of paste should be placed on the brush.

D. **Tetracycline stain** presents as a gray to brown to yellow intrinsic stain of permanent teeth caused by systemic tetracycline prescribed during crown formation, a process that begins early in the first year of life. The physician should defer use of systemic tetracycline until age 6 years. Infrequent 7-day courses, however, most likely will not cause staining.

V. **Dental caries** is a preventable condition. Daily supervised brushing with fluoride toothpaste and regular meal times plus two to three snacks per day minimize the risk of caries. Sleeping with a bottle and, if breast-fed, with the mother are high-risk behaviors for nursing caries and should be discouraged.

A. **Early recognition.** White, demineralized lines in enamel near the gingiva represent early, reversible dental caries. If plaque has accumulated in this area, it should be wiped away so these white lines will be visible. If demineralization is observed, the physician should suspect bedtime bottle-feeding, nighttime breast-feeding, or frequent eating and drinking and ask the appropriate questions. Parents should be reminded about daily brushing to remove plaque.

B. **Advanced caries** occurs as early as age 12 months when high-risk behaviors are either not recognized by health care providers or the caretaker does not comply with oral health recommendations. It presents as tan-colored holes in the enamel surface; dental referral is indicated.

C. **Toothache.** When dental caries goes unrecognized or untreated, the pulp becomes infected and painful. Treatment with pain medication and emergent dental referral are necessary.

D. **Facial cellulitis** results when pulpal infection spreads from the tooth, through surrounding bone, and into the facial tissues. The patient presents with facial swelling and may be quite ill-appearing. Facial cellulitis secondary to an infected tooth should be treated with antibiotics (usually penicillin or amoxicillin alone), pain medication, and immediate dental referral. Facial cellulitis of dental origin must be differentiated from primary bacteremic facial (buccal) cellulitis seen in infants and young children (3 months–3 years of age), which requires different evaluation and management.

VI. **Trauma.** When infants begin to walk, they are at risk for accidental oral trauma. The clinician must be alert to physical abuse as part of the differential, as oral injuries are seen in half of physically abused children. Principles of oral trauma management include evaluation and treatment as soon as possible.

A. **A loose tooth** is the most frequent injury of the primary dentition. Patients with loose teeth should be referred to a pediatric dentist for evaluation and long-term follow-up.

B. An **intruded tooth** occurs when traumatic force pushes the tooth deeper into its socket. In some instances, the tooth is pushed in so deep that the crown is no longer visible. If the crown is not visible, the clinician always must rule out ingestion or aspiration. Dental referral is indicated.

C. **Fractured teeth** should be evaluated by a pediatric dentist within a day of the injury. Lip lacerations, frequently associated with crown fractures, may contain tooth fragments, which should be removed before suturing.

D. **Avulsed teeth.** Replacing avulsed primary teeth generally is not indicated. Avulsed permanent teeth, however, should be replaced as soon as possible, as prognosis is best when the tooth is replaced quickly. The avulsed tooth should be held by the crown, and any foreign material should be rinsed from the root. The tooth should then be returned to the empty socket. If the avulsed permanent tooth cannot be replaced, it should be brought in milk or saline with the child to the dentist. If the avulsed tooth cannot be found, rule out aspiration, ingestion, or intrusion.

E. **Mandibular fracture.** Children with chin-tip trauma are at risk for unilateral or bilateral subcondylar fracture. They may present with pain and swelling anterior to the tragus, pain on swallowing, or drooling onto the chin and chest from guarding (not swallowing saliva). In a unilateral subcondylar fracture, the mandible deviates to the side of the fracture. If both condyles are fractured, an anterior open bite often is seen. A panoramic dental film and Towne projection of the mandible are helpful in confirming the diagnosis.

Mandibular body fractures always are accompanied by a hematoma in the floor of the mouth. Frequently seen are vertical tears in the gingiva and, on palpation of the inferior border of the mandible, a bony step defect. Emergent referral to an oral surgeon is recommended.

VII. **Acute herpetic gingivostomatitis** is seen predominantly in children younger than 6 years and is caused by herpes simplex virus (*Herpes hominis*, type I). The initial symptoms are fever, fretfulness, cervical lymphadenopathy, and refusal to eat. Several days later, the gingiva becomes red and painful. Mucosal surface vesicles develop on and around the lips, the gingiva, the tongue, and hard palate. The vesicles ulcerate and form lesions 1–3 mm in diameter that may coalesce to form larger ulcers. Therapy is symptomatic with cold liquids, ice cream, cold pudding, Popsicles, and so forth plus acetaminophen or ibuprofen. Children with gingivostomatitis occasionally may have pain so severe that they are unable to keep themselves hydrated orally and require other methods of hydration. The ulcerations usually resolve in 1–2 weeks.

## Selected Readings

Neville BW, Damm DD, White DK et al. *Color Atlas of Clinical Oral Pathology*. Philadelphia: Lea & Febiger, 1991.

Pinkham JR. *Pediatric Dentistry Infancy Through Adolescence*. Philadelphia: Saunders, 1994.

C

# Lower Respiratory Tract Disorders

# Asthma

Christine L. McHenry

Asthma is responsible for more days of missed school and restricted activity than any other chronic childhood disease. Asthma has three components: (1) airway obstruction that is completely or partially reversible, (2) airway inflammation, and (3) airway hyperresponsiveness. Airway obstruction is responsible for the clinical symptoms of asthma such as dyspnea and wheezing. This obstruction is compounded by an inflammatory response resulting from the release of mediators from bronchial mast cells. These mediators produce immediate smooth-muscle contraction followed by recruitment of macrophages, neutrophils, and eosinophils 4–12 hours after the initial environmental exposure. The macrophages, neutrophils, and eosinophils secrete their own vasoactive substances that disrupt the integrity of the respiratory epithelium and increase bronchial hyperresponsiveness. The result is both an early- and late-phase reaction to an environmental stimulus.

I. **History.** In assessing a patient with asthma, current symptoms and medications, precipitating factors, past medical history, and family history are important areas to explore. In addition, the number of missed school days may indicate both the severity of the disease and how well it is controlled. Finally, the impact of the patient's disease on the family should not be ignored.

  A. **Current symptoms and medications.** The physician should note the onset of symptoms, cough, wheezing, dyspnea, chest tightness, and pain and ask about medications used, including doses and frequency, most recent dose, and recent systemic steroid use.

  B. **Precipitating factors.** The physician should determine if there were any precipitating factors, such as upper respiratory infection (URI), tobacco smoke, changes in the weather, exercise, emotions, drugs (e.g., aspirin, nonsteroidal anti-inflammatory drugs), foods, or contact with animals.

  C. **Past medical history.** The physician should ask about the patient's past medical history, such as hospitalizations for asthma (including intensive care unit [ICU] admission), history of bronchiolitis or bronchopulmonary dysplasia, history of gastroesophageal reflux, and history of recurrent otitis media or chronic or seasonal rhinitis or sinusitis.

  D. **Family history.** The physician should ask if any other family members have asthma, allergies, eczema, hay fever, or chronic sinusitis.

II. **Physical examination.** The physical examination begins with a general assessment of the patient. Is the patient in severe respiratory distress, or is he or she sitting comfortably on the examination table? Vital signs are noted. The chest examination begins with observation for increased anterior-posterior diameter, accessory muscle use, flaring of the alae nasi, and skin color. On auscultation, the physician should listen for the character of breath sounds (normal, decreased), wheeze (expiratory, inspiratory, both), inspiration-expiration ratio, rales, and focality of findings. If the patient is old enough to cooperate, a peak flow (PF) measurement when compared to the standard table or the patient's own best PF as measured when not symptomatic is a much better indicator of airway obstruction than physical findings, especially in mild to moderate obstruction. Other evidence of allergy or infection such as eczema, rhinitis, or sinusitis also should be noted.

**III. Outpatient management**

**A. Crisis management.** Mild to moderate exacerbations of asthma often can be managed at home or in the physician's office. Parents and patients should be instructed as part of the child's routine care about how to assess the severity of airway obstruction, ideally including some quantitative measurement such as PF if the child is old enough. The physician should provide the patient or parent with the following general guidelines regarding when to call the physician and when to go directly to the emergency department for acute care:

1. **Mild exacerbations.** With a mild exacerbation (PF 70–90% of baseline, minimal accessory muscle use, mild dyspnea, normal speech, good color, expiratory wheeze only), the parent can begin treatment at home with an inhaled $beta_2$-agonist delivered by a metered dose inhaler or nebulizer. This can be given every 15–20 minutes up to three times. If this fails, the physician should be contacted to determine the next step.
2. **Moderate exacerbations.** In moderate exacerbations (PF 50–70% of baseline, moderate accessory muscle use, moderate dyspnea, pale color, inspiratory and expiratory wheezing), the patient should be given a single inhaled treatment, and the physician should be contacted to determine where the patient should be seen. When to begin systemic steroids for mild to moderate exacerbations is somewhat controversial. Factors to consider when deciding to use steroids include recent systemic steroid use, inhaled steroid use, how long symptoms have been present, and previous hospitalizations for asthma. Patients managed in the outpatient setting should be reassessed by phone or office or clinic visit in 24 hours and again in 3–4 days.
3. **Severe exacerbations.** In severe exacerbations (PF <50% of baseline, accessory muscle use, nasal flaring, severe dyspnea, single-word speech, pale color to cyanotic, inaudible breath sounds), the patient should be given one or more inhaled treatments and immediately transported to the emergency department.

**B. Chronic mild asthma** is defined as intermittent brief episodes of wheezing and dyspnea lasting less than 1 hour and occurring up to two times per week. For children younger than 5 years, a nebulized or oral beta$_2$-agonist such as albuterol usually is effective. For children older than 5 years, an inhaled beta$_2$-agonist is best. The beta$_2$-agonist should be used for the duration of the symptoms.

C. **Chronic moderate asthma** is defined as symptoms occurring more than once or twice a week that may last for days and occasionally result in emergency department care. Therapy consists of an inhaled beta$_2$-agonist prn to tid–qid *and* cromolyn. If symptoms persist, inhaled steroids are used. Once the patient is stabilized on inhaled steroids, cromolyn may be discontinued. Alternative management is to use an inhaled beta$_2$-agonist prn to tid–qid *plus* theophylline *or* an oral beta$_2$-agonist.

D. **Chronic severe asthma** is defined as continuous symptoms with frequent exacerbations resulting in decreased activity level and occasional emergency department visits and hospitalizations. Therapy includes an inhaled beta$_2$-agonist tid–qid *and* inhaled steroids with or without cromolyn. In addition, theophylline, an oral beta$_2$-agonist, or both may be added. Alternate-day systemic steroids should be considered.

E. **Exercise-induced asthma.** Approximately 35–40% of patients with allergic rhinitis and up to 90% of patients with asthma have bronchoconstriction with exercise. Exercise-induced asthma usually is easily controlled by using an inhaled beta$_2$-agonist (two puffs) or cromolyn (two puffs) before exercise followed by prn use. If the patient still wheezes with the above regimen, four puffs of a beta$_2$-agonist or cromolyn or two puffs of each can be used before exercise.

## Selected Readings

Committee on Sports Medicine and Fitness. Metered-dose inhalers for young athletes with exercise-induced asthma. *Pediatrics* 94:129, 1994.

Excerpts from the NAEP executive summary. Guidelines for the diagnosis and management of asthma. *Pediatr Ann* 21:537, 1992.

McFadden ER, Gilbert IA. Exercise-induced asthma. *N Engl J Med* 330:1362, 1994.

Plant TF. Helping asthma patients breathe easier. *Contemp Pediatr* October 1989, Pp 59–76.

Provisional Committee on Quality Improvement. Practice parameters: The office management of acute exacerbations of asthma in children. *Pediatrics* 93:119, 1994.

Shapiro GG. Childhood asthma: update. *Pediatr Rev* 13:403, 1992.

Shapiro GG. Let's help kids with asthma lead normal lives. *Contemp Pediatr* November 1990, Pp 105–123.

# 23

# Bronchiolitis

Robert M. Siegel

Bronchiolitis is an acute, febrile, clinical syndrome of infants and young children associated with a lower respiratory tract infection and characterized by cough and wheeze.

I. **Etiology and pathophysiology**. The most common cause of bronchiolitis is respiratory syncytial virus (RSV). Other pathogens associated with the syndrome are the parainfluenza and influenza viruses, rhinovirus, adenovirus, and *Mycoplasma pneumoniae*. Bronchiolitis occurs most often during the winter months in infants younger than 12 months (80%). The disease's natural course is an upper respiratory tract infection with fever and rhinorrhea that progresses over 2–5 days to lower tract involvement with wheezing and some degree of respiratory distress manifested by tachypnea, nasal flaring, and retractions. In RSV infection, the virus invades the epithelial cells of the respiratory tract, moving cell-to-cell from the upper to lower tract. The result is necrosis of the epithelium with subsequent sloughing and obstruction of the small airways, leading to the characteristic findings of wheezing and hyperinflation.

II. **Clinical course**. Two-thirds of children with bronchiolitis have fever. Physical examination often reveals an irritable infant with tachypnea and tachycardia. Wheezing is the hallmark of the disease. Infants with bronchiolitis may be unable to take adequate oral fluids and become dehydrated. Other complications of bronchiolitis include hypoxemia, respiratory failure, apnea, and bacterial superinfection. Apnea can be a presentation in infants younger than 6 months. Some factors associated with more severe disease include a history of prematurity, young chronological age, chronic lung disease (especially bronchopulmonary dysplasia), and congenital heart disease. Ten to twenty percent of infants with bronchiolitis develop significant respiratory compromise necessitating hospitalization. The mortality for bronchiolitis caused by RSV is 0.5–1.5% for hospitalized patients (as high as 37% for infants with congenital heart disease).

III. **Evaluation.** The outpatient evaluation should begin with a good history and physical exam, since bronchiolitis is a clinical diagnosis. A chest x-ray should be considered to rule out other causes of wheezing in this age group such as foreign body aspiration, congenital anomalies, or bacterial pneumonia. The chest x-ray usually shows hyperinflation and peribronchial thickening; the presence of atelectasis may indicate a more severe course. Pulse oximetry determination of oxygen saturation may reveal hypoxemia, which is common even in the absence of clinically detectable cyanosis. If the infant is extremely tachypneic or in moderate respiratory distress, capillary blood gases should be analyzed to rule out carbon dioxide retention, a sign of respiratory failure. A CBC is generally not helpful.

**Table 23-1. Indications for ribavirin therapy**

| |
|---|
| Complicated congenital heart disease |
| Bronchopulmonary dysplasia |
| Cystic fibrosis |
| Other chronic lung conditions |
| Premature infants |
| T cell immune deficiency |
| Infants with significant respiratory compromise (e.g., $PaO_2$ <65 mm Hg, $SaO_2$ <90%, $PaCO_2$ >40 mm Hg) |

IV. **Diagnosis**. Although bronchiolitis is a clinical diagnosis, a specific etiology can be determined with a nasal wash for culture and RSV antigen. All infants admitted to the hospital should have a nasal wash to help determine isolation procedures.

V. **Treatment** for most children is largely supportive. Oxygen should be given to those with hypoxia and IV fluids to those without adequate oral intake.

The decision to admit a child with bronchiolitis to the hospital is a difficult one. It should be based on (1) general appearance (whether a child looks toxic or appears happy and playful), (2) age (infants younger than 3 months of age or of gestational age of less than 34 weeks are at greater risk for apnea and should be observed closely in the hospital), (3) tachypnea (an infant consistently breathing more than 60–70 times/minute is likely to tire and needs monitoring), (4) oral intake (if an infant is unable to take adequate oral fluids because of tachypnea or respiratory distress, IV hydration is necessary), and (5) hypoxemia (a resting oxygen saturation of <95%; saturation is likely to decrease with crying or sucking, and such infants should be admitted with supplemental oxygen).

The efficacy of bronchodilator therapy in bronchiolitis is questionable and depends on the degree of bronchospasm present. Some infants with a positive family history for atopic disease may have a significant degree of bronchospasm, and the current illness represents the first episode of reactive airways disease secondary to lower respiratory tract infection. Other infants have a predominantly viral lower respiratory tract infection component to the disease with little to no bronchospasm present. The latter commonly have significant rales present on physical examination. Beta-agonist aerosols may be tried and continued if there is improvement with therapy.

Ribavirin is a broad-spectrum antiviral agent that has been used for the treatment of RSV infection in more than 100,000 patients. The drug has proved safe and effective in some studies, but some experts still question its efficacy. Because ribavirin is expensive, its use should be limited to children at high risk for severe disease (Table 23-1). The drug is administered by a small-particle generator and is given for 12–18 hours continuously, daily.

VI. **Prevention.** RSV has a high potential for spread in the daycare and hospital setting. Since the infection is spread person-to-person by large droplets of respiratory secretions, the mainstay of prevention is good handwashing. The hospitalized patient should be put in contact isolation. Caretakers should wear goggles and gloves to help prevent the spread of this agent.

## Selected Readings

American Academy of Pediatrics. Respiratory Syncytial Virus. In G Peter (ed), *1994 Red Book: Report of the Committee on Infectious Diseases* (23rd ed). Elk Grove Village, IL: American Academy of Pediatrics, 1994.

La Via W, Marks MI, Stutman HR. Respiratory syncytial virus puzzle: Clinical features, pathophysiology, treatment, and prevention. *J Pediatr* 121:503, 1992.

Shaw KN, Bell LM, Sherman N. Outpatient evaluation of infants with bronchiolitis: Predictors of serious morbidity. *Am J Dis Child* 142:388, 1988.

Welliver R, Cherry JD. Bronchiolitis and Infectious Asthma. In RD Feigin, JD Cherry (eds), *Textbook of Pediatric Infectious Diseases* (3rd ed). Philadelphia: Saunders, 1992.

24

# Croup (Acute Viral Laryngotracheobronchitis)

Raymond C. Baker

**I. Description.** Croup (acute viral laryngotracheobronchitis) is a lower respiratory tract infection caused by parainfluenza viruses (most common), respiratory syncytial virus, adenovirus, influenza viruses A and B, and measles virus. It is seen more commonly in young children 6 months–3 years of age during the fall and winter months. Croup begins with viral upper respiratory infection (URI) symptoms of fever, runny nose, and cough in a non–toxic-appearing child. These symptoms are followed in 1–4 days by hoarseness; a resounding, seal-like cough; inspiratory stridor and intercostal retractions; and, in unusually severe cases, restlessness (hypoxia) progressing to cyanosis.

The laboratory is rarely helpful in the diagnosis, which is almost exclusively clinical. Airway films reveal subglottic stenosis on anterior-posterior view (steeple sign) but are not usually necessary to make the diagnosis.

Viral croup must be differentiated from two other serious illnesses that may present similarly—epiglottitis and bacterial tracheitis (membranous croup). Features that distinguish **epiglottitis** are age (usually older—in the age range of 3–7), the absence of cough as a significant symptom, the presence of a severe sore throat, very acute onset with septic appearance and rapid progression, and a muffled voice. Respiratory distress is a sign of advanced disease that requires immediate airway management. As this disease has a predominantly *Haemophilus influenzae* type B etiology, it is rapidly disappearing along with *H. influenzae* meningitis since the advent of universal immunization with conjugate *H. influenzae* vaccine.

Bacterial croup probably begins as viral croup with similar symptoms, but then the child develops increasing toxicity and respiratory distress as the airway becomes occluded with pus resulting from *Staphylococcus aureus* (and less commonly *H. influenzae*) superinfection.

**II. Treatment** of mild croup is largely supportive. A cool mist humidifier may help reduce subglottic edema, although the effect of a cool mist humidifier is probably mostly placebo in that it gives the parents "something to do." The child should be observed closely for progression of symptoms that might require hospitalization. In the hospital, treatment may include oxygen, racemic epinephrine (0.5 ml in 2.5 ml saline administered by aerosol), steroids (dexamethasone 0.6 mg/kg initially), and, rarely, intubation.

Several factors help determine whether a child should be hospitalized: (1) age younger than 12 months, (2) patient making a second, unplanned visit to the physician or emergency department, (3) questionable compliance or follow-up,

**Table 24-1. Croup score**

| Finding | Score 0 | 1 | 2 | 3 |
|---|---|---|---|---|
| Stridor | None | Only with agitation | Mild at rest | Severe at rest |
| Retraction | None | Mild | Moderate | Severe |
| Color | None | — | — | Cyanotic |
| Level of consciousness | Normal | Restless when disturbed | Restless when undisturbed | Lethargic |
| Severity | Mild | Mild to moderate | Moderate | Severe |
| Total score | ≤ 4 | 5–6 | 7–8 | ≥ 9 |

Source: Adapted from GR Fleisher, S Ludwig (eds). *Textbook of Pediatric Emergency Medicine* (3rd ed). Baltimore: Williams & Wilkins, 1993.

(4) distance the patient lives from hospital, and (5) the presence of any of the following: somnolence, poor oral intake, cyanosis, stridor at rest, dehydration from refusal of oral liquids, and croup score higher than 7 (Table 24-1).

## Selected Readings

Denny FW, Murphy TF, Clyde WA et al. An 11-year study in a pediatric practice. *Pediatrics* 71:871, 1984.

Fleisher GR, Ludwig S (eds). *Textbook of Pediatric Emergency Medicine* (3rd ed). Baltimore: Williams & Wilkins, 1993.

Kairys SW, Olmstead EM, O'Connor GT. Steroid treatment of laryngotracheitis: A meta-analysis of the evidence from randomized trials. *Pediatrics* 83:683, 1989.

Knott AM, Long CE, Hall CB. Parainfluenza viral infections in pediatric outpatients: Seasonal patterns and clinical characteristics. *Pediatr Infect Dis J* 13:269, 1994.

Ruddy RM. Croup—Has management changed? *Contemp Pediatr* October 1993, Pp 21–32.

Singer OP, Wilson WJ. Laryngotracheobronchitis: 2 years' experience with racemic epinephrine. *Can Med Assoc J* 115:132, 1976.

Tunnessen WW, Feinstein AR. The steroid-croup controversy: an analytic review of methodologic problems. *J Pediatr* 96:751, 1980.

# 25

# Pertussis

Raymond C. Baker

Pertussis is an acute respiratory tract infection caused by *Bordetella pertussis*, a small, gram-negative pleomorphic rod. A lower respiratory tract illness resembling pertussis also may be caused by *Bordetella parapertussis, Chlamydia trachomatis*, and certain adenoviruses.

**I. Epidemiology.** Pertussis, especially during the early catarrhal stage, is extremely contagious and transmitted by the respiratory route. It occurs during all seasons of the year. All ages can be infected and symptomatic, but the greatest incidence and highest morbidity and mortality occur in infants and children. The mortality is as high as 1.3% in infants less than 1 month of age and 0.3% in the age range of 1 month–1 year. Complications in young infants include pneumonia in 20%, seizures in 3%, and encephalopathy in about 1%. The incidence of pertussis declined dramatically with the introduction of a vaccine, but several thousand cases still occur each year in the United States, with a significant increase in the last 2–3 years.

**II. Description.** Following an incubation period of 6–20 days (mean 7 days), the disease usually runs a course characterized by three stages.

**A. Catarrhal.** The catarrhal stage lasts 1–2 weeks with mucous rhinorrhea, mild cough, conjunctival injection, and low-grade fever. The mucus produced during this stage is characteristically stringy and viscous, resulting in young infants producing "nose bubbles" and older infants, who are able to sit, producing ropy strings of mucus.

**B. Paroxysmal.** In the paroxysmal stage, which lasts 2–4 weeks, the cough becomes more frequent and severe, occurring in paroxysms that cannot be suppressed. The classic pertussis cough is a series of staccato-like coughs followed by a sudden, forceful inspiration that produces a characteristic whoop (inspiratory stridor). Post-tussive vomiting is common. Infants younger than 6 months old may have a severe, persistent cough with post-tussive vomiting without the whoop.

**C. Convalescent.** The convalescent stage consists of coughing and vomiting episodes that gradually diminish over 1–2 weeks, although the cough may persist for months. Physical findings are nonspecific during this stage.

**III. Laboratory.** The WBC count commonly is elevated (between 20,000 and 50,000/μl) with a marked predominance of lymphocytes. The chest radiograph may show perihilar infiltrates ("shaggy heart"), atelectasis, or both. A positive fluorescent antibody test of nasopharyngeal secretions suggests the diagnosis; however, false-positives are frequent. A positive nasopharyngeal culture on Bordet-Gengou medium confirms the diagnosis (80% positive). The yield is greatest during the catarrhal phase, which corresponds with the period of greatest infectivity.

IV. **Treatment** of pertussis is erythromycin (30–50 mg/kg/day in 4 divided doses for 14 days; maximum 2 g/day), which may modify the illness if administered during the catarrhal stage. It has no effect on the course of illness once paroxysms are established, but it is recommended to limit the spread of the organism. Otherwise, treatment is supportive. Infants, especially those younger than 6 months old and those with potentially severe disease, should be hospitalized to anticipate complications such as apnea, seizures, encephalopathy, and pneumonia. Respiratory isolation should be continued until the child completes 5 days of antibiotics or until 3 weeks after the onset of paroxysms in the untreated child.

Close contacts, including household and day-care contacts, should receive erythromycin in the above dosage as prophylaxis regardless of vaccination status. In addition, previously immunized contacts younger than 7 years old should receive a booster dose of pertussis vaccine unless they received a booster dose on schedule within the previous 3 years. Unimmunized contacts younger than 7 years old should be started on an immunization schedule. The current vaccine probably provides protection in about 80% of children who have received at least three doses of vaccine.

## Selected Readings

Binkin NJ, Salmaso S, Tozzi AE et al. Epidemiology of pertussis in a developed country with low vaccination coverage: the Italian experience. *Pediatr Infect Dis J* 11:653, 1992.

Christie CDC, Marx ML, Marchant CD et al. The 1993 epidemic of pertussis in Cincinnati. *N Engl J Med* 331:16, 1994.

Gordon M, Davies HD, Gold R. Clinical and microbiologic features of children presenting with pertussis to a Canadian pediatric hospital during an eleven-year period. *Pediatr Infect Dis J* 13:617, 1994.

Heininger U, Stehr K, Schmitt-Grohe S et al. Clinical characteristics of illness caused by *Bordetella parapertussis* compared with illness caused by *Bordetella pertussis*. *Pediatr Infect Dis J* 13:306, 1994.

# 26

# Pneumonia in Infants and Children

Raymond C. Baker

There are multiple etiologies of pneumonia in infants and children, although viruses predominate. The more common viral etiologies are respiratory syncytial virus, parainfluenza virus, rhinovirus, adenovirus, and influenza virus. Bacterial pneumonia is less common; etiologies may include (in decreasing order of importance) *Streptococcus pneumoniae, Haemophilus influenzae* type B, *Staphylococcus aureus, Streptococcus pyogenes, Klebsiella pneumoniae, Escherichia coli* (and other gram-negatives), *Bordetella pertussis,* and *Mycobacterium tuberculosis.* Miscellaneous infectious agents include *Mycoplasma pneumoniae* and *Chlamydia (trachomatis* and *pneumoniae).* Less common infectious agents include various fungal and parasitic organisms, including *Pneumocystis carinii.* Pneumonia also may result from aspiration (foreign bodies, vomitus, hydrocarbons, meconium, lipids).

I. **Symptoms** of pneumonia vary from fever alone to a combination of symptoms that might include fever, chills, cough, vomiting, abdominal pain, pleuritic chest pain, decreased activity, and decreased appetite.

II. On **physical examination**, fever usually is present in association with any combination of tachypnea, grunting respirations, retractions, rales, wheeze, decreased or bronchial breath sounds, and dullness to percussion. In children, there may be little on physical examination other than fever and tachypnea to suggest pneumonia. The presence of fever and abdominal pain with a normal abdominal examination sometimes suggests lower-lobe pneumonia in the young child.

III. The **laboratory** often is not helpful in establishing the diagnosis and etiology (the exception is a culture when a specimen is available). Laboratory work-up may include a CBC, blood culture, and chest x-ray. The degree of illness may dictate other laboratory parameters to determine acuity, such as arterial blood gases, oxygen saturation, thoracentesis, or tracheal aspirate for culture.

IV. **Etiology.** The history, examination, CBC with differential, and chest x-ray may sometimes suggest an etiology to the pneumonia that is helpful to direct therapy.

- A. **Bacterial**. Children with bacterial pneumonia usually have an abrupt onset of symptoms; appear toxic with tachypnea and high fever; have an elevated WBC count; and have chest x-ray findings of unilobar disease, alveolar infiltrate, effusion, or pneumatoceles. The latter is especially associated with *S. aureus*.
- B. **Viral.** Infants and children with viral pneumonia tend to have a more gradual onset, appear less ill, wheeze, and have any of the following on chest x-ray: multilobar disease, pneumonitis, and hyperinflation.

C. **Mycoplasma**. In the older child and adolescent, headache, sore throat, wheeze, and a history of other family members with a similar illness suggest mycoplasma pneumonia ("walking pneumonia").

D. ***Chlamydia***. Chlamydial pneumonia is seen in the infant who is afebrile and mildly to moderately ill and has a staccato cough. There may be conjunctivitis on examination (or history of conjunctivitis). On examination, the chest usually sounds worse (rales) than the child appears; the chest x-ray shows hyperinflation with a diffuse, reticulonodular appearance. The CBC may show eosinophilia.

E. **Pertussis**. Paroxysms of cough with color change and the presence of inspiratory stridor (whoop) are characteristic of pertussis (see Chap. 25). The WBC count characteristically is elevated with a pronounced lymphocytosis.

V. **Admission to hospital.** The following clinical situations suggest a need for hospitalization:

A. **Children who are vomiting significantly and unable to take oral medications** may require a brief period of parenteral therapy.

B. **Infants with a presumed bacterial etiology** usually require parenteral antibiotics.

C. **Infants with probable pertussis** should be hospitalized initially because of the significant complications in this age range.

D. **Very young infants in whom sepsis cannot be ruled out** clinically **and immunocompromised children** usually are hospitalized pending culture results.

E. **Infants and children with recurrent pneumonias** may require hospitalization for evaluation.

F. **Other possible indications** for hospitalization include septic-appearing infants, pyogenic complications, significant pleural effusion, and significant respiratory distress or impending respiratory failure.

VI. **Treatment.** Besides symptomatic and supportive therapy, antibiotics commonly are used empirically in the treatment of pneumonia because a specific etiology is usually unknown. Also, the physician prefers bacterial coverage, especially in the patient who is being treated as an outpatient. Nonetheless, pneumonia at any age is most commonly viral. Some general guidelines for antibiotic therapy follow.

A. **Outpatient antibiotic therapy**

1. **Wheeze present.** No antibiotic therapy may be considered in the infant with typical bronchiolitis during a period of RSV prevalence. Otherwise, oral erythromycin estolate for 10 days is appropriate, which would provide coverage for mycoplasma (and chlamydia) as a treatable cause of pneumonia with wheeze (primarily older children and adolescents). Bronchodilators may be indicated, especially if reactive airways disease is suggested by family history or past medical history.

2. **Wheeze absent.** In the absence of a wheeze, oral amoxicillin for 10 days should be adequate coverage if bacterial disease is present. In the older child and adolescent, oral erythromycin estolate is also acceptable and covers both bacterial and mycoplasmal disease.

**B. Inpatient antibiotic therapy**

1. **Younger than 3 months old.** Supportive therapy with humidified oxygen and hydration in infants younger than 3 months old should be provided. Bronchodilators may be indicated if wheezing is present, especially if the family history is positive for asthma. The antibiotic choice might include IV ampicillin and gentamicin or IV nafcillin (instead of ampicillin) and gentamicin if *S. aureus* is suspected. Oral erythromycin may be added or substituted if chlamydia or pertussis is suspected.
2. **3–6 months of age.** Provide supportive therapy plus IV ampicillin alone in infants 3–6 months of age. Cefuroxime should be used instead of ampicillin if *H. influenzae* or *S. aureus* is suspected or if the infant appears septic. Oral erythromycin may be added if chlamydial or pertussis infection is suspected.
3. **6 months–6 years of age.** Administer ampicillin alone. Oral erythromycin may be added if pertussis or *Mycoplasma* is suspected. Cefuroxime should be substituted for ampicillin if *H. influenzae* or *S. aureus* is suspected.
4. **Older than 6 years.** Give penicillin G; give oral erythromycin if *Mycoplasma* is suspected.

## Selected Readings

Cohen GJ. Management of infections of the lower respiratory tract in children. *Pediatr Infect Dis J* 6:317, 1987.

Denny FW, Clyde WA. Acute lower respiratory tract infections in nonhospitalized children. *J Pediatr* 108:635, 1986.

Gordon ES, Jacobs RF. Management of community-acquired bacterial pneumonia in hospitalized children. *Pediatr Infect Dis J* 11:160, 1992.

Teele D. Pneumonia: Antimicrobial therapy for infants and children. *Pediatr Infect Dis J* 4:330, 1985.

Turner RB, Lande AE, Chase P et al. Pneumonia in pediatric outpatients: Cause and clinical manifestations. *J Pediatr* 111:194, 1987.

D

# Gastrointestinal Disorders

# 27

# Acute Gastroenteritis

Raymond C. Baker

I. **Etiology.** Acute gastroenteritis (AGE) with diarrhea, vomiting, and fever is a common illness presenting to the primary care physician year-round. Multiple etiologies exist for infectious enteritis, but a relatively small number of organisms account for the majority of cases. Among viral etiologies, *Rotavirus* and Norwalk-like viruses predominate during cold winter months; other viral etiologies include enteric adenovirus, pestivirus, astroviruses, caliciviruses, parvoviruses, and nongroup A *Rotavirus*. Bacterial etiologies are less common but tend to be more severe and have more complications. These include *Salmonella*, *Escherichia coli*, *Shigella*, *Campylobacter*, *Yersinia*, *Aeromonas*, and *Plesiomonas*. Less common bacterial etiologies are *Clostridium difficile*, *Vibrio parahemolyticus*, *Staphylococcus aureus*, and *Clostridium perfringens*. *Giardia* is the only common parasitic cause of AGE, although *Cryptosporidium* is seen in immunosuppressed individuals.

II. **Evaluation.** The evaluation of infants and children with AGE begins with a history, which might suggest an etiology (e.g., foodborne illness, exposure, time of year, underlying illness, associated symptoms), and a historical assessment of hydration, including urine output; stool quality, quantity, and frequency; and the ability to maintain hydration. The physical examination should focus on the state of hydration (Table 27-1), degree of illness, and physical features that might suggest an etiology (e.g., associated rash).

In the majority of AGE cases, no laboratory work-up is needed, and the disease is treated supportively with appropriate oral rehydration and maintenance fluids and diet. Stool cultures should be considered for any of the following: (1) blood or mucus in the stool, (2) significant fever, or (3) sudden onset of diarrhea without vomiting or with vomiting that came on after the diarrhea. In febrile infants younger than 12 months old in whom a bacterial etiology is suspected, a blood culture also should be obtained because of the tendency toward bacteremia of *Salmonella* species.

III. **Treatment.** In mild diarrhea ($\leq 5\%$ dehydration) of short duration (1–2 days), simple oral rehydration and maintenance can be achieved with temporary (usually 24 hours) cessation of routine diet and replacement with nonformulated clear liquids. The electrolyte content of rehydration solutions for treating mild diarrhea is relatively unimportant. Fluids might include beverages at home such as soft drinks, Kool-Aid, Gatorade, or broth followed by a return to regular diet. Follow-up examination (other than by telephone) is probably unnecessary.

In more significant diarrhea, attention should be paid to electrolyte replacement, and formulated rehydration fluids should be used for rehydration and maintenance (e.g.,

**Table 27-1. Physical signs of dehydration**

| | Mild (3–5%) | Moderate (5–10%) | Severe (>10%) |
|---|---|---|---|
| General condition | Well, alert | Restless, irritable | Lethargic, unconscious, floppy |
| Eyes | Normal | Sunken | Very sunken and dry |
| Tears | Present | Absent | Absent |
| Mouth and tongue | Moist | Sticky | Dry |
| Thirst | Normal | Thirsty, drinks eagerly | Drinks poorly, unable to drink |
| Skin retraction following pinch | Immediate | Slow | Very slow |
| Heart rate | Normal | Somewhat increased | Increased |
| Blood pressure | Normal | Normal | Decreased |

Rehydralyte, Pedialyte, Ricelyte) with appropriate follow-up examination. Oral rehydration can be initiated in an emergency department or hospital setting making IV resuscitation unnecessary except in more severe dehydration with hemodynamic instability. The duration of treatment with formulated rehydration fluids should not exceed 24–48 hours to avoid prolonged calorie deprivation. Refeeding following the initial period of rehydration probably should consist of a non–lactose-containing soy formula until gastrointestinal recovery has occurred (7–10 days); the latter is unnecessary if the infant is breast-fed. Follow-up is necessary to ensure compliance and resolution of the illness.

Other important features of the treatment of AGE include advice to parents concerning infection control measures (handwashing), especially when the infant is still in diapers.

IV. **Bacterial gastroenteritis.** In bacterial AGE, further work-up and antibiotic therapy may be appropriate as follows:

A. ***Salmonella***. In infants younger than 6 months old, further evaluation for sepsis may be indicated in documented *Salmonella* infection (with bacteremia) followed by parenteral antibiotic therapy with ampicillin. In older infants, antibiotic therapy is not indicated. Close attention to infection control measures should be instituted, especially if the infant is in a day-care setting or if the occupation of any of the caregivers is in public food handling.

B. ***Shigella***. All infants and children with documented *Shigella* AGE should be treated with antibiotics to prevent person-to-person spread and shorten the course of the illness, as a very small inoculum of *Shigella* can cause infection. Trimethoprim-sulfamethoxazole, 0.5 ml/kg PO bid for 5 days, is usually effective.

C. ***Campylobacter***. Treatment with erythromycin, 8–10 mg/kg PO qid, may shorten the course of the illness and the period of excretion. This treatment is especially appropriate if the child is in day-care or family members are involved with public food handling.

**D.** ***Yersinia, Aeromonas,*** **and** ***Plesiomonas***. Treatment with trimethoprim-sulfamethoxazole may be indicated if the child is in day-care or members of the family are involved with public food handling.

## Selected Readings

Ashkenazi S, Cleary TG. Antibiotic treatment of bacterial gastroenteritis. *Pediatr Infect Dis J* 10:140, 1991.

Lew JF, Glass RI, Petric M et al. Six-year retrospective surveillance of gastroenteritis viruses identified at ten electron microscopy centers in United States and Canada. *Pediatr Infect Dis J* 9:709, 1990.

Lifshitz F (ed). Management of acute diarrheal disease, proceedings of a symposium. *J Pediatr* 118:S25, 1990.

Richard L, Claeson M, Pierce NF. Management of acute diarrhea in children: lessons learned. *Pediatr Infect Dis J* 12:5, 1993.

Geme JW III, Hodes HL, Marcy SM et al. Consensus: Management of *Salmonella* infection in the first year of life. *Pediatr Infect Dis J* 7:615, 1988.

28

# Chronic Abdominal Pain in Children

## Michael K. Farrell

I. **Chronic abdominal pain** is a problem frequently encountered by the primary care physician. It affects about 10–15% of the school-age population. A reasonable definition is one proposed by Apley: three or more episodes of abdominal pain within 3 months severe enough to interfere with the child's activities. Evaluation of the child with chronic abdominal pain requires time and patience; it cannot be done in the brief office visit. The purpose of the evaluation is to exclude serious abdominal disorders and explain the natural history of chronic abdominal pain to the child and family.

There are three patterns of pain: dyspepsia, paroxysmal periumbilical pain, and crampy lower abdominal pain associated with altered defecation. Dyspepsia is a vague epigastric pain often associated with meals; related GI symptoms such as nausea, bloating, early satiety, and flatulence are common. Crampy lower abdominal discomfort associated with altered bowel habits is more common in adolescents and equivalent to irritable bowel syndrome.

II. The specific **etiology** of chronic abdominal pain is usually unknown. In multiple series, no organic cause for the pain can be found in 90–95% of cases. Current theory is that the pain is the result of a GI stimulus such as peristalsis that is perceived as pain in a sensitized host. The response to stress as a sensitizing factor plays a critical role in the syndrome. The goals of the initial evaluation are to exclude serious organic GI pathology and help the child and family understand the cause of the pain.

III. **History** is crucial to the diagnosis and management of chronic abdominal pain. The history should be obtained whenever possible from both the child and parents in an unhurried manner that encourages sharing of psychosocial issues. In addition to the usual medical questions, time must be spent discussing the child's personality and response to stressors. The two most common stresses in a child's life are family and school. Children with chronic abdominal pain tend to be "high-strung" perfectionistic worriers. In Apley's words, "They take the little issues of life too much to heart." The parent and child's concerns must be discussed to explore their fears and ideas. Two common concerns are the fear of cancer and concern about appendicitis or ulcers. The family history is useful in excluding serious familial GI disease and eliciting a positive history of stress-related disease. "Red flags" in the history that suggest organic disease are listed in Table 28-1.

IV. The **physical examination** should be meticulous, complete, and discussed with family and child. It should include a digital rectal examination to exclude constipation, which may be a great masquerader. At the end of the evaluation, certain

**Table 28-1. "Red flags" suggesting organic etiology in chronic abdominal pain**

| |
|---|
| Decentralized pain |
| Nocturnal pain |
| Diarrhea (with or without occult blood) |
| Hematemesis |
| Hematochezia |
| Weight loss or growth failure |
| Perianal lesions |

**Table 28-2. Most common organic etiologies of recurrent abdominal pain**

| Disease | Clue |
|---|---|
| Urinary tract infection | Vomiting, flank pain, dysuria, enuresis |
| Inflammatory bowel disease | Poor growth; perianal disease; systemic symptoms; anemia; lower abdominal pain, tenderness, or mass |
| Peptic disease | Family history of peptic disease, nocturnal pain, epigastric tenderness |
| Pancreatitis | Radiation of pain to back, vomiting |
| Constipation | Left-lower quadrant pain, palpable stool, symptoms relieved by defecation |
| Esophagitis | Burning epigastric pain, substernal pain |
| Giardiasis | Diarrhea, distention, and flatulence |
| Lactose intolerance (excessive sorbitol/fructose ingestion) | Diarrhea, distention, symptoms related to meals |

baseline laboratory studies may be indicated; the most common are a CBC, sedimentation rate, urinalysis and culture, and stool for occult blood. If these, the history, and physical examination are normal, there is little likelihood of serious abdominal pathology. Radiographic studies are rarely helpful; the upper GI series misses superficial mucosal lesions and does not detect *Helicobacter pylori* disease. The barium enema is insensitive to mucosal disease and results in significant gonadal radiation. The abdominal and pelvic ultrasound, though rarely positive, does view the genitourinary and biliary systems and occasionally may be indicated to rule out disease in these organ systems. Table 28-2 lists the most frequent organic causes of chronic abdominal pain and diagnostic clues.

V. **Treatment** should consist first of explanation and reassurance. The goal is to educate the family and child about the physiologic response to stress. The pain must be acknowledged as real and not "in the head." Pertinent examples relevant to the family and child's experiences may be helpful. For example, most children and adults have experienced abdominal discomfort ("butterflies in the stomach") prior to an important exam or participation in a pivotal sporting event. The clinician must be confident and avoid the "one more test" trap, which undermines the family's confidence. Specific stressors that have been identified should be discussed, and psychological intervention occasionally is indicated. Stress reduction techniques are useful.

There are no data to support a pharmacologic approach to chronic abdominal pain; $H_2$-blockers are useful only in acid peptic disease. If evidence of *H. pylori* infection is present, it should be treated appropriately. One study has suggested that increasing dietary fiber may be helpful. Constipation should be treated vigorously.

If concerns are recognized, a complete and thorough evaluation done, and an honest discussion of the findings allowed, most children respond well. The physician should emphasize his or her continued availability and schedule follow-up appointments to monitor the child's progress.

## Selected Readings

Apley J. *The Child with Abdominal Pain* (2nd ed). Oxford, England: Blackwell, 1975.

Apley J, Naish N. Children with recurrent abdominal pains: A field survey of 1,000 school children. *Arch Dis Child* 33:165, 1957.

Boyle JT. Chronic Abdominal Pain. In WA Walker, PR Durie, JR Hamilton et al. (eds), *Pediatric Gastrointestinal Disease*. Philadelphia: Decker, 1991. Pp 45–54.

Coleman WL, Levine MD. Recurrent abdominal pain: The cost of aches and the aches of the cost. *Pediatr Rev* 8:143, 1986.

# 29

# Encopresis

## Raymond C. Baker

Encopresis (fecal soiling) is seen in 1–2% of children—boys more commonly than girls—and is usually associated with chronic constipation. The disorder typically begins after stool continence has been achieved for 1 or more years (secondary encopresis). The etiology of encopresis usually is related to a period of painful defecation, which may be due to multiple causes, including rectal fissures, chronic constipation with painful stool passage due to large-caliber stools, and, occasionally, psychological factors. Over time, the subsequent voluntary withholding of stool passage causes colon distention with hard stool, loss of tone and sensation (of fullness) of the colon, and finally, liquid stool leakage around the impaction through a lax anal sphincter.

I. **History.** The typical presenting history of encopresis is frequent fecal soiling of small amounts of soft stool and periodic (every 2–4 weeks) painful defecation of a large quantity of large-caliber stool. Typically, the parent may report that the stool's quantity and size may stop up the toilet and have to be broken up to flush it down. Following passage of an extremely large stool, there is usually a short period of decreased symptoms, and then the cycle repeats. Children may deny the process, hide soiled underwear, and commonly have secondary psychological problems from the intolerance of their peers.

II. The **physical examination** is usually normal except for lax anal sphincter tone and the presence of a large quantity of hard stool in the ampulla. Hard stool also may be palpable on abdominal exam. The primary differential is Hirschsprung's disease and behavioral or psychological encopresis. In the former disorder, an aganglionic segment of distal colon functionally obstructs passage of stool. Children with Hirschsprung's disease tend to be small in size, pass small-caliber stools, and have an empty ampulla on examination. Most have had abnormal stool patterns from birth. In encopresis of psychological origin, the tendency is to be periodically incontinent of larger quantities of normal-appearing stool.

III. The **treatment** of encopresis requires the physician to fully explain to the parents the condition's pathogenesis, especially since the treatment (laxatives) may seem paradoxical to parents whose perception is that their child has frequent liquid or very soft stools. It is important that parents understand that the end result of encopresis, namely incontinence, is involuntary.

At the initial visit, the bowel needs to be emptied—either as part of the visit (with enemas) or with careful instructions to the parent regarding the procedure to be carried out at home. Colonic evacuation may be accomplished with a combination of enemas (one-to-one mixture of milk and molasses, soap suds, or Fleet's) and osmotic laxatives and stimulants (e.g., milk of magnesia, Dulcolax) as needed. Subsequently, the child should be started on a combination of (1) regular stool softeners with or without stimulants to maintain very soft stools that are passed easily and without pain at least daily and (2) defecation retraining.

**A. Stool softeners.** In the cooperative older child, mineral oil is very effective and inexpensive (over-the-counter) as a stool softener. It should be given in progressively larger doses on a regular basis until the desired very soft stool consistency is achieved. That dose is given regularly 1–2 months as necessary to maintain stool softness. The dose is usually in the range of 1–2 oz qd–bid. Since mineral oil may decrease absorption of fat soluble vitamins in food, it should not be given at mealtime. Some children also may require a mild stimulant laxative, such as Senokot Syrup or Senokot Granules, to aid evacuation during the retraining period (see sec. **III.B**). Another effective stool softener is lactulose (which requires a prescription) given regularly in increasing doses of 0.5–1.0 ml/kg PO bid (maximum dose 45 ml bid) until the desired consistency of stool is achieved. The starting dose for adolescents is 15 ml PO bid for adolescents. The dose is titrated to maintain a very soft consistency to the stools.

**B. Defecation retraining.** Children with encopresis often have long-standing habits of voluntary fecal retention resulting in loss of normal colonic tone and may require extensive defecation retraining. Retraining consists of taking advantage of the gastrocolic reflex by having the child sit on the toilet 10–15 minutes after the two largest meals of the day and encouraging him or her to try to have a bowel movement. It should be clear to the child that sitting on the toilet is not an option, yet it should not be presented in a negative or disciplinary manner. The parent may want to give the child something to do while he or she sits on the toilet, such as reading or playing with toys or books. Over a period of days, a pattern will develop in which the child defecates once or twice after one or both of these meals.

At the same time stool softeners are added, the parent should add fiber to the child's diet, such as that found in popcorn, grains, fruits, and vegetables. Stool softeners should be continued for several months until regular stooling is established. A very important aspect of the retraining program is to provide positive reinforcement for stools passed in the toilet and lack of soiling. This may be in the form of new underwear (especially those that are brightly colored with cartoon characters), a trip to the local "fast food" restaurant, and so forth. Parents should be educated about the possibility of the recurrence of impaction and vigorous intervention with laxatives if the child goes more than 48–72 hours without a bowel movement.

**C. Follow-up.** A most important aspect of therapy is frequent follow-up, some of which may be by telephone. Regular visits are needed to document progress, reinforce the regimen, and ensure compliance and success. It is important for the physician to talk directly to the child, praising for successes and empathizing with relapses with carefully worded, understandable aids for the child.

## Selected Readings

Hatch TF. Encopresis and constipation in children. *Pediatr Clin North Am* 35:257, 1988.

Levine MD. Encopresis: Its potentiation, evaluation, and alleviation. *Pediatr Clin North Am* 29:315, 1982.

Schmitt BD, Mauro RD. 20 common errors in treating encopresis. *Contemp Pediatr* May 1992, Pp 47–65.

# 30

# Hyperbilirubinemia in the Term Infant

Christine L. McHenry

Most full-term infants appear jaundiced during the first few days of life. As a primary care physician, it is important to determine whether the jaundice is secondary to physiologic jaundice of the newborn or whether it is of pathologic origin. This task has been made somewhat more difficult because of early discharge programs from newborn nurseries. Any infant discharged from the nursery who is less than 48 hours old should be evaluated by a health care professional (home nurse, physician) within 48 hours of discharge for evidence of jaundice.

**I. History and physical examination**

**A. History**

1. **Maternal**. When evaluating an infant for jaundice, the physician should consider the mother's ethnic background, blood type and rhesus factor (Rh), and serology. In addition, the physician should ask about any previous deliveries of jaundiced infants, illness, and drug use during pregnancy.
2. **Delivery**. The physician should determine whether oxytocin was administered during delivery, whether the newborn was extracted with a vacuum, whether membranes ruptured prematurely, and the infant's Apgar score.
3. **Infant**. The physician should determine the infant's age when the jaundice occurred; the infant's feeding pattern; the color of the infant's urine and stools; and whether the infant has had vomiting, fever, irritability, or lethargy.

**B. Physical examination**. When evaluating an infant for jaundice, the physician should consider his or her general impression of the infant (awake and alert, irritable, or lethargic) and look for congenital anomalies, evidence of enclosed hemorrhage, and signs of infection (congenital or acquired).

**II. Classification of hyperbilirubinemia**

**A. Classification**. Hyperbilirubinemia can be classified as indirect (unconjugated) when the direct (conjugated) component is less than 15% of the total, direct (conjugated) when the direct component is greater than 30% of the total, and indeterminate when the direct component is 15–30%.

**B. Criteria for investigation**

1. Infants who are **jaundiced within the first 24 hours of life**
2. Infants who have a **rapid rise in bilirubin** (>5 mg/dl/day)
3. **Full-term infants with a total bilirubin greater than 13 mg/dl**

4. Infants **older than 7 days who are jaundiced**
5. **Infants who have direct (conjugated) hyperbilirubinemia**

**III. Physiologic jaundice of the newborn**

**A. Definition and etiology.** Physiologic jaundice of the newborn, a transient elevation of unconjugated bilirubin, usually is evident between 48 and 72 hours of age and resolves by 1 week of age. The etiology of physiologic jaundice is a complex interplay among several factors, including increase bilirubin load from decreased red cell survival, decreased bilirubin uptake by the hepatocyte, decreased glucuronyl transferase activity, and defective bilirubin excretion.

**B. Treatment**. The use of phototherapy and exchange transfusion to treat physiologic hyperbilirubinemia is controversial. Most studies of hyperbilirubinemia and kernicterus have included only babies with hemolytic disease, particularly Rh incompatibility. Studies of hyperbilirubinemia and other neurologic problems have shown mixed results. Reasonable recommendations for the full-term infant with hyperbilirubinemia secondary to physiologic jaundice are to institute phototherapy at a bilirubin level of 18–20 mg/dl and perform an exchange transfusion at greater than 25 mg/dl. The major consideration is whether phototherapy, exchange transfusion, or both is of greater benefit than risk to the infant with hyperbilirubinemia.

**IV. Indirect (unconjugated) hyperbilirubinemia**

**A. Differential diagnosis**

1. **Isoimmune hemolysis** (ABO and Rh incompatibility)
2. **Nonisoimmune hemolysis** (G6PD deficiency, pyruvate kinase deficiency, spherocytosis, elliptocytosis)
3. **Polycythemia** (from delayed cord clamping, infant small for gestational age, infant of a diabetic mother)
4. **Enclosed hemorrhage (e.g., cephalohematoma)**
5. **Swallowed maternal blood**
6. **Increased enterohepatic circulation from small-bowel obstruction**
7. **Asphyxia**
8. **Sepsis**
9. **Hypothyroidism**
10. **Crigler-Najjar syndrome**
11. **Physiologic jaundice**
12. **Breast-feeding or breast milk jaundice**

**B. Evaluation**. The evaluation of "clinically significant" indirect hyperbilirubinemia in an otherwise healthy full-term infant should consist of (1) mother's blood type and Rh, (2) direct Coombs' test on the infant blood, and (3) infant's total serum bilirubin. Additional tests to consider if the history and physical examination are suggestive include a sepsis work-up, blood count with a platelet count, reticulocyte count, G6PD screen, hemoglobin electrophoresis, thyroid function studies, and an abdominal film or upper GI study.

**C. Treatment**. The level of total serum bilirubin at which to consider phototherapy or exchange transfusion varies somewhat according to the infant's age. In general, the treatment guidelines given under physiologic jaundice (see sec. **III.B**) are reasonable.

**V. Direct (conjugated) hyperbilirubinemia**

**A. Differential diagnosis**. Conjugated hyperbilirubinemia is always pathologic and always requires an investigation into the etiology. The differential diagnosis includes the following:

1. **Extrahepatic obstruction** (extrahepatic biliary atresia, choledochal cyst)
2. **Intrahepatic cholestasis** (intrahepatic biliary atresia, drugs)
3. **Neonatal hepatitis and infection** (hepatitis B, syphilis, toxoplasmosis, rubella, cytomegalovirus, herpes virus, echovirus, coxsackievirus, bacterial sepsis)
4. **Genetic and metabolic disorders** (cystic fibrosis, $alpha_1$-antitrypsin deficiency, galactosemia, fructosemia, tyrosinemia, Gaucher's disease, hypothyroidism, hypopituitarism)
5. **Dubin-Johnson and Rotor's syndromes**

**B. Evaluation**. The initial evaluation of an infant with direct hyperbilirubinemia should include a measurement of fractionated serum bilirubin level, serum transaminases and alkaline phosphatase levels, prothrombin time, congenital infection evaluation (TORCH titers), and urine for reducing substances. It also is important to look at stool color to see if it is pigmented. Most, if not all, infants with direct hyperbilirubinemia should be evaluated by a gastroenterologist for a more detailed diagnostic evaluation and therapeutic intervention.

**C. Treatment** consists of supportive measures and specific treatment directed at the underlying etiology of the direct hyperbilirubinemia.

**VI. Jaundice associated with breast-feeding.** In healthy term newborns, interruption of breast-feeding for clinical jaundice should be discouraged. Mothers should be encouraged to breast-feed 8–10 times a day. Supplemental water or glucose water has not been shown to decrease the bilirubin concentration in such infants.

## Selected Readings


Ahlfors CE. Criteria for exchange transfusion in jaundiced newborns. *Pediatrics* 93:488, 1994.

Maisels MJ, Gifford K, Antle CE et al. Jaundice in the healthy newborn infant: A new approach to an old problem. *Pediatrics* 81:505, 1988.

Newman TB, Maisels M. Evaluation and treatment of jaundice in the term newborn: A kinder, gentler approach. *Pediatrics* 89:809, 1992.

Oski FA. Hyperbilirubinemia in the term infant: An unjaundiced approach. *Contemp Pediatr* April 1992, Pp 148–154.

Provisional Committee for Quality Improvement and Subcommittee on Hyperbilirubinemia. Practice parameter: Management of hyperbilirubinemia in the healthy term newborn. *Pediatrics* 94:558, 1994.

Rosenthal P, Sinatra F. Jaundice in infancy. *Pediatr Rev* 11:79, 1989.

# 31

# Infantile Colic

Raymond C. Baker

Infantile colic is a difficult management problem for the primary care physician, a problem usually without easy solutions. A colicky infant can be very stressful even in the most stable of homes. When the caregivers are young parents, a single parent, parents with a large family with several young children, parents with poor coping skills, or parents without outside support, the stress can disrupt the entire household. More attention has been focused on the problem of colic in recent years, resulting in a clearer understanding of the problem. More descriptive terms for colic are **paroxysmal fussing** and **primary excessive crying**.

**I. Definition.** To define colic, one first must consider what normal crying behavior is in infants. Brazelton studied 80 middle-class healthy infants and found that 2-week-old infants spent an average of 1.75 hours a day crying; 4-week-old infants, 2 hours; 6-week-old infants, 2.75 hours; 8-week-old infants, 2 hours; 10-week-old infants, 1.5 hours; and 12-week-old infants, about 1 hour. In the same study, he noted that the majority of crying at all ages occurred during the early evening hours.

Abnormal crying behavior, or colic, may therefore be defined as an exaggeration of normal crying time, usually peaking during the early evening hours. Practically speaking, however, the physician also must accept that the perception of abnormal depends somewhat on the caregiver's expectations and tolerance of and reaction to crying behavior. What constitutes colic and intolerable crying to one parent may be viewed as merely a fussy infant requiring extra cuddling to another.

Illingworth defined colic as rhythmic attacks of screaming during the first 3 months of life, usually in the evenings, that cannot be explained by any known cause of crying. Adams described colic as crying time greater than the seventy-fifth percentile above "normal" crying time. Carey defined the colicky infant as one crying "full force" (not just fussing) for more than 3 hours a day for at least 4 days a week.

A minority of infants with colicky symptoms may indeed have an underlying medical condition such as true formula intolerance (e.g., cow's milk allergy or lactose intolerance); these conditions usually are suggested by the history. The majority of infants with colic have no medical cause for their prolonged crying; therefore, infant temperament is a likely explanation for colic. Infants with colic tend to have heightened responses to external stimuli, especially noxious stimuli. For example, abdominal distention is a noxious stimulus that may result from overfeeding and results in a spectrum of infant behavior ranging from mild fussiness in the more "laid back" baby to vigorous and prolonged crying in the colicky baby. The latter behavior unfortunately also exacerbates distention with the swallowing of air.

II. **The natural history of colic** is that of a term infant following a normal pregnancy, labor, and delivery who has onset of symptoms at 2–3 weeks of age that peak at 1–2 months and resolve by 3–4 months. Colicky infants tend to be overweight rather than small as a result of parents' frequent feeding in an attempt to decrease the crying. Resolution corresponds with the normal development of the infant's ability to self-stimulate (hands to midline); increased interaction with the environment, parents, and siblings (smiling, cooing); and increased maturation of self-regulating mechanisms (dampening responses to external stimuli).

III. **The evaluation and treatment** of colic begin with a careful history focusing on a medical or physical explanation for crying and should include accurate measurements of height, weight, and head circumference. It is important for the physician to perform a careful physical examination *in front of parents* to assure them he or she is taking their complaints seriously. In classic colic (primary excessive crying is a good descriptive synonym, which implies the absence of a medical condition causing the crying behavior), the physical examination is entirely normal except for the infant's tendency to be overweight.

For the most part, colic is treated by listening to parents' concerns, showing empathy for their distress, and counseling regarding the problem's self-limiting nature. The physician should emphasize several important points in his or her discussion with parents about their infant's health, including the following:

A. **The infant is physically healthy.**

B. **Parents are not doing anything to cause the colic.**

C. **The infant has normal or excessive weight gain,** which implies that the formula "agrees with the baby." (It may be helpful to tell parents that an infant cannot gain weight on a formula to which he or she is intolerant, whether it be due to lactose intolerance, protein intolerance, or milk allergy.)

This should be followed by an explanation about infant temperament and infants' differing reactions to noxious stimuli (such as an overly full stomach from too frequent feeding). Presenting a scenario of the "colicky family" often brings nods of agreement from parents as they hear a description of the disrupted family life a colicky infant can cause.

D. **Some specific suggestions** for treating (tolerating) the colicky infant may include the following:

1. **Limit external stimuli to the infant** (e.g., choosing a quiet area to feed the infant, adherence to a feeding schedule rather than demand feeding to avoid overfeeding and abdominal distention).
2. **Check the infant for avoidable causes of crying,** such as wet diaper, hunger, being too hot or cold, or boredom (need for cuddling).
3. **Increase non-nutritive sucking (pacifier).**
4. **Increase carrying time** by using slings, back carriers, and so forth.
5. **Discuss the need to "get away from the baby once in a while,"** especially with single parents, who are usually the sole primary caregivers.

6. **Assure parents there is "a light at the end of the tunnel."** Colic usually subsides around 3 months of age when the infant attains the ability to self-stimulate and interact with his or her environment.
7. **Consider formula changes only if weight gain has been inadequate or the family insists on trying another formula.** In this circumstance, a trial of a soy-based formula may be appropriate.

The key to successful treatment of colic is frequent follow-up by office visits or telephone. It is important for the physician to be empathetic and positive in assuring the family. Drug therapy is almost never appropriate at the first visit and seldom plays an important role once appropriate counseling has been performed. If needed, simethicone may be used; its placebo effect may be more efficacious than its true effect.

## Selected Readings

Adams LM, Davidson M. Present concepts of infant colic. *Pediatr Ann* 16:817, 1987.

Barr RG, Rotman A, Yaremko J et al. The crying infants with colic: A controlled empirical description. *Pediatrics* 90:14, 1992.

Brazelton TB. Crying in infancy. *Pediatrics* 29:579, 1962.

Carey WB. "Colic"—primary excessive crying as an infant-environment interaction. *Pediatr Clin North Am* 31:993, 1984.

Carey WB. The difficult child. *Pediatr Rev* 8:39, 1986.

Hewson P, Oberklaid F, Menahem S. Infant colic, distress, and crying. *Clin Pediatr* 26:69, 1987.

Mones RL, Asnes RS. The colicky baby: Helping parents cope. *Contemp Pediatr* April 1986, P 86.

Parkin PC, Schwartz CJ, Manuel BA. Randomized controlled trial of three interventions in the management of persistent crying of infancy. *Pediatrics* 92:197, 1993.

Taubman B. Clinical trial of the treatment of colic by modification of parent-infant interaction. *Pediatrics* 74:998, 1984.

Wolke D, Gray P, Meyer R. Excessive infant crying: A controlled study of mothers helping mothers. *Pediatrics* 94:322, 1994.

E

# Genitourinary Disorders

# 32

# Primary Nocturnal Enuresis

## Raymond C. Baker

Primary nocturnal enuresis may be defined as nighttime urinary incontinence in the absence of urinary pathology that occurs continually from birth to beyond the age at which the majority of children achieve nocturnal continence. The definition must be vague regarding age because the age of achieving nighttime urinary continence varies. By the age of 3 years, 65% of children are continent, and about 80% are at age 6. However, by age 15 years, as many as 1–2% of teen-agers still have occasional nighttime urinary incontinence.

I. **History.** Most physicians would not consider nocturnal incontinence "abnormal" or consider medical evaluation for nocturnal incontinence until the child reaches the age of 6 years. The evaluation should begin with a complete history to rule out anatomic or infectious abnormalities. Specific symptoms that suggest infection are dysuria, frequent urination, urgency, daytime incontinence, and dribbling. Additional history that might suggest an etiology are associated congenital anomalies in the patient or family, incontinence in other family members, a history of constipation, psychological or social problems, and a history of sexual abuse. The physician should ask what efforts parents or other health care providers have made to manage the incontinence. Obvious causes of incontinence also should be sought, such as fear of a dark room or inability to manipulate the pajamas.

II. **Physical examination and laboratory evaluation.** The physical examination should include blood pressure, growth parameters, and a general examination with attention to the abdomen, genitalia, and rectum. From a laboratory perspective, only a urinalysis with or without urine culture is indicated in most circumstances unless the history and physical examination suggest other etiologies for the enuresis.

III. **Treatment** of primary nocturnal enuresis varies according to the child's age and cognitive abilities. Before age 6 years, no treatment is recommended other than counseling regarding normal development of the urinary tract and continence. The physician should emphasize to parents that the child is not bedwetting consciously; therefore, punishment is not indicated. A discussion of practical issues, such as the use of plastic sheets (or plastic garbage bags) beneath the sheets, may help the parent cope with the inconvenience of the enuretic child. Prolonged use of diapers beyond bowel incontinence usually is not recommended, especially if it encourages teasing by siblings and peers.

   A. **6–8 years.** From 6–8 years, positive reinforcement with an incentive calendar, praise for dry mornings, having the child be responsible for changing bed linens, and bladder exercises are appropriate. Bladder exercises consist of having the child practice holding in urine during the day for a few minutes beyond when the urinary urge begins. Then, while voiding, the child is encouraged to start and stop the urinary stream voluntarily.

**B. 8–10 years.** From 8–10 years, the above should be continued, and consideration should be given to an enuresis alarm, which makes a loud noise when the first few drops of urine complete an electrical circuit on a sensor sewn into the child's underwear. Alarms can be purchased by mail for $30–50 (e.g., Wet-stop from Palco Industries, 8030 Soquel Ave., Santa Cruz, CA 95062) and can be very effective unless the child is a very sound sleeper. More recently, alarms have become available that vibrate on completion of the circuit (Potty Pager, Ideas for Living, 1285 N. Cedarbrook, Boulder, CO 80304).

**C. Over 10 years of age.** If incontinence continues and the above has failed, drug therapy may be considered. By this age, many children are increasingly embarrassed by their incontinence, especially if peers share the knowledge. (Overnight stays at friends' houses are common at this age, which present potentially embarrassing situations for the incontinent child.) Two drugs have been used to treat nocturnal enuresis: imipramine, a tricyclic antidepressant, which is given at bedtime (usually 25 mg), and desmopressin, a synthetic analog of vasopressin, starting at one spray in each nostril at bedtime (at a cost of $2–3 per day). Both are successful; however, both have a considerable relapse rate when discontinued.

## Selected Readings

Crawford JD. Treatment of nocturnal enuresis, proceedings of a symposium. *J Pediatr* 114:687, 1989.

Maizels M, Gandhi K, Keating B et al. Diagnosis and treatment for children who cannot control urination. *Curr Probl Pediatr* 23:402, 1993.

Moffatt MEK, Harlos S, Kirshen AJ et al. Desmopressin acetate and nocturnal enuresis: How much do we know. *Pediatrics* 92:420, 1993.

Schmitt, BD. Nocturnal enuresis: Finding the treatment that fits the child. *Contemp Pediatr* September 1990, Pp 70–97.

# Urinary Tract Infections in Children

Robert M. Siegel

Urinary tract infection (UTI) occurs in about 1% of boys and 3% of girls. Because symptoms may be nonspecific in young children, the diagnosis can be elusive and should be considered in all young children with fever without a source.

I. **Pathophysiology.** The most common predisposing factor for UTI in children is an underlying anatomic abnormality. Obstructive lesions such as posterior urethral valves are common in boys, vesicoureteral reflux in girls. Poor hygiene and colonization with aggressive coliform organisms may play a role in UTI. Not being circumcised increases an infant boy's chances of UTI over 30-fold compared to being circumcised. The most common organism isolated in children with a UTI is *Escherichia coli*, although other organisms such as *Klebsiella, Enterobacter,* and *Proteus* may be isolated, particularly in those with recurrent disease, history of instrumentation, or obstructive lesions.

II. **Clinical presentation.** The signs and symptoms of UTI in the older school-age child are similar to those of adults—dysuria and increased urinary frequency. Fever and flank pain may be present with upper-tract disease. In the younger child, however, signs are nonspecific and may include fever, poor feeding, vomiting, and irritability. There are no reliable clinical indicators to differentiate lower- and upper-tract disease in the younger child.

III. **Evaluation of a child suspected of having UTI**

A. The **history** should include questions to determine if there are any conditions that may predispose the child to UTI (dysuria, frequency, enuresis, previous history of UTI, family history of UTI); nonspecific signs (fever, irritability, poor feeding, vomiting); and other possible etiologies (the use of products that can cause urethral irritation [bubble bath], sexual activity [sexually transmitted diseases], genitourinary hygiene, and sexual abuse [post–sexual abuse syndrome]).

B. **Physical examination.** The child's temperature, blood pressure, weight, and state of hydration should be recorded. Signs of upper-tract disease may be indicated by focal abdominal pain or flank tenderness. Genitalia should be examined for any abnormalities, including increased erythema, discharge, foreign body, or injury.

C. **Laboratory tests.** A definitive diagnosis of UTI is made by urine culture. While a urinalysis with microscopic examination may be helpful, the presence of pyuria is neither sensitive nor specific. A positive nitrite test as part of the urinalysis is 90% specific and 70% sensitive for UTI. In freshly obtained urine, more than 1 bacterium per high-power field in unspun urine also correlates with UTI. Half of infants under 2 months of age with UTI have a normal urinalysis.

Opinions vary about how a urine sample is best obtained. Suprapubic aspiration remains the gold standard, and growth with any colony count represents infection. Many practitioners find the technique too invasive, however, and prefer bladder catheterization. Colony counts of greater than $10^3$ colonies/ml represent infection. Clean-catch midstream collection in the continent older child produces an acceptable specimen for urine culture, particularly in males, in whom the result is equivalent to catheterization. In females, the risk of contamination is greater but can be minimized if the child is cleaned well and the specimen is obtained with the child sitting backward on the toilet, which causes the labia to separate. If this is not possible, two specimens from two separate voids are satisfactory alternatives. Colony counts of greater than $10^5$ of one organism suggest a true infection. Bag specimens of both boys and girls are too likely to represent contamination and are not recommended except as a screen.

Routine laboratory tests cannot distinguish between cystitis and pyelonephritis; therefore, in the febrile younger infant, a blood culture should be obtained to rule out urosepsis.

**IV. Treatment**

**A. Supportive.** The decision to admit a child with UTI to the hospital depends on the child's age and clinical status. In the older child who is not vomiting or dehydrated and by whom compliance seems likely, outpatient management is a reasonable choice. Several factors, however, may suggest hospitalization: infants under 6 months of age; infants and children with significant systemic symptoms of fever, toxicity, and flank tenderness suggestive of pyelonephritis; children requiring IV fluids secondary to poor intake and vomiting; and children unable to take oral medications.

**B. Antibiotic therapy** should be directed toward the most likely causative organisms, pending culture and sensitivity results. For outpatient therapy, trimethoprim-sulfamethoxazole or amoxicillin is a good first-line oral agent. For the hospitalized patient, ampicillin and gentamicin should be given until the organism is identified. A broad-spectrum cephalosporin is a reasonable IV alternative. Duration of antibiotic therapy is 7–10 days.

**V. Follow-up**

**A. Laboratory tests.** A urine culture should be obtained after treatment to document urine sterility. A urine culture after 48 hours of therapy is preferable; however, this is not feasible in most circumstances, and telephone contact at 48–72 hours to document the disappearance of symptoms is sufficient. Children with a UTI are at risk for recurrence; 75% are within 1 year of infection. Following a UTI, a urine culture should be obtained within 1 week of stopping therapy and then about every 3 months for 1 year.

**B. Radiologic evaluation.** Girls under 7 years of age and boys of any age with a UTI should be evaluated for the presence of an underlying abnormality. Initial evaluation can be a renal ultrasound and voiding cystourethrogram (VCUG). (A nuclear cystogram may be substituted for the traditional VCUG in girls because they are at low risk for posterior urethral valves and the procedure involves less radiation exposure.) Both ultrasound and VCUG may be done during the acute illness. A dimercaptosuccinic acid (DMSA) scan detects nonfunctioning and poorly functioning renal tissue such as seen with pyelonephritis and may be appropriate in certain circumstances.

C. **Chemoprophylaxis.** Recurrent UTIs are common (30% after the first UTI). In patients at risk for renal damage secondary to reflux of bacteria (significant reflux present on cystography), prophylactic antibiotic therapy (nitrofurantoin, trimethoprim-sulfamethoxazole) should be considered. Urologic referral may be considered for children with recurrent UTIs or anatomic abnormalities, including grade III, IV, or V reflux. Siblings of children with renal abnormalities, including vesicoureteral reflux, are also at risk for urinary tract abnormalities and should be monitored for symptoms of UTI.

## Selected Readings

Andrich MP, Majd M. Diagnostic imaging in the evaluation of the first urinary tract infection in infants and young children. *Pediatrics* 90:436, 1992.

Belman AB. Urinary imaging in children. *Pediatr Infect Dis J* 8:548, 1989.

Durbin WA, Peter G. Management of urinary tract infections in infants and children. *Pediatr Infect Dis J* 3:564, 1984.

Edelmann CM. Urinary tract infection and vesicoureteral reflux. *Pediatr Ann* 17:568, 1988.

Hellerstein S, Wald E. Consensus: Roentgenographic evaluation of children with urinary tract infections. *Am J Radiol* 144:815, 1985.

Hellerstein S. Recurrent urinary tract infections in children. *Pediatr Infect Dis J* 1:127, 1982.

McCracken GH. Diagnosis and management of acute urinary tract infections in infants and children. *Pediatr Infect Dis J* 6:107, 1987.

McCracken G. Prevention of genitourinary infections. *Pediatr Infect Dis J* 4:429, 1985.

Shapiro ED. Infections of the urinary tract. *Pediatr Infect Dis J* 11:165, 1992.

Wiswell TE, Roscelli JD. Corroborative evidence from the decreased incidence of urinary tract infection in circumcised male infants. *Pediatrics* 78:96, 1986.

# Sexually Transmitted Diseases

Robert M. Siegel

The incidence of sexually transmitted diseases (STDs) continues to rise in children and adolescents. As many as half of adolescents are sexually active by age 16 years, putting them at risk for STDs. Groups at particularly high risk for STDs include (1) those beginning sexual activity younger than age 16 years, (2) those abusing alcohol or other drugs, (3) children who have been sexually abused, (4) adolescents with multiple sex partners, (5) adolescents with a previous history of an STD, and (6) adolescents practicing "survival sex" (e.g., runaways, homeless children, and prostitutes).

The subject of sexual abuse in children is addressed in Chap. 49. About half of rapes occur in teen-agers; therefore, all teens who are evaluated for STDs should be questioned as to whether their sexual activity was consensual.

Symptoms of STDs vary depending on the infectious agent, stage of the infection, and the host. An STD evaluation should be considered in a child or adolescent if (1) there are genital complaints such as discharge or dysuria, (2) there is a history of sexual activity, particularly if there are multiple sex partners, (3) there is a history of STD exposure, or (4) if the teen is pregnant.

## I. Specific etiologies

**A. Gonococcal infection in adolescents.** Gonorrhea may present as asymptomatic infection, cervicitis, urethritis, pelvic inflammatory disease, or disseminated disease. The diagnosis is made by culturing the organism on a chocolate agar such as Thayer-Martin medium. Treatment for gonorrhea depends on the site of infection and clinical syndrome.

1. **Uncomplicated gonorrhea.** Any of the following single-dose regimens are adequate to treat adolescents for uncomplicated disease:
   a. **Ceftriaxone,** 125 mg IM
   b. **Cefixime,** 400 mg PO
   c. **Ciprofloxacin,** 500 mg PO
   d. **Ofloxacin,** 400 mg PO

   All adolescents with gonorrhea also should be evaluated for *Chlamydia* infection and syphilis. It should be noted that quinolones have no activity against syphilis, and there are no definitive data on the effectiveness of cefixime on incubating syphilis.
2. **Disseminated gonorrhea** results from gonococcal bacteremia and can yield petechial skin lesions, arthralgias, tenosynovititis, or septic arthritis. Treatment is for a minimum of 7 days. Initial therapy should be ceftriaxone, 1 g IM q24h; cefotaxime, 1 g IV q8h; ceftizoxime, 1 g IV q8h; or spectinomycin, 2 g IM q24h. The regimen is continued until there is clinical improvement (usually 24–48 hours) and then changed to oral

therapy as follows: cefixime, 400 mg PO bid, or ciprofloxacin, 500 mg PO bid.

**B. Gonococcal infections in children.** Any child outside of the newborn period with gonorrhea should be evaluated for sexual abuse. Treatment of uncomplicated disease is similar to that of adults except that quinolones should not be used in children younger than age 16 years and the efficacy of cefixime has not been proved in clinical trials. Ceftriaxone, 125 mg IM as a single dose, may be given in children. It is reasonable to presume that cefixime in a dose of 8 mg/kg (maximum 400 mg) is also effective. In infants with ophthalmia neonatorum, ceftriaxone at 25–50 mg/kg IM or IV (not to exceed 125 mg/day) once daily for 7 days may be given. Infants with disseminated disease should be given ceftriaxone at 25–50 mg/kg IM or IV once daily for 10–14 days.

**C. Chlamydial infection in adolescents.** *Chlamydia trachomatis* is the most common cause of nongonococcal urethritis and cervicitis and a frequent copathogen in pelvic inflammatory disease. Diagnosis can be made by culture of the suspected site or a rapid antigen test (note that rapid antigen tests are not accurate enough for sexual abuse evaluation). There is such a high prevalence of *C. trachomatis* coinfection in individuals with gonococcal infection that those treated for gonorrhea also should be treated for *C. trachomatis*. First-line treatment in adolescents is either doxycyline, 100 mg PO bid for 7 days, or azithromycin, 1 g PO in a single dose. Alternative regimens include any of the following:

1. **Erythromycin base,** 500 mg PO qid for 7 days,
2. **Erythromycin ethylsuccinate,** 800 mg PO qid for 7 days,
3. **Sulfisoxazole,** 500 mg PO bid for 10 days, **or**
4. **Amoxicillin,** 500 mg PO tid for 7–10 days (in pregnant teens)

**D. Chlamydial infections in children.** Chlamydial infection from maternal-infant transmission is well described. Most experts agree that this is an unlikely route beyond 3 years of age; therefore, any infection with *C. trachomatis* beyond this age is likely from sexual activity. Culture is the only test for *C. trachomatis* accurate enough for a sexual abuse evaluation. Perinatal transmission of the organism from mother to infant can lead to conjunctivitis or pneumonitis. Treatment in infants and children is erythromycin, 30–50 mg/kg PO divided qid for 10–14 days.

**E. Syphilis.** The diagnosis and treatment of syphilis depend on the patient's age and the stage of the disease. A definitive diagnosis can be made by identifying spirochetes on dark-field microscopy or direct fluorescent antibody test of a specimen. The diagnosis, however, usually is made by serology, either with a nontreponemal test, such as the Venereal Disease Research Laboratories test (VDRL) or RPR, or a specific treponemal test, such as the fluorescent treponemal antibody absorption (FTA-ABS) test.

1. **Congenital syphilis.** All pregnant women should be screened with a nontreponemal test prior to delivery,

and both infant and mother ideally should be tested after delivery. An infant should be evaluated for congenital syphilis after delivery if the infant's mother:

a. **Had untreated syphilis**
b. **Had syphilis and was treated with erythromycin**
c. **Was treated for syphilis within 1 month of delivery**
d. **Was treated for syphilis and did not demonstrate an adequate reduction in nontreponemal antibody titer**
e. **Did not have a well-documented history of treatment**

Evaluation should include serology, long-bone x-ray for evidence of metaphysitis, and measurement of cerebrospinal fluid for VDRL testing and cytology. Chest x-ray and liver function tests also may be indicated.

Treatment for congenital syphilis consists of aqueous crystalline penicillin G, 50,000 units/kg per dose IV q12h during the first 7 days of life then q8h for a total course of 10–14 days. If more than 1 day of therapy is missed, the entire course should be restarted. If diagnosis is delayed and the child is treated after 4 weeks of age, treatment consists of aqueous crystalline penicillin G, 200,000–300,000 units/kg/day IV divided q6h for 10–14 days.

2. **Syphilis in teen-agers**
   a. **Early acquired syphilis**. Syphilis of less than 1 year's duration (primary, secondary, or early latent) should be treated with benzathine penicillin G 2,400,000 units IM in a single dose. For those who are allergic to penicillin, doxycycline, 100 mg PO bid, or tetracycline, 500 mg PO qid for 2 weeks, is an alternative.
   b. **Syphilis of greater than 1 year's duration** (or if duration is unknown) should be treated with benzathine penicillin 2,400,000 units IM weekly for 3 consecutive weeks.
   c. **Neurosyphilis**. CNS involvement with syphilis may occur at any stage of illness. Any patient with CNS symptoms should have the cerebrospinal fluid examined. The recommended regimen is aqueous penicillin G 12,000,000–24,000,000 units/day divided q4h for 10–14 days. Procaine penicillin, 2,400,000 units IM daily, plus probenecid, 500 mg PO qid for 10–14 days, is an alternative.

F. **Trichomoniasis**. Infection with *Trichomonas vaginalis* is frequently asymptomatic, particularly in males. Symptoms in women often are most severe just prior to menstruation. The diagnosis is made by examination of a wet mount preparation of vaginal discharge or microscopic examination of the urine for the organism. Treatment consists of metronidazole, 15 mg/kg/day divided tid with a maximum of 250 mg/dose. Alternative regimens in adolescents are 2 g of metronidazole as a single oral dose or 500 mg bid for 7 days. Many clinicians empirically treat individuals for

*Trichomonas* infection when treating for suspected gonococcal infection or *Chlamydia.*

**G. Genital herpes simplex virus.** Approximately 30 million Americans have genital herpes infection. Primary disease is often the most severe and may even require hospitalization, and painful recurrences may occur. Although there is no cure, antiviral therapy can reduce the illness's severity. For primary illness, therapy is acyclovir, 200 mg PO five times a day for 7–10 days. For those requiring hospitalization, IV acyclovir at 5–10 mg/kg q8h for 5–7 days may be required. Treatment regimens for recurrences are acyclovir at 200 mg PO five times a day or 400 mg tid or 800 mg bid for 5 days.

**H. Bacterial vaginosis (BV)** is caused by the replacement of *Lactobacillus* species by anaerobic bacteria, such as *Gardnerella vaginalis* and *Mycoplasma hominis.* BV gives a white, homogenous discharge. Diagnosis is made by the presence of clue cells on a wet mount of vaginal discharge or a fishy odor with the addition of 10% KOH to the discharge. Treatment regimens are metronidazole, 500 mg PO bid for 7 days; metronidazole, 2 g PO once; or clindamycin, 300 mg PO bid for 7 days.

**I. Pelvic inflammatory disease (PID),** infection of the upper genital tract, is most frequently caused by *Neisseria gonorrhoeae, C. trachomatis* or vaginal flora such as anaerobic bacteria. Empirical treatment for PID should be initiated if the following criteria are met in the absence of another explanation: (1) lower abdominal pain, (2) adnexal tenderness, and (3) cervical motion tenderness. Some experts suggest that all teen-agers with PID be hospitalized to ensure compliance and minimize the risk of complications such as infertility. Hospitalization clearly is indicated if any of the following factors are a concern: (1) pelvic abscess, (2) peritonitis, (3) pregnancy, (4) an intrauterine device in place, (5) the patient's intolerance of oral therapy, or (6) no response to outpatient therapy after 48 hours. The initial regimens recommended by the Centers for Disease Control (CDC) are the following:

1. **Inpatient**
   - **a.** Cefoxitin, 2 g IV q6h (or cefotetan, 2 g IV q12h) and doxycyline, 100 mg IV or PO q12h **or**
   - **b.** Clindamycin, 900 mg IV q8h, plus gentamicin loading dose of 2 mg/kg IV followed by 1.5 mg/kg IV q8h.
2. **Outpatient**
   - **a.** Cefoxitin, 2 g IV, and probenecid, 1 g PO, **or** ceftriaxone, 250 mg IM, and doxycycline, 100 mg PO bid, **or**
   - **b.** Ofloxacin, 400 mg PO bid, and either clindamycin, 450 mg PO qid, or metronidazole, 500 mg PO bid.

Therapy, regardless of the regimen, should last 14 days.

**J. General considerations.** Any adolescent with an STD is engaging in high-risk sexual activity and is at risk for pregnancy and other STDs. All teens treated for an STD should be counseled on risk reduction. Human immunodeficiency virus (HIV) testing also should be considered in those who are diagnosed with an STD. If possible, the patient's sexual contacts should be evaluated and treated.

## Selected Readings

Centers for Disease Control and Prevention. 1993 sexually transmitted diseases guidelines. *MMWR* 42(RR–14), 1993.

Ingram DL. *Neisseria gonorrhoeae* in children. *Pediatr Ann* 23:341, 1994.

Peter G (ed). *1994 Red Book: Report of the Committee on Infectious Diseases* (23rd ed). Elk Grove Village, IL: American Academy of Pediatrics, 1994.

Starling SP. Syphilis in infants and young children. *Pediatr Ann* 23:334, 1994.

F

# Endocrine/Growth Disorders

35

# Assessment of Pubertal Development Variations

Anita Cavallo

Puberty depends on the activation of the hypothalamic-pituitary-gonadal axis, resulting in the maturation of the gonads and increased steroidogenesis. The increased secretion of sex steroids causes the development of secondary sexual characteristics. A disturbance in the hypothalamus, pituitary gland, or gonad can alter the onset and cadence of puberty. Pubarche is the development of pubic and axillary hair, normally dependent on the activation of the pituitary-adrenal axis (adrenarche), with increased secretion of a weak adrenal androgen, dehydroepiandrosterone sulfate (DHEAS). Although puberty and adrenarche normally occur in close temporal proximity, they may be dissociated when there is an abnormality in either axis. The adrenal gland also can produce other androgens and estrogens; thus, abnormal sex steroid production by the adrenal gland may result in the clinical signs of puberty.

**I. Definitions**

A. **Precocious puberty** is the onset of puberty before age 7.5 years in girls or 9 years in boys as a result of premature activation of the hypothalamic-pituitary-gonadal axis (**central precocious puberty**) or as a result of sex steroid production without activation of the hypothalamic-pituitary-gonadal axis ("**pseudopuberty**"). Pseudopuberty is related to exogenous sources of sex steroids (e.g., ingestion of oral contraceptives) or a gonadal or adrenal lesion (e.g., tumor). Precocious puberty also may occur because of gonadal maturation independent of the hypothalamic-pituitary axis, such as found in McCune-Albright syndrome (characterized by polyostotic fibrous dysplasia, abnormal pigmented skin lesions, and precocious puberty), familial male precocious puberty (testotoxicosis), and human chorionic gonadotropin (HCG)–secreting tumors.

B. **Premature pubarche** is the onset of pubic hair before age 7.5 years in girls and 9 years in boys, which may be due to premature activation of the pituitary-adrenal axis by increased secretion of DHEAS (premature adrenarche) or increased androgen secretion by either the adrenal gland or the gonad (virilization). The distinction between adrenarche and virilization is described below.

C. **Premature thelarche** is the isolated appearance of breast development in girls younger than 7.5 years old without other signs of sexual maturation.

D. **Gynecomastia** is the presence of glandular breast tissue in the male.

E. **Menarche** is the onset of menses, which usually is preceded by breast development but may be the first manifestation of puberty in a girl.

F. **Delayed puberty** is the lack of pubertal signs in a girl 13 years old or older or in a boy 14 years old or older.

G. **Virilization** is the abnormal appearance of signs of androgen excess in either sex characterized by accelerated linear growth, increased muscle mass, advanced bone maturation, acne, hirsutism, pubic hair, and clitoral or penile enlargement.

**II. Normal puberty**

A. **Sequence of the physical changes of puberty.** The first sign of puberty is breast enlargement in girls and testicular enlargement in boys (>2.5 cm in length). The Tanner staging of puberty describes the progression of these changes (see Appendix G). Pubarche generally begins after onset of breast or testicular development. See Appendix H for the normal sequence of physical maturation.

B. **Common misconceptions by patients and parents**

1. **Pubertal onset.** Most people relate puberty to the appearance of pubic hair, acne, facial hair, or change in voice in boys and to the appearance of pubic hair or onset of menses in girls. As a result, puberty may be quite advanced without the child's awareness.
2. **Breast development.** Initial breast development may be unilateral, causing great but needless anxiety in the child and parents.
3. **Subareolar mass.** Initial breast development may be rather firm, described as a hard lump and often feared to be a tumor or an abscess. Referral for biopsy or excision is not indicated.
4. **Delayed puberty.** Pubarche in boys generally does not occur until genital development is at about stage 3; thus, parents and child may be concerned needlessly about delayed puberty.
5. **Pubic hair.** Frequently, normal body hair in the pubic area is mistaken for pubic hair. The physician should compare the texture and density of hair in the pubic area with that of other body areas, mainly in the lumbosacral area and the legs. Pubic hair is thicker and darker than body hair and is curly. Hypertrichosis (excess body hair) is not related to abnormal sex steroid production, although it may be found in Cushing's syndrome.

C. **Physiologic pubertal gynecomastia.** About two-thirds of normal males during midpuberty develop some degree of subareolar breast tissue, which may be transiently tender. The tissue may be unilateral or bilateral and resolves without intervention within months to 1–2 years. The patient and his parents should be advised of the condition's physiologic and transient nature and counseled that the majority of boys at similar ages and pubertal stages experience the same condition.

**III. Assessment of precocious puberty.** Rapid progression of precocious pubertal maturation is accompanied by considerable advancement in bone maturation and significantly reduced adult height in boys and girls. Noncentral causes of precocious puberty often need immediate referral for surgery due to the possibility of pathologic origin (e.g., an adrenal or ovarian tumor). Hence, the diagnostic approach is aimed first at distinguishing among central causes of sexual precocity, peripheral causes of sexual precocity, and the characterization of gonadotropin-independent precocious puberty (McCune-Albright syndrome or testotoxicosis).

**A. History.** Important information to be included in the history taking is age of onset of puberty, rapidity of changes, and associated symptoms (e.g., headaches, abdominal symptoms). It is important to search the family history for early maturers, neurofibromatosis, familial testotoxicosis, and congenital adrenal hyperplasia.

**B. Physical examination.** At each visit, the physical examination should include calculation of the growth rate (see Chap. 36), staging of genital or breast development and pubic hair development, a search for signs of virilization (clitoral enlargement, facial hair, acne, hirsutism), and description of the vaginal mucosa's appearance. (Immature mucosa is thin and bright red; estrogenized mucosa is thicker and pale pink with a pearly appearance.) Optic disks and visual fields should be examined for signs of an intracranial tumor. The skin should be examined for abnormal pigmentation (McCune-Albright syndrome, neurofibromatosis). In boys with central precocious puberty or familial testotoxicosis, testicular enlargement is bilateral; unilateral enlargement should be evaluated for an androgen-secreting tumor.

**C. Laboratory and other tests.** The initial history and physical examination determine the need and scope of additional evaluations.

1. **Bone age.** A baseline bone age is helpful in most cases. A significant advancement at the initial evaluation dictates an immediate, more extensive laboratory evaluation.
2. **Sex steroid and gonadotropin levels.** There is still significant variability in the quality of assays for gonadotropins and sex steroids. It is important to have reliable laboratory measures of the pediatric ranges of these hormones. Pubertal levels of estradiol or testosterone are important diagnostic findings but do not localize the abnormality's source (central versus gonadal or adrenal abnormality). Pubertal levels of luteinizing hormone (LH) and follicle-stimulating hormone (FSH) indicate central precocious puberty; however, prepubertal levels do not exclude central precocious puberty, and a luteinizing hormone–releasing hormone (LHRH) stimulation test may be necessary.

**D. Pelvic and abdominal ultrasound.** A pelvic ultrasound in girls shows uterine development (fundus, cervix, endometrium) and the ovaries. A pubertal-appearing uterus with bilateral ovarian enlargement indicates central precocious puberty or gonadotropin-independent precocious puberty. Ovarian cysts are nonspecific, as they may be found in healthy girls. Hence, it is important to review the ultrasound study with a radiologist experienced in pediatric ultrasound. Children with large ovarian cysts should not be referred to surgery; instead, observation and frequent re-evaluation are indicated. An ovarian tumor can be detected by ultrasound; a child with an ovarian tumor should be referred immediately for surgery. An abdominal ultrasound also may detect an adrenal mass, which requires immediate referral to surgery and endocrinology.

A significant advancement in bone age, pubertal levels of sex steroids or gonadotropins, or rapid acceleration of growth in a child with signs of precocious sexual maturation should prompt immediate referral to an endocrinologist.

IV. **Assessment of precocious thelarche.** Onset of breast development before age 7.5 years may be the first sign of central precocious puberty. The evaluation's approach and extent depend on the child's age and associated findings (vaginal bleeding, pubic hair, virilization, cushingoid features).

A. **Infancy**. Transient breast development that may be present over several months frequently is observed in infants. It generally becomes more evident when the child slims down during the second year of life. The physician must search for exposure to exogenous sources of estrogen, such as cosmetic creams, vitamins, other nutritional supplements, or the use of a progestin or progestin-estrogen combination oral contraceptive in a nursing mother. Note that oral contraceptives generally are not indicated for the nursing mother; however, if used, a progestin alone is preferred over a combination product. The physician should determine growth velocity and examine the infant for associated findings, mainly pubic hair, virilization, or cushingoid features. External genitalia are examined for estrogenization. The typical infant with idiopathic precocious thelarche has a normal growth rate, breast budding that may be sizable with no areolar changes or associated abnormal features, and immature vaginal epithelium. In such case, no additional evaluations are necessary at the initial presentation, but the infant should be re-examined in 3–4 months. The physician should instruct the parent to return with the infant for another check-up if the infant's breast size enlarges rapidly or pubic hair, vaginal discharge, spotting, or bleeding develops.

B. **Childhood.** Beyond infancy, the appearance of isolated breast development must be evaluated thoroughly. Initial assessment should include determination of serum estradiol and gonadotropin levels and bone age. Pubertal levels of estradiol or gonadotropins or advanced bone age in a child with precocious onset of breast development require further evaluation immediately, which generally is in consultation with an endocrinologist. In the absence of rapid progression of breast development and with normal bone age and prepubertal levels of estradiol and gonadotropins, re-examinations at 4- to 6-month intervals are recommended until the child is close to the normal age of pubertal onset. Acceleration in growth rate, sexual maturation, and bone age dictate the need for repeat laboratory evaluations or referral.

V. **Assessment of precocious pubarche**

A. **Age.** Onset of pubic hair development in infancy is always abnormal and requires prompt and thorough investigation, which is best done by referral to an endocrinologist. Although precocious pubarche is the onset of pubic hair before age 7.5 years in girls and 9 years in boys by definition, onset of pubic hair appears to be somewhat earlier in black children, particularly in girls.

B. **Associated findings.** The child's evaluation depends on the presence or absence of signs of virilization in either sex, precocious puberty, or cushingoid features.

1. **No associated findings.** The physician should obtain a bone age and serum DHEAS level. If the child has idiopathic precocious adrenarche, bone age will not be advanced more than a year and the DHEAS level will be pubertal. The child should be re-examined in 3–4 months to determine rapidity of progression and to monitor for associated signs of puberty, virilization, or cushingoid features. Precocious adrenarche usually is accompanied by slight acceleration in growth velocity and bone maturation.

2. **Virilization.** The presence of pubic hair and signs of virilization in a young child require immediate and thorough evaluation and referral. The physician should look for a discrepancy between penile development and testicular size. Pubic hair in a prepubertal-age boy accompanied by testicular enlargement suggests central precocious puberty. Pubic hair and virilization in either sex could be related to abnormal sex steroid production by the gonad (e.g., due to a tumor) or the adrenal gland (e.g., due to a tumor, hyperplasia, or congenital adrenal hyperplasia). Serum testosterone, DHEAS, and 17-OH progesterone levels help in the differential diagnosis.

3. **Cushingoid features.** The presence of associated obesity with round facies, hypertrichosis, hypertension, and virilization in infancy or childhood requires urgent evaluation for adrenal hyperplasia or tumor. In addition to the laboratory tests above, serum cortisol, 24-hour urinary cortisol, and dexamethasone suppression tests should be performed, usually with an endocrinology consultation.

VI. **Assessment of delayed puberty.** Pubertal delay is defined as lack of breast development by age 13 years or of menses by age 15 years in a girl, or lack of testicular enlargement by age 14 years in a boy, irrespective of the presence or absence of pubic hair. As in precocious puberty, the initial task is to distinguish between central and peripheral causes. Central causes include constitutional delay and hypogonadotropic hypogonadism; peripheral causes include all forms of primary gonadal failure.

A. **History.** Important information to obtain in the history includes the child's nutrition, body image, general well-being, ability to smell, headaches, visual problems, GI symptoms, excessive exercise, previous heights and weights, and growth rate. Family history should focus on delayed puberty and chronic illness; it is usually positive for delayed puberty in cases of constitutional delay.

B. **Physical examination.** In particular, the physician should establish the child's growth rate and weight gain, determine body proportions (arm span, upper-lower ratio), stage breast or genital development and pubic hair development, and examine the optic discs and visual fields.

C. **Laboratory and other tests**

1. **Bone age.** A baseline bone age is helpful in the diagnostic evaluation and estimation of final adult height. In constitutional delay, bone age is usually 2 or more years delayed relative to chronologic age.
2. **Sex steroids, gonadotropins, and other hormonal levels.** The hormonal events of puberty precede the physical changes. Hence, pubertal levels of testosterone or estradiol and of LH and FSH may be found a clinically prepubertal child. Prepubertal levels, however, are not diagnostic and may require a follow-up LHRH test to determine whether the hypothalamic-pituitary axis is activated to pubertal levels. In contrast, LH and FSH levels above the normal range in a pubertal-age child without signs of sexual maturation indicate primary gonadal failure, such as in Turner's syndrome, anorchia, and Klinefelter's syndrome. Serum prolactin, thyroxine, and thyroid-stimulating hormone (TSH) levels may be needed when there is concern about acquired hypogonadotropic hypogonadism.
3. **Other studies.** A CBC with differential, erythrocyte sedimentation rate (ESR), and a renal panel should be obtained to rule out other possible chronic illness, such as inflammatory bowel disease or other causes of malabsorption or chronic renal failure. Serum thyroxine and TSH testing may be indicated if there is diminished growth rate or other signs of hypothyroidism. A CT scan or MRI of the brain may be necessary when there are associated neurologic symptoms (e.g., headaches and visual field defects) and in case of possible acquired hypogonadotropic hypogonadism.

VII. **Constitutional delay of puberty** may be indistinguishable from hypogonadotropic hypogonadism and primary gonadal failure. A careful history should be obtained, including the presence of headaches, visual problems, anosmia, chemotherapy, or radiation therapy. Chronic illness, such as regional ileitis or chronic renal failure, also must be excluded before considering constitutional delay of puberty. In children with constitutional delay of puberty, short stature is often the presenting complaint in the prepubertal years. Typically, growth rate is normal for the first 2–3 years; the height then crosses percentiles and follows a growth curve below what is expected for midparental height. Thus, the pubertal growth spurt fails to occur at the expected age. The family history is usually positive for delayed puberty, and all screening laboratory tests are normal. Bone age is delayed by 1.5 or more years, and serum testosterone or estradiol, LH, and FSH levels are all prepubertal. The approach may then be expectant depending on the child's height and level of anxiety. The growth rate and pubertal progression should be monitored every 4–6 months. Constitutional delay commonly causes social adjustment problems in boys, and testosterone treatment may be indicated. In such cases, a referral to a pediatric endocrinologist should be made.

## Selected Readings


Grumbach MM, Styne D. Puberty: Ontogeny, Neuroendocrinology, Physiology, and Disorders. In JD Wilson, DW Foster (eds), *Williams Textbook of Endocrinology*. Philadelphia: Saunders, 1992.

Kaplan SA. Growth and Growth Hormone: Disorders of the Anterior Pituitary. In SA Kaplan (ed), *Clinical Pediatric and Adolescent Endocrinology*. Philadelphia: Saunders, 1982.

Kelch RP. Management of precocious puberty. *N Engl J Med* 312:1057, 1985.

Lee P, O'Dea LStL. Primary and secondary testicular insufficiency. *Pediatr Clin North Am* 37:1359, 1990.

Marshall WA, Tanner JM. Variations in the pattern of pubertal changes in girls. *Arch Dis Child* 44:291, 1969.

Marshall WA, Tanner JM. Variations in the pattern of pubertal changes in boys. *Arch Dis Child* 45:13, 1970.

Tanner JM, Davies PW. Clinical longitudinal standards for height and height velocity for North American children. *J Pediatr* 107:317, 1985.

Wheeler M, Styne D. Diagnosis and management of precocious puberty. *Pediatr Clin North Am* 37:1255, 1990.

# 36

# Assessment of Abnormal Linear Growth

Anita Cavallo

The assessment of growth at each pediatric visit provides important information about the child's well-being. Generally, a normal velocity of linear growth and weight gain is indicative of a healthy child. Conversely, deviations from normal velocities of growth and weight gain should alert the primary care physician to a possible medical problem, such as nutritional deficiency, recurrent or chronic illness, or endocrine disorders. Deviation from normal growth may be the only manifestation of an underlying medical problem in a healthy-appearing child.

I. **Charting and interpreting growth data.** Standard growth charts (see Appendix E) are based on **supine length measurements** up to age 3 years for the charts labeled "Birth–36 Months" and **standing height** for the charts labeled "2–18 Years."

A. **Common pitfalls in the measurement of length (height)**

1. **In measuring standing height and plotting it on the length chart**, there may be a loss of as much as 2.2 cm from the supine to the upright measurement of a young child. Hence, both the appropriate technique and the correct chart must be used.
2. **Poor technical skills in measuring**, such as failing to position the child properly or leaving on the child's shoes during the measurement, commonly result in inaccurate measurements.

II. **Shifting growth during infancy.** The correlation between birth size and ultimate mature size is notoriously poor. Crossing percentiles on a growth chart during infancy may be normal as the infant shifts growth curves based on genetic potential. Other causes of apparent shifting growth during infancy are the following:

A. **"Catch-up growth,"** which begins shortly after birth (e.g., in an infant born small for gestational age)

B. **Slow down in growth,** which tends to begin at 3–6 months of age

C. By age 2–3 years, most children have reached the growth curve for their genetic potential. After 3 years of age, the child maintains a steady growth velocity until the onset of the **pubertal growth spurt**.

III. **Normal growth.** Besides plotting growth parameters on the growth chart, it is important to calculate **growth velocity**. Generally, an interval of 3–4 months between two measurements permits the physician to estimate accurately the annualized growth velocity.

A. **Normal growth velocity.** Table 36-1 summarizes the average expected growth velocities for both sexes. In eval-

**Table 36-1. Normal range of growth velocity for boys and girls**

| Age | Inches/year | Centimeters/year |
|---|---|---|
| 0–12 mos | 9–11 | 18–26 |
| 12–24 mos | 4–5 | 10–13 |
| 24–36 mos | 2.25–4.25 | 6–11 |
| 3–6 yrs | 2–3.25 | 5–8 |
| 6 yrs–puberty | 1.6–3 | 4.5–7.5 |
| Peak puberty | 2.5–4.25 | 7.5–11 |

Source: Adapted from JM Tanner, PW Davies. Clinical longitudinal standards for height and height velocity for North American children. *J Pediatr* 107:317, 1985; and PVV Hamill et al. Physical growth: National Center for Health Statistics percentiles. *Am J Clin Nutr* 32:607, 1979.

uating possible growth disorders, the physician should consult a sex-specific growth velocity chart.

**B. Abnormal growth velocity**

1. **Decreased growth velocity.** In a child 3 years of age or older, a growth velocity of consistently less then 5 cm a year is worrisome; 4 cm a year or less is definitely abnormal and requires investigation.
2. **Increased growth velocity.** Although decreased growth velocity is a considerably more common event, increased growth velocity above the expected norm also warrants investigation.

**IV. Genetic influence on stature.** Numerous factors can alter a child's height (e.g., nutrition, age of pubertal onset, intercurrent illnesses). Genetic influence is also notably important and must be considered in each child's growth evaluation. The child's target height based on genetic potential is estimated based on the biological parents' heights as follows:

**A. Determining the target height in centimeters for girls.** [(father's height + mother's height − 13)/ 2] ± 5

**B. Determining the target height in centimeters for boys.** [(father's height + mother's height + 13)/2] ± 5

Children whose growth varies from the projected pattern based on parental height need to be monitored closely—for example, a prepubertal girl who has a normal growth velocity but is too short for her genetic potential (not necessarily below the third percentile on the height curve) should be evaluated for Turner's syndrome even in the absence of obvious stigmata.

**V. Decreased growth velocity.** The expected growth deceleration in infancy for adjustment to the genetic potential has been described in sec. **II**, and Chap. 37 addresses growth problems in the infant and young child. The remainder of this chapter briefly outlines an approach to growth problems beyond infancy. As a rule, a child's growth stabilizes for genetic potential by age 3 years; hence, persistently decreased growth velocity after this age should be investigated.

**A. Common causes of decreased growth velocity**

1. **Nutrition.** Nutritional causes for poor growth are important even after age 3 years, and a good nutrition-

al history should be obtained. Nutrition is also important for the preteen and teen-age child who may not have had dramatic weight loss but instead has failure to gain weight adequately with subsequent deceleration of linear growth. Examples of children with decreased growth velocity due to nutrition are children with anorexia nervosa and boys who want to remain in a lower weight category for wrestling.

2. **Chronic illness.** Chronic renal failure, malabsorption, and recurrent illnesses also may cause significant linear growth delay. Generally, weight gain in these cases also is compromised, and the child tends to be underweight for height.
3. **Endocrine disorders** associated with poor growth generally cause increased weight for height.
4. **Constitutional delay.** Children with constitutional delay have a normal growth velocity after the second year of life, but their height is generally below the fifth percentile or within the normal range for age but below the projected height based on midparental height. At the time of puberty, they fail to have the growth spurt that most of their peers exhibit, and puberty is delayed.
5. **Rigorous physical training.** Strict training in gymnastics for more than 18 hours a week beginning before puberty may decrease growth velocity to the extent that the expected height may not be reached.

**B. General approach to a child with decreased growth velocity**

1. **History and physical examination.** A good medical history to screen for risk factors of chronic illness is essential. The physical examination should include a neurologic exam, visualization of the optic fundi, and assessment of the visual fields.
2. **Screening tests.** Generally useful tests to rule out a systemic disorder are a CBC with differential, erythrocyte sedimentation rate, serum chemistries (for renal function), and serum thyroxine and thyroid-stimulating hormone (TSH) determinations. A baseline bone age is often helpful to determine the current status and assess the child's progression. Other tests, such as metabolic screening tests, cardiac evaluation, sweat test, or tests for malabsorption, are performed on an individual basis. Presently, certain tests such as for insulin growth factor 1 (IGF-1) (previously named somatomedin C) or IGF-binding proteins are not yet standardized sufficiently to be considered valuable screening tools for growth hormone deficiency. If screening tests exclude another system disorder, referral to an endocrinologist should be considered for the child with decreased growth velocity.

**VI. Accelerated growth velocity**

**A. Genetic potential.** Growth acceleration in infancy to reach the genetic potential has been described in sec. **II**.

**B. Caloric excess.** Overfeeding in infancy may cause acceleration in linear growth and excessive weight gain. Although most infants grow appropriately with "feeding on demand" approach, this feeding technique often is misinterpreted by parents and health care providers. When a bottle of formula routinely is offered to a crying infant in place of other comforting measures, the baby accepts the bottle even when not hungry, with resultant obesity. Acceleration of linear growth frequently accompanies continued excessive weight gain.

C. **Endocrine disorders.** Acceleration of linear growth without excessive weight gain should alert the physician to other endocrine disorders. Excess growth hormone production is rare in the young child but should be considered in the older child or adolescent with abnormally rapid growth. Excess thyroid hormone occasionally causes significant growth acceleration, but the symptoms and signs of hyperthyroidism are usually evident. More commonly, excess sex steroids are implicated in growth acceleration—for example, in both boys and girls, excess androgens may be present due to congenital adrenal hyperplasia or a virilizing adrenal, testicular, or ovarian tumor. Precocious puberty also causes growth acceleration (see Chap. 35).

## Selected Readings

Hamill PVV et al. Physical growth: National Center for Health Statistics percentiles. *Am J Clin Nutr* 32:607, 1979.

Kaplan SA. Growth and Growth Hormone: Disorders of the Anterior Pituitary. In SA Kaplan (ed), *Clinical Pediatric and Adolescent Endocrinology*. Philadelphia: Saunders, 1982.

Ounsted M, Moar V, Scott A. Growth in the first four years. II. Diversity within groups of small-for-dates and large-for-dates babies. *Early Hum Dev* 7:29, 1982.

Smith DW (ed). *Growth and Its Disorders*. Philadelphia: Saunders, 1977.

Tanner JM, Davies PW. Clinical longitudinal standards for height and height velocity for North American children. *J Pediatr* 107:317, 1985.

Theintz GE, Howald H, Weiss U et al. Evidence for a reduction of growth potential in adolescent female gymnasts. *J Pediatr* 122:306, 1993.

# 37

# Failure to Thrive

## Julie Jaskiewicz

Failure to thrive may be defined as growth deficiency due to inadequate nutrition. Determining the exact cause often is complicated, and treatment poses a challenge to the primary care physician. It has been reported that 3–5% of pediatric hospitalizations are related to failure to thrive. About 80% of cases occur in children less than 18 months of age, and the incidence is higher in lower socioeconomic groups.

I. **Growth deficiency** may be broadly defined as growth below two standard deviations for age and sex, including weight, height, and head circumference. Two operational definitions of growth deficiency are (1) weight persistently below the third percentile for age and out of proportion to height (the most common type of growth deficiency) and (2) weight drop across two major percentile lines in 6 months. Depressed weight for age alone usually suggests acute malnutrition (for weeks to months); depressed weight and height for age suggest chronic malnutrition. The best way to express growth parameters is as a percentage of the median (fiftieth percentile) weight for age. Table 37-1 relates the degree of malnutrition to the percentage of median weight for age.

II. **Differential diagnosis.** It is important to distinguish true growth deficiency from other conditions associated with being small.

A. **Constitutional short stature** is associated with an average or above average weight for height and may reflect a genetic tendency to be short for age. Assessment of mean parental height may be useful in distinguishing this condition from true growth deficiency. Parental height also may reflect the nutritional status of parents, who may not have reached their own full genetic growth potential.

B. **Prematurity.** Premature infants may be well below the third percentile for all three growth parameters and should be plotted on a special growth chart for premature infants (see Appendix E) for the first year of life.

C. **Congenital syndromes.** Some children have limited growth potential associated with particular syndromes, including congenital cytomegalovirus (CMV) infection, Down's syndrome, and fetal alcohol syndrome. These children may never "fit" on the standard growth curve even though they may not be truly growth deficient.

III. **Pathogenesis.** Failure to thrive is a complex and interactive problem involving the biomedical, environmental, and psychosocial features of a child's experience. Most cases of growth deficiency encountered in the outpatient setting are related primarily to aberrations in the home and psychosocial environment, but rarely is the process simply a matter of parental deprivation alone. Some infants and children without an overt medical illness may have subtle neurologic conditions or behaviors that render them particularly difficult to

**Table 37-1. Classification of growth failure**

| Degree of malnutrition | Median weight for age |
|---|---|
| Mild | 75–85% of fiftieth percentile |
| Moderate | 60–74% of fiftieth percentile |
| Severe | <60% of fiftieth percentile |

Source: Adapted from WG Bithoney, H Dubowitz, H Egan. Failure to thrive/growth deficiency. *Pediatr Rev* 13:453, 1992.

feed. If these children are cared for in a disorganized environment by a stressed or psychosocially limited caregiver, the potential for growth deficiency is enhanced. Growth deficiency results from insufficient calories to meet the body's needs and may occur by several mechanisms.

A. **Inadequate intake of calories**
   1. **Insufficient calories may be provided,** resulting from formula mixing errors, inadequate feeding frequency, lactation problems, parental neglect, or extreme poverty.
   2. **Insufficient caloric intake** may result from anorexia or oral-motor dysfunction (e.g., cleft palate, cerebral palsy).

B. **Excessive caloric loss** usually is associated with GI abnormalities, such as vomiting, reflux, rumination, malabsorption, or diarrhea.

C. **Increased caloric requirements** commonly are seen with chronic infections and cardiac, respiratory, or metabolic abnormalities.

D. **Inadequate caloric use.** The most common example of inadequate caloric use is insulin-dependent diabetes mellitus.

IV. **Risk factors.** Neither the child nor the environment alone determines the child's growth outcome; however, each affects and is affected by the other. Most cases of growth deficiency involve the relationship between the child's demands and the capabilities of the child's caregiver. Sorting out the relative contributions of each can be very difficult. Potential risk factors for growth deficiency include the following:

A. **Biologic conditions** that may place a child at risk for growth deficiency include congenital anomalies (cleft palate, microcephaly), pre- and postnatal undernutrition syndromes (fetal alcohol syndrome, congenital infections), medically compromised prematurity (congenital heart disease, bronchopulmonary dysplasia), ongoing medical conditions (cardiac, respiratory, infection with the human immunodeficiency virus [HIV]), and behavioral or neurologic problems (attention deficit-hyperactivity disorder).

B. **Environmental features** that increase a child's risk for growth deficiency include child issues (difficult temperament—irritable and fussy or withdrawn and passive infant), caregiver issues (easily frustrated and anxious caregiver), disturbed interaction between child and caregiver (both show withdrawal; negative, demanding behaviors; or both toward one another), abnormal feeding behaviors in the child (disinterest; bizarre maneuvers with food), and psychosocial stressors in the family (frequent moves, single-parent family, isolation, recent traumatic events, poor marital relationship).

**V. Diagnostic approach.** The evaluation of a child suspected of inadequate growth begins by determining whether the child is really growth-deficient or "just small." The physician should remember that 3% of all children at any age have a weight below the third percentile (by definition). A diagnosis of growth deficiency should be based on positive historical and physical findings after careful clinical assessment and observation. Growth deficiency secondary to nonmedical causes is not a diagnosis of exclusion; both biological and environmental factors need to be addressed at the same time. The primary caregivers are key to providing an accurate history and ensuring successful long-term management; thus, they must be approached in a caring, nonjudgmental manner to ensure their complete cooperation in the assessment of their child's nutritional state and to avoid giving them the impression that they are responsible.

**VI. Clinical assessment**

**A. Age.** Feeding behaviors of children are related closely to their developmental abilities, including motor, cognitive, and psychosocial skills. Problems with attachment, separation, and individuation may lead to maladaptive feeding and abnormal interactive behaviors between child and caregiver that may exacerbate poor nutrition. By knowing when a child began to demonstrate growth deficiency, the stage of psychosocial development for that child may be determined. Recognizing the developmental stage of a child with growth deficiency is useful in determining appropriate intervention.

**B. History.** The single most important diagnostic procedure in determining the etiology of growth deficiency in a child is the history. It is optimal to have both parents present to observe their attitudes and interactions with each other, both verbal and nonverbal (supportive versus detached, angry, impersonal). The physician should observe each parent's interaction with the child (affectionate and encouraging versus negative or demanding) and look for symptoms in the child often associated with family dysfunction (irritability, excessive crying, and sleep or discipline problems). The physician should pay attention to the parents' attitudes toward the history-taking process (tense, hostile, depressed, in a hurry to leave). A second, third, or fourth history may be more revealing than the first, especially if some trust has been established. The following are important components of the history:

1. **The child's age at growth decline onset** by parental history or growth chart
2. **Birth history**, including maternal age; health; pre- or postnatal depression; prenatal care; drug, alcohol, or tobacco use; length of gestation; birth weight; initial feeding pattern; stool pattern; and early weight gain
3. **Developmental milestones**, including delays and previous interventions

4. **Medical history** of previous illnesses, hospitalizations, and chronic illnesses (otitis media, pneumonia, diarrhea)
5. **Review of systems**, especially GI symptoms and CNS
6. **Family history**, including parents' and siblings' growth, familial disease (especially endocrine), and congenital abnormalities
7. **Psychosocial issues**, including family constellation, finances, extended family, social supports, substance abuse, physical or sexual abuse, recent changes in lifestyle, death of a family member, divorce, recent move, or job change
8. **Diet**, including child's caloric intake, 24-hour dietary recall, 3-day food diary, bizarre or fad diets, parental (mis)perceptions of the child's needs, formula preparation, frequency of feedings, who feeds the child and how the infant feeds, bottle propping, parental anxiety, forced feeding, and consistency between the child's age and feeding behavior

C. **Physical examination.** A thorough general physical examination is crucial. Signs and symptoms of vitamin, protein, or calorie deficiencies or a specific medical condition may be present. The physician also should note the following during the physical examination:

1. **General appearance**, including appearing acutely ill versus chronically ill, signs of poor hygiene or inflicted trauma, or disturbed affect (apathetic, scared)
2. **Growth.** The physician should plot the following on the appropriate growth charts: weight (unclothed), height, head circumference, weight for height, and triceps skinfold thickness.
3. **Development.** If possible, the physician should administer the Denver Developmental Screening Test, which should be delayed if the child is acutely ill or dehydrated.

D. **Careful observation** of the child's behaviors, especially during feeding, and the child's interactions with caregivers, other children, and adults often provides clues to interaction difficulties between the child and his or her environment that contribute to growth deficiency. Behaviors thought to be associated with disturbed psychosocial functioning as the primary etiology of growth deficiency include "radarlike gaze," "frozen watchfulness," minimal smiling, decreased vocalization, resistance to being held, tonic immobility of the arms (arms up and back with elbows flexed), and self-stimulating rhythmic movements.

E. **Laboratory.** If the history and physical examination do not suggest an underlying medical illness or organic cause of growth deficiency, there is no rationale for doing an extensive laboratory assessment. A limited number of laboratory tests may be appropriate in certain circumstances, including screens for iron deficiency and lead exposure (especially if there is a history of pica or the child lives in a high-risk area for lead exposure), urinalysis to look for chronic urinary tract infection, tuberculin skin testing,

HIV testing if suggested by history or high risk, and thyroid function if height is affected primarily. All other laboratory tests should be done only if suggested by history, physical examination, or both.

**VII. Management.** The primary goal in managing the growth-deficient child is to restore adequate nutrition. Nutritional rehabilitation involves several concurrent processes.

**A. Determining caloric requirements.** To determine the child's caloric requirements to restore growth, the child's length is measured, and ideal weight is determined for that height (fiftieth percentile for that height). The normal daily caloric intake needed to maintain that weight is determined and increased by 50% to provide for an accelerated rate of "catch-up growth."

**B. Providing dietary counsel.** Once caloric requirements are established, the physician or nutritionist should counsel caregivers about the appropriate dietary intake to meet those needs, emphasizing particularly the quality and quantity of foods. Often, the parent can provide the necessary calories by increasing the caloric density of liquids and foods offered (e.g., high-calorie supplemental drinks) rather than increasing the volume of liquids. If the parent and child do not already participate in the Women, Infants, and Children (WIC) program but qualify, they should be referred for enrollment to help supply the needed nutrition.

**C. Managing medical illness.** Underlying medical disease, such as infection or lead toxicity, should be addressed concurrently with nutritional support.

**D. Supporting the family.** The primary care physician is often a case manager and can serve as a liaison between the family and other professionals, such as a community health nurse, social worker, dietitian, and mental health worker. The physician should provide guidance for parents concerning appropriate developmental tasks for age, especially as they relate to feeding. Successful management of any growth-deficient child means sustained weight gain once the child has returned home. Frequent follow-up, often every week initially, is essential. Frequent weight checks help document progress but are just as important as an opportunity for the physician to provide ongoing support and guidance for the family and to build with them a relationship of trust.

**E. Hospitalization.** The decision to hospitalize a growth-deficient child is not an easy one. Sometimes even a child from a disturbed psychosocial environment may fail to gain weight in the hospital, away from familiar surroundings.

1. **Recommendations.** Hospitalization should be strongly considered when the physician is concerned about active abuse or neglect, severe (grade II or III) malnourishment (weight <60% of median weight for age), the presence of a significant medical illness that requires intensive inpatient management, failure of intensive outpatient management to provide adequate catch-up growth over a 6-month period, the family's unreliability to follow through with outpatient plans, or the child becoming lost to follow-up.

2. **Goals** of hospitalization include providing adequate calories for catch-up growth; documentation of sustained weight gain; providing better observation of child and parent-child behaviors that may contribute to growth deficiency; providing an organized program of stimulation for the child; and providing interdisciplinary evaluation with nutrition, social services, nursing, and child-life services.
3. **Expectations.** Documented weight gain in the hospital is not conclusive evidence that psychosocial problems alone cause poor growth. Children with and without specific medical illness have been shown to gain weight in the hospital, though weight gain is often not immediate. Parents need to be cautioned against expecting a quick solution. Often, infants require from a few days to a week before establishing satisfactory weight gain.

**VIII. Prevention.** Ideally, physicians can prevent growth deficiency in children by identifying risk factors early. This requires ongoing anticipatory guidance for families of infants and children concerning development, behavior, and feeding practices. The physician should ask about biological and environmental stressors at each regular well-child visit. Parents should be counseled at each visit about appropriate feeding according to the child's age and until the next visit. They should learn not only what the child should be eating, but *how* the child should be eating (e.g., it is appropriate for a 1-year-old to try to feed himself or herself and make a mess). The physician continually should monitor the psychosocial attachment between parent and child, especially as it relates to feeding, and keep abreast of new changes in the family (new baby on the way, recent separation of parents) as warning signs for the potential for feeding problems to begin. Finally, it is important for the physician to remember that a child with primary environmental reasons for growth deficiency may at some point develop a medical illness that may be missed if the focus is exclusively on the psychosocial aspects.

## Selected Readings

Bithoney WG, Dubowitz H, Egan H. Failure to thrive/growth deficiency. *Pediatr Rev* 13:453, 1992.

Chatoor I, Schaeffer S, Dickson L et al. Non-organic failure to thrive: A developmental perspective. *Pediatr Ann* 13:829, 1984.

Ellerstein NS, Ostrov BE. Growth parameters in children hospitalized because of caloric-deprivation failure to thrive. *Am J Dis Child* 139:164, 1985.

Frank DA, Silva M, Needlman R. Failure to thrive: Mystery, myth and method. *Contemp Pediatr* 2:114, 1993.

Goldbloom RB. Failure to thrive. *Pediatr Clin North Am* 29:151, 1982.

Goldbloom RB. Growth failure in infancy. *Pediatr Rev* 9(2):57, 1987.

Sills RH. Failure to thrive. *Am J Dis Child* 132:967, 1978.

Sills RH, Sills IN. Don't overlook environmental causes of failure to thrive. *Contemp Pediatr* 3:25, 1986.

# 38

# Obesity

Julie Jaskiewicz

Childhood obesity is a complex and increasingly common problem. Between 15% and 25% of all children in the United States are obese, a 50% increase in prevalence since the 1960s. Multiple etiologies have been suggested, and experts still disagree about the magnitude of influence of the many genetic and environmental contributors. Unfortunate misconceptions about the etiology and natural history of obesity exist, and many physicians erroneously assume that nothing can be done for the obese child.

I. **Measures of body fat.** Obesity is defined as an excess of body fat. Evidence in studies of adults suggests that the predominant distribution of body fat (abdominal versus pelvic) may be more important in predicting obesity-related morbidity than simply the degree of absolute fatness.

   A. **Weight** alone is not a good measure of body fat. It is an easy and reproducible measure that can be compared to population standards but does not indicate body fat distribution. Using weight alone, a very muscular child may be mislabeled as obese.

   B. **Body mass index (BMI).** The BMI (weight/[height$^2$]) is preferable to weight when measuring body fat content. BMI can be compared to population standards, but like weight, it does not indicate body fat distribution.

   C. **Skinfold thickness (SFT)** is the preferred measure of body fat content. Using skinfold calipers, a direct measure of subcutaneous fat mass (usually in the triceps or subscapular skinfolds) is obtained. The measurements are reproducible, can be compared to population standards, and indicate body fat distribution.

II. **Definitions of obesity**

   A. **Obesity** is weight for height greater than 120% of the ideal (controlling for sex and age) or a triceps SFT greater than the eighty-fifth percentile.

   B. **Superobesity** is weight for height greater than 150% of the ideal or a triceps SFT greater than the ninety-fifth percentile.

III. **Classification of obesity**

   A. **Exogenous** (simple) obesity represents about 99% of cases of childhood obesity and is characterized by obese children who are tall for their age (usually height above the fiftieth percentile for age) and have a normal to advanced bone age, normal mentality, no physical abnormalities, and often a family history of obesity.

   B. **Endocrine and genetic.** Less than 1% of childhood obesity is associated with an endocrine or genetic syndrome. These children are short for their age, have a delayed bone age, may be mentally limited, often have associated physical abnormalities, and rarely have a family history of obesity.

1. **Endocrine syndromes** include the following:
   a. **Hypercortisolism** (Cushing's syndrome)
   b. **Hypothyroidism**
   c. **Primary hyperinsulinism**
2. **Genetic syndromes** include the following:
   a. **Prader-Willi syndrome** is characterized by severe hyperphagia, hypotonia, mental retardation, and occasionally the pickwickian syndrome.
   b. **Bardet-Biedl syndrome.** This autosomal recessive syndrome is characterized by predominantly truncal and proximal limb obesity, polydactyly, and genital hypoplasia.
   c. **Cohen's syndrome** is characterized by mid-childhood onset of obesity, dysmorphic facial features, and mental retardation.
   d. **Alstrom's syndrome** is similar to the Prader-Willi syndrome but with the onset of insulin-resistant diabetes commencing during puberty.

**IV. Etiology of exogenous obesity**

**A. Energy homeostasis.** Obesity results from excess energy stored in the adipose tissue as fat and represents an imbalance between excess energy and energy expenditure. Obesity is a problem of energy homeostasis rather than a primary abnormality of the fat itself; obese people do not have a different kind of fat than lean individuals.

**B. Genetics versus environment.** The problem of energy homeostasis in obesity is more than simply consuming too much food without expending adequate amounts of energy. The idea that obesity is simply the result of an individual's lazy lifestyle and poor dietary choices has exacerbated the widely held belief that nothing can help the obese person, who is destined to remain overweight. Such assumptions have not been substantiated in the literature. Diet and exercise are important considerations in the development of obesity, but multiple associated factors (e.g., gender, genetics, family constellation, geography, and even season of the year) probably play an important role as well. How much of a role each factor plays for a particular individual, however, is often very difficult to determine.

**V. Natural history.** Most obese children do not become obese adults; childhood obesity accounts for only 10–30% of adult obesity. The persistence of childhood obesity into late childhood and adolescence increases the likelihood obesity will continue into adulthood. Some believe that obese children with early, rapid weight gain in the first few years of life; who have obese parents, siblings, or both; or who have obese family members who are continuing to gain weight may be at greater risk for continuing to be obese into adulthood.

**VI. Consequences.** Obese children experience many of the same morbidities associated with excess fat stores as do obese adults. Almost all of these morbidities can be reversed with weight loss.

**A. Cardiovascular abnormalities.** Obesity is the most common identifiable cause of hypertension in children.

**B. Pulmonary abnormalities associated with obesity** include the pickwickian syndrome (hypoventilation, obesity, and congestive heart failure) and sleep apnea.

C. **Common orthopedic abnormalities associated with obesity** are coxa vara, slipped capital femoral epiphysis, Blount's disease, and Legg-Calvé-Perthe disease.

D. **Endocrine.** Hyperinsulinemia and resistance to insulin-mediated glucose transport commonly are associated with obesity. Chemical diabetes is rare. Increased adrenocorticotropic hormone (ACTH) can lead to premature adrenarche, and an increase in somatomedin may accelerate bone age.

E. **Integument.** Overlapping skinfolds in obese individuals are frequent sites for intertrigo and furunculosis.

F. **Psychiatric.** There are no conclusive studies to show that obese children have a poor self-image, are more depressed than their peers, or have other identifiable psychiatric disorders. Whether or not obese children are discriminated against by their peers, teachers, or other adults is not entirely known and is a source of great controversy.

VII. **Outpatient approach.** Physicians should identify obese children and children at greatest risk for becoming obese so timely intervention can be initiated.

A. **History.** The physician should note the following in the history when evaluating an obese child:

1. **Complete past medical history**, including birth weight, weight gain pattern in infancy and early childhood, height pattern, developmental delays, and chronic conditions
2. **Family history** may help identify exogenous obesity. The physician should determine the weight and height of parents and siblings and cardiovascular risk factors and morbidities in parents, especially if parents are obese.
3. **Dietary and nutritional history**, including intake, type of foods, mealtime behavior and structure, snacking habits, and parental and child concerns about weight (worried or nonchalant)
4. **Psychosocial issues.** The physician should look for evidence that parents use food as a reward or to control the child's behavior and for signs and symptoms of depression, anxiety, or boredom.

B. **Physical examination.** The physician should determine the following during the physical examination:

1. **Growth patterns**, including weight, height, weight for height, and triceps SFT plotted on the appropriate growth charts as well as distribution of body fat.
2. **Development.** The physician should determine if stigmata are associated with endocrine or genetic obesity and note any mental deficiency, genital abnormalities, or dysmorphic features.
3. **Blood pressure**

C. **Laboratory**

1. **Urinalysis.** Glycosuria is the most common abnormality associated with obesity.
2. **Nutritional indices.** Cholesterol, triglycerides, low-density lipoprotein (LDL), and high-density lipoprotein (HDL) should be measured. Abnormal levels require further testing (e.g., fasting cholesterol).

3. **Other.** Additional studies should be performed if indicated by the history or physical examination (e.g., dysmorphic appearance, mental deficiency) and might include an oral glucose tolerance test, thyroid studies, or karyotype.

D. **Classification.** The physician should determine whether obesity is exogenous or endocrine/genetic.

E. **Identification of morbidities**

VIII. **Management.** The primary goal of managing the child with exogenous obesity is to minimize morbidity without causing untoward effects from the treatment. Dietary restriction is required in most cases, but the physician should be aware of very restricted, low-energy diets in children, which may cause side effects such as headaches, nausea, fatigue, or constipation. Severe measures for weight control in children, such as jaw wiring or gastric stapling, are never recommended. Severely restricting caloric intake in young infants may cause statural or brain growth impairment and is not appropriate.

A. **Morbidities.** The first priority of managing the obese child is to identify and treat any morbidity associated with the condition. Hypertension is usually mild and should respond to dietary changes and weight reduction; significant hypertension should be treated with medication. Orthopedic problems, especially slipped capital femoral epiphysis and sleep apnea, require immediate attention.

B. **Diet** varies depending on the child's age and the severity of the obesity and should be designed to provide sufficient quantities of carbohydrates, fat (especially essential fatty acids), protein, minerals, and vitamins to fully meet lean body mass and linear growth requirements. Fad diets, such as protein-sparing diets, which are very low in calories, should be avoided. An outpatient referral to a dietitian specialist often is warranted.

C. **Activity.** People who increase their activity levels maintain weight loss better than those who do not. There is no evidence that obese children are less active than their lean peers, but an exercise plan is recommended for all obese children. Parents also should be involved in the exercise program. When beginning an exercise program, it is helpful to start slowly and reward the child's progress for even modest increases in activity. Such positive reinforcement can be a strong motivator for even more activity and helps the child's and the parents' morale.

D. **Behavior modification** can help ensure long-term success in the management of obesity. Older children can learn to monitor their own food intake and activity and how to obtain rewards other than food for their changed behavior. It is helpful to explore with the children alternatives to overeating. Psychotherapy is usually not necessary.

E. **Family.** The success of any weight control program depends on family involvement. Parents are responsible for most of the foods brought into the home, and they model both eating and activity behaviors for their children. Parents must be involved in the management plan from the beginning and may need as much support and encouragement as the child. The physician should provide frequent follow-up in the office and use the opportunity to educate parents and their children about healthy, lifelong dietary habits.

## Selected Readings

Agras W, Kraemer H, Berkowitz R et al. Influence of early feeding style on adiposity at 6 years of age. *J Pediatr* 116:805, 1990.

Bandini L, Dietz W. Myths about childhood obesity. *Pediatr Ann* 21:647, 1992.

Dietz W, Gortmaker S. Do we fatten our children at the television set? Obesity and television viewing in children and adolescents. *Pediatrics* 75:807, 1985.

Giorgi PL, Suskind RM, Catassi (eds). The Obese Child. In *Pediatric Adolescent Medicine*. Basel, Switzerland: Karger, 1992

Gortmaker S, Dietz W, Sobol M et al. Increasing pediatric obesity in the United States. *Am J Dis Child* 141:535, 1987.

Kaplan K, Wadden T. Childhood obesity and self-esteem. *J Pediatr* 109:367, 1986.

Ravussin E, Lillioja M et al. Reduced rate of energy expenditure as a risk factor for body weight gain. *N Engl J Med* 318:467, 1988.

Robinson T, Hammer L et al. Does television viewing increase obesity and reduce physical activity? Cross-sectional and longitudinal analyses among adolescent girls. *Pediatrics* 91:273, 1993.

Rosenbaum M, Leibel R. Obesity in childhood. *Pediatr Rev* 11:43, 1989.

Stunkard A, Sorensen T et al. An adoption study of human obesity. *N Engl J Med* 31:193, 1986.

# 39

# Contraception

## Julie Jaskiewicz

Adolescent sexual activity is increasing in the United States. Today, more than half of all adolescents 15–19 years of age have been sexually active. Unfortunately, many teen-agers delay seeking contraception until they have been coitally active for many months and then often use contraception inconsistently and ineffectively. It is important for the adolescent's primary care physician to counsel sexually active adolescents about the prevention of unplanned pregnancy and sexually transmitted diseases (STDs).

I. **The primary care physician's role.** The physician must identify adolescents at risk for sexual activity, counsel them about sexual behaviors, educate them about suitable contraceptive methods and protection against STDs, and provide access to contraception if requested. It is best to discuss sexual interest, attitudes, and behaviors with an adolescent in an open and nonjudgmental way, preferably before the young person has initiated sexual intercourse. The benefits of delaying coital activity should be stressed and reasons for the adolescent's desire to begin sexual activity discussed (e.g., peer pressure, expectations). The physician then can help the adolescent identify his or her own goals for safe sexual behavior and emphasize that taking responsibility for sexual decisions is a part of overall adult, responsible behavior. It is important to encourage sexually active teens to involve their partners in decisions regarding coital activity and contraception and to consider the effect of their sexual activity on relationships with partners and family. For the adolescent who already has begun coital activity, the physician should provide appropriate reproductive health care, including information about contraceptive methods and prevention of STDs.

II. **Evaluation.** Evaluating the adolescent for birth control requires a careful history and physical examination to determine if the adolescent is at risk for and wants to prevent pregnancy, STDs, or both and can understand and accept responsibility for appropriate contraceptive methods.

A. **History.** Adolescents and parents should be informed at the beginning of the office visit that the adolescent has a right to confidentiality except in life-threatening circumstances. The sexual history should determine the adolescent's sexual interest, knowledge about pregnancy, contraception and STDs, current sexual behaviors, and use of contraception. The physician can help choose the best birth control option for an adolescent by identifying any risk factors associated with available contraceptive methods. The sexual history should include the following:

1. **General sexual history**
   a. **Age**
   b. **Reason for the visit**
   c. **Current sexual behaviors**

**Table 39-1. Contraindications for oral contraceptive use**

| Absolute | Relative |
|---|---|
| Pregnancy | Hypertension |
| Coronary artery disease | Vascular or migraine headache |
| Cerebrovascular disease | Sickle cell disease |
| Thrombophlebitis and thrombotic disease | Hyperlipidemia |
| Breast and uterine cancer | Collagen vascular disease |
| Active liver disease | Lactation |
| Benign or malignant liver tumor | |
| Previous cholestasis with pregnancy | |
| Undiagnosed uterine bleeding | |

Source: Adapted from JA Jaskiewicz, ER McAnarney. Pregnancy during adolescence. *Pediatr Rev* 15:32, 1994.

d. **Reasons for wanting contraception** (desire to prevent pregnancy and STDs)
e. **Partners, involvement of partners in contraceptive decisions, parental or guardian involvement, values about sexuality or sexual activity**
f. **Past and present use of contraception** (e.g., type, perceived benefits, problems)
g. **Knowledge about contraceptive choices, concerns, perceived negative effects**
h. **Type of contraceptive desired, perceived willingness of partner to use contraceptive method**
i. **Ability to comply with contraceptive method**

2. **Medical and gynecologic history**
   a. **Menstrual history** (menarche, frequency and duration of menses, dysfunctional bleeding, dysmenorrhea, date of last menstrual period, date of last pelvic examination, history of abnormal Papanicolaou smear)
   b. **Prior sexual history (pregnancy, abortion, STDs, and treatment of partners)**
   c. **Psychosocial problems,** including depression and alcohol and drug use
3. **Review of systems** should focus on the following when considering oral contraceptives:
   a. **Absolute and relative contraindications** (Table 39-1)
   b. **Conditions influenced by use of oral contraceptives** (acne, contact lenses)
   c. **Medications and drug allergies**
   d. **Cardiovascular risk factors** (familial hyperlipidemia, family history of early heart disease, smoking, obesity)
   e. **Psychiatric problems**, including depression and alcohol and drug use
4. **Psychosocial development and maturity**

**B. Physical examination.** A careful physical examination should be performed with special attention given to abnormalities that may limit contraceptive choices.

1. The **general examination** should include the following:
   - a. **Height and weight**
   - b. **Thyroid examination**
   - c. **Breast examination**
   - d. **Examination of the cardiovascular system** (for edema, pulses)
   - e. **Examination of the GI system** (for liver size, tenderness, evidence of chronic disease)
   - f. **Examination of the skin** (for acne, xanthomata)
   - g. **Tanner staging** (for sexual maturity)
2. **Pelvic examination of the female** should include the following:
   - a. **External, bimanual, and speculum examinations**
   - b. **Specimen for Papanicolaou smear**
   - c. **Cultures of specimens for *Neisseria gonorrhoeae, Chlamydia trachomatis*,** and others as appropriate
3. **Genital examination of the male** should include the following:
   - a. **Testicular and penile examination**
   - b. **Cultures of specimens for STDs** as above

**C. Laboratory.** All females should have a pregnancy test before a birth control method is prescribed. Additional laboratory tests should be done on an individual basis. Some tests to consider include urinalysis, CBC, lipid screen, liver function tests, sickle cell screen, and serologic test for syphilis.

**III. Contraceptive methods.** The best contraceptive method for an adolescent is one that he or she and partners will accept and use consistently. Physicians should familiarize themselves with contraceptive methods suitable for adolescents and be prepared to help the adolescent make an informed choice for his or her situation. Contraceptive needs and preferences may change over time, so the physician should continue to provide follow-up to make adjustments as necessary. Table 39-2 gives the expected failure rates of some of the most frequently used birth control methods for adolescents.

**A. Abstinence.** Any discussion of contraception with an adolescent should start with abstinence, the most effective and safe form of birth control available. Adolescents can be encouraged to choose abstinence, but the provider must be ready to discuss alternative contraceptive methods with the teen-ager who desires to be sexually active.

1. **Advantages.** Abstinence is the only 100% safe and effective birth control method. It has no side effects and is the best protection against STDs ("easy" to use).
2. **Disadvantages.** Abstinence has no disadvantages or contraindications.

**B. Oral contraceptives.** The combined estrogen-progestogen oral contraceptive pill frequently is used by adolescents. Combined oral contraceptives inhibit ovulation by

**Table 39-2. Contraceptive methods: Lowest expected first-year failure rates**

| Type of contraceptive | Failure rate (%) |
|---|---|
| Abstinence | 0.0 |
| Norplant | 0.04 |
| Oral contraceptives (combined) | 0.1–0.5 |
| Condom | 2 |
| Vaginal spermicides | 3 |
| Coitus interruptus (withdrawal) | 4 |
| Diaphragm and cervical cap | 6 |
| Vaginal sponge | 6–9 |
| Rhythm method | 1–9 |

Source: Adapted from PK Braverman, VC Strasburger. Adolescent sexuality. II. Contraception. *Clin Pediatr* 32:728, 1993.

inhibiting the gonadotropin-releasing hormone (GnRH) in the hypothalamus, resulting in secondary ovarian suppression. More than 30 brands of oral contraceptives are available, including low-dose estrogen pills, which contain 30–35 μg of estrogen, and triphasic pills, which contain varying amounts of hormones throughout the menstrual cycle. The primary contraceptive estrogen is ethinyl estradiol.

1. **Advantages.** Oral contraceptives are highly effective when used correctly, safe, and reversible; decrease menstrual blood flow, the risk of ovarian and endometrial cancer, the incidence of fibrocystic breast disease and ovarian cysts, and the incidence of dysmenorrhea; and provide some protection against salpingitis.
2. **Disadvantages.** Oral contraceptives require compliance with a daily pill and do not protect against STDs. Common side effects (often reduced after a few cycles) include nausea, weight gain, breast tenderness, leg cramps, fluid retention, depression, breakthrough bleeding, headache, and acne. Rare side effects include corneal edema (contact lens wearers), thromboembolic events, stroke, and hypertension. Table 39-1 lists the contraindications for using oral contraceptives.

C. **Mini-pill (progestin-only pill).** The mini-pill is similar to the combined oral contraceptive pill but contains only progestin. Side effects and reduced efficacy limit its use in adolescents, but this method could be considered in situations in which estrogen is contraindicated.

1. **Advantages** of using the progestin-only pill include fewer estrogen-related side effects, such as reduced risk of thromboembolic events and hypertension. Lactation is not a contraindication.
2. **Disadvantages** of using the progestin-only pill include increased failure rate and higher incidence of breakthrough bleeding, amenorrhea, and hirsutism. It provides no protection against STDs.

D. The **condom** is a mechanical barrier that covers the penis during sexual intercourse. Only latex condoms should be recommended because natural membrane condoms do not protect against STDs. When used with a spermicide (e.g., nonoxynol-9), protection against pregnancy is close to that of oral contraceptives. Proper use of condoms should be discussed with the adolescent, including using only water-based lubricants and not using torn, damaged, or previously used condoms.

1. **Advantages.** Condoms are easily accessible and inexpensive, do not require a prescription, and have few side effects. Condom use involves the male partner in contraception choices and is the best method after abstinence for protection against STDs.
2. **Disadvantages.** Condom use requires male participation in contraception and planning for sexual activity in advance. Latex allergy occurs occasionally.

E. **Vaginal spermicides** are chemical contraceptives available in a variety of forms, such as creams, gels, foams, tablets, and suppositories. (Nonoxynol-9 is the most frequently used chemical.) Spermicides are most effective when used with barrier contraceptives.

1. **Advantages.** Spermicides are easily accessible and inexpensive and do not require a prescription; they have few side effects.
2. **Disadvantages.** The efficacy of spermicides is limited when used alone; there are no absolute contraindications.

F. **Diaphragm and cervical cap.** The diaphragm is a rubber cap with a metal spring in the rim designed to fit over the cervix and provide a physical barrier to sperm entering the cervix. The cervical cap is a small, flexible latex cap that uses suction to fit over the cervix. Both methods are used with a vaginal spermicide. These methods are most successfully used by older adolescents.

1. **Advantages.** Diaphragms and cervical caps used with spermicide are effective and used only when needed, protect against STDs, and have few side effects. Spermicide is available without a prescription.
2. **Disadvantages.** Proper fit of diaphragms and cervical caps is required, and the adolescent must feel comfortable inserting the device herself. Diaphragms and cervical caps require planning for sexual activity in advance and increase the risk of urinary tract infection. Occasional vaginal malodor and discharge are associated with this contraception method. Contraindications are a severely retro- or anteverted uterus, allergy to latex (cervical cap), and history of toxic shock syndrome.

G. The **vaginal sponge** is a disposable, doughnut-shaped polyurethane sponge with a retrieval loop that contains 1 g of nonoxynol-9. Water is added prior to insertion, and the device swells within the vagina to cover the cervix.

1. **Advantages.** The sponge does not require a prescription and is easier to insert than the diaphragm or cervical cap; it is effective for 24 hours.
2. **Disadvantages.** The sponge has a variable failure rate; can be difficult to remove; and is associated with

toxic shock syndrome (reported one case/2 million users), vaginal malodor, and candidiasis.

H. **Norplant** is a new, subdermal progestin-only implant that provides continuous contraception for up to 5 years. Six Silastic capsules that release 30 $\mu$g of levonorgestrel a day are inserted under local anesthesia in the upper arm.

1. **Advantages.** Norplant is highly effective and has no estrogen side effects. Its effectiveness does not depend on compliance, and fertility returns quickly after removal.
2. **Disadvantages.** Norplant's initial cost is high, and it provides no protection against STDs. Norplant's side effects include irregular menstrual bleeding, weight gain, and headaches.

I. **Other methods.** Two methods commonly used by adolescents are **coitus interruptus** (male partner withdrawal before ejaculation) and the **rhythm method** (periodic abstinence around the time of anticipated ovulation). Neither method is indicated for adolescents to prevent pregnancy. Adolescents do not use these methods consistently or correctly, and failure rates can be high (see Table 39-2). Most important, neither method provides protection against STDs. Adolescents who desire to be sexually active should be advised to use other forms of birth control.

## Selected Readings

American Academy of Pediatrics Committee on Adolescence. Contraception and adolescents. *Pediatrics* 86:134, 1990.

Braverman PK, Strasburger VC. Contraception—adolescent sexuality: II. *Clin Pediatr* 32:725, 1992.

Greydanus DE, Patel DR. Contraception. In ER McAnarney (ed), *Textbook of Adolescent Medicine*. Philadelphia: Saunders, 1992.

Jaskiewicz JA, McAnarney ER. Pregnancy during adolescence. *Pediatr Rev* 15:32, 1994.

Woods ER. Contraceptive choices for adolescents. *Pediatr Ann* 20:313, 1991.

# G

# Neuromusculoskeletal Disorders

# 40

# Genu Varum and Genu Valgum

**Raymond C. Baker**

I. **Genu varum (bow legs).** During growth and development of the lower extremities in children, physiologic bowing of the lower extremities is common and usually resolves by age 24 months. Coexisting internal tibial torsion exaggerates the appearance of bowing. The physician should anticipate questions about physiologic bowing and tell parents that this is usually normal and requires no treatment. It is important, however, to quantitate the degree of deformity at each visit to document correction, which usually begins by age 18–24 months. A simple clinical method of quantitation is measuring the distance between the medial aspects of the knees while the child lies in the supine position with thighs and legs adducted to the midline and the medial malleoli touching (Fig. 40-1). If more than 10 cm is measured or the condition does not improve by age 24 months, the physician should consider orthopedic referral or radiographs of the knees to rule out other conditions such as rickets or tibia vara (Blount's disease).

II. **Genu valgum (knock knees).** Genu valgum is less common than genu valgum and occurs in the older child 3–6 years of age. Although its etiology is not entirely clear, several factors may contribute to genu valgum, including abnormal development of the femoral condyles, lax medial collateral ligaments, pes varus, and obesity. Genu valgum is quantitated clinically by placing the child in the supine position with thighs and legs adducted and measuring the distance in centimeters between the medial malleoli of the ankles with the medial aspects of the knees touching (Fig. 40-2). A distance greater than 10 cm at any age indicates orthopedic referral. Genu valgum usually resolves by age 6–8 years and rarely requires orthopedic intervention. Again, the physician should anticipate questions from parents and discuss the transient nature of the condition.

## Selected Readings

Bunnell WP, Shook JE. Orthopaedics in the pediatric office. *Curr Prob Pediatr* 22:13, 1992.

Scoles PV. *Pediatric Orthopedics in Clinical Practice* (2nd ed). Chicago: Year Book, 1988.

Wilkins KE. Bowlegs. *Pediatr Clin North Am* 33:1429, 1986.

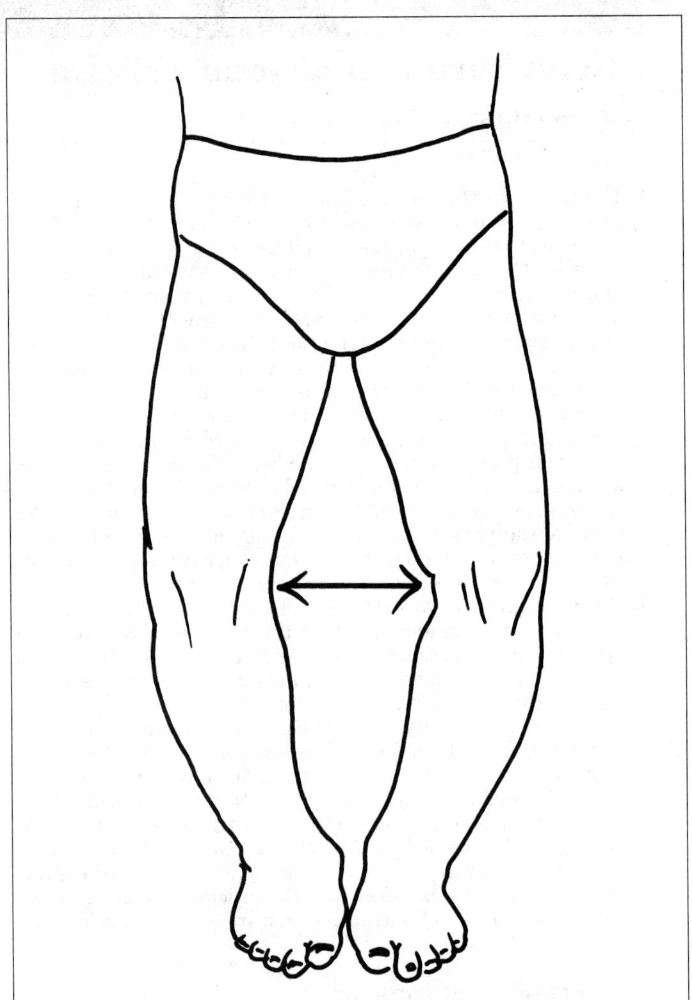

**Fig. 40-1. Quantitation of genu varum (bow legs).**

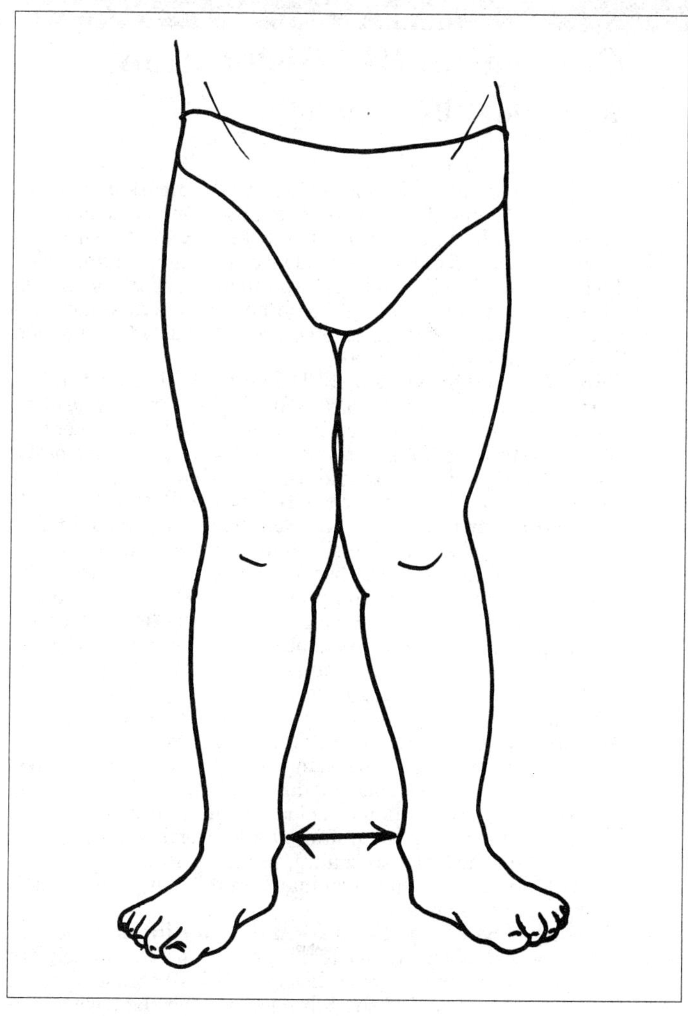

**Fig. 40-2. Quantitation of genu valgum (knock knees).**

# 41

# Congenital Hip Dislocation

**Raymond C. Baker**

Congenital hip dysplasia/dislocation (CHD) occurs in approximately 0.1% of infants, with a predilection for females to males of 5:1. In infants with a family history (first-degree relative affected) of CHD, the incidence is 10 times higher. The incidence of CHD is also higher in infants born in the breech position and infants with certain other congenital abnormalities, including torticollis, clubfoot, metatarsus adductus, and hyperextension of the knee.

I. **Diagnosis** and prevention of CHD in the newborn depend on demonstrating hip instability. (Hip instability may lead to frank dislocation or subluxation.) Since early treatment of CHD is crucial, infants must be screened on a regular basis, especially those at increased risk as above. Instability is demonstrated by means of the Ortolani and Barlow tests.

   A. **Ortolani test.** In this maneuver, the infant is examined in the supine position. The examiner holds the infant's pelvis with one hand to stabilize it during manipulation. The examiner then slowly and gently abducts the infant's opposite hip with the other hand, pulling the femur forward and using the greater trochanter as a fulcrum as in Fig. 41-1. In the infant with an unstable hip, the examiner will feed a sudden shifting sensation and may hear or feel a "clunk" simultaneously as the hip reduces anteriorly.

   B. **Barlow test.** In this maneuver, the infant is examined in the supine position. The examiner holds the infant's pelvis with one hand to stabilize it during manipulation. With the other hand, the examiner holds the infant's opposite hip in the adducted, flexed position while exerting gentle pressure over the lesser trochanter as in Fig. 40-2. In the infant with an unstable hip, a similar "clunk" may be felt as the hip subluxes posteriorly.

   C. **Diagnosis of hip dislocation in older infants.** Beyond 6–8 weeks of age, the Ortolani and Barlow tests likely are negative in infants with dislocated hips because the soft tissues surrounding the hip have become tight with contractures. In the older infant, signs of dislocation are the following:

      1. **Incomplete or asymmetric abduction of the hips** (normal hip abduction is almost 90 degrees)
      2. **Leg length discrepancy** with apparent shortening of the affected side as measured either with the infant's thighs and legs extended or the infant supine with hips and legs flexed and legs adducted as the examiner looks for asymmetry of the height of the knees
      3. **Thigh fold asymmetry**
      4. **Trendelenburg's sign** (due to shortening and weakening of hip stabilizing muscles)

II. **Confirmation and treatment.** The diagnosis of hip instability and dislocation are confirmed by hip ultrasound in the

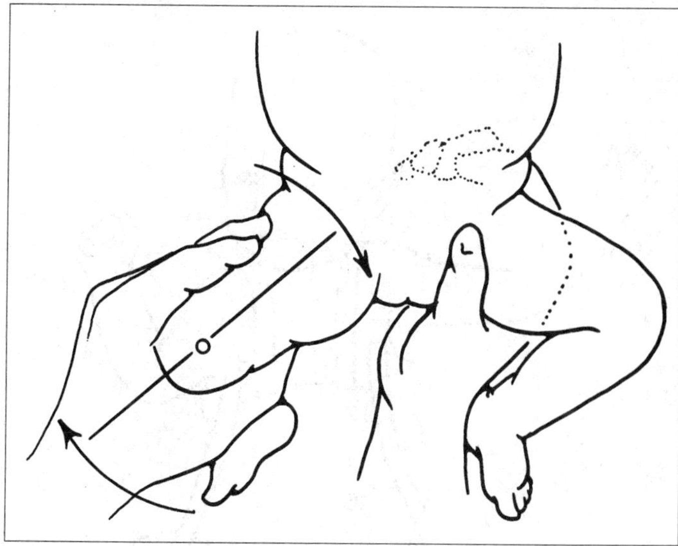

**Fig. 41-1. The Ortolani test for hip instability.**

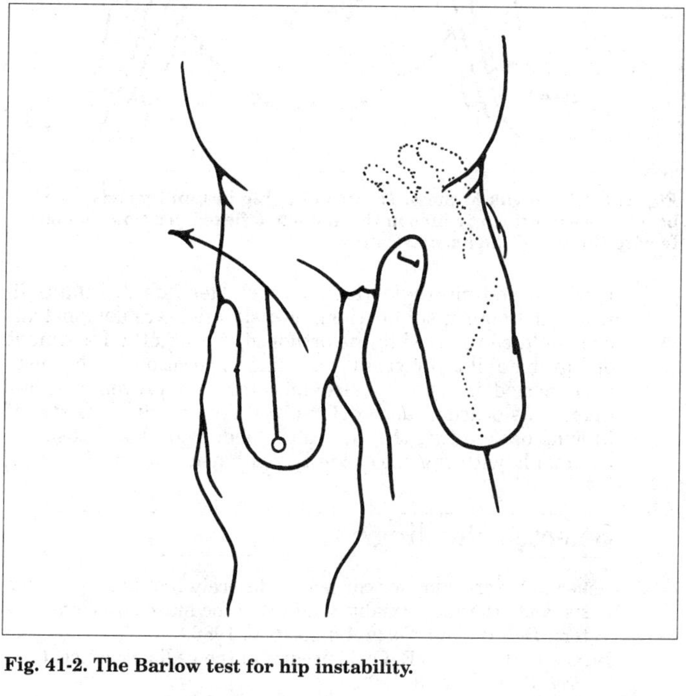

**Fig. 41-2. The Barlow test for hip instability.**

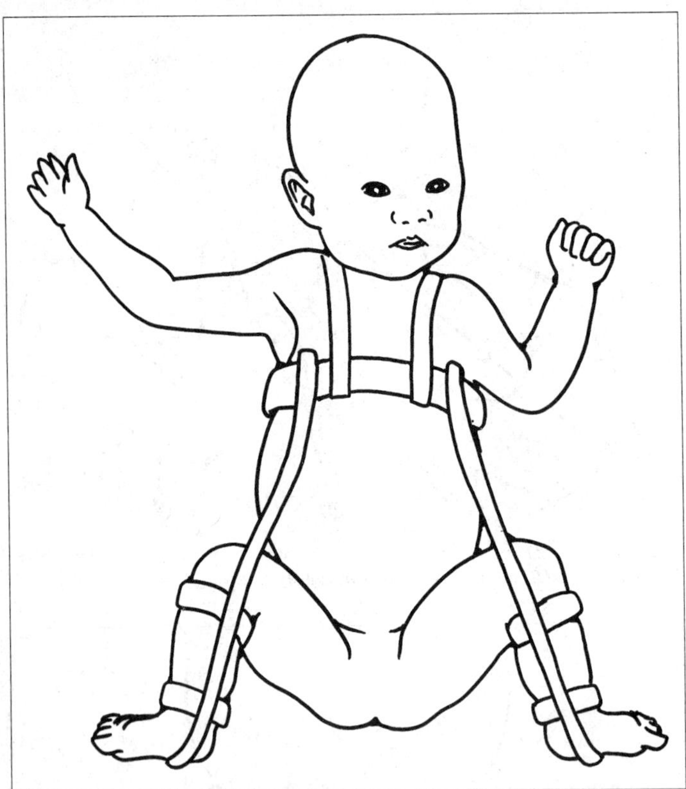

**Fig. 41-3. The Pavlik harness. Treatment of hip instability consists of bracing or splinting the hips in the abducted, flexed position, commonly with the use of the harness.**

newborn and hip radiographs in the older infant. Infants in whom instability, subluxation, or dislocation are demonstrated should be referred to the orthopedist promptly. Treatment of hip instability or easily reducible dislocation in the newborn period is usually uncomplicated and prevents subsequent dislocation and deformity. Treatment consists of bracing or splinting the hips in the abducted, flexed position, commonly with the use of the Pavlik harness as in Fig. 41-3.

## Selected Readings

Asher MA. Screening for congenital dislocation of the hip, scoliosis, and other abnormalities affecting the musculoskeletal system. *Pediatr Clin North Am* 33:1336, 1986.

Bunnell WP, Shook JE. Orthopaedics in the pediatric office. *Curr Prob Pediatr* 22:13, 1992.

Scoles PV. *Pediatric Orthopedics in Clinical Practice* (2nd ed). Chicago: Year Book, 1988.

# Evaluation of the Patient with Intoeing

Raymond C. Baker

Intoeing ("pigeon toes") in the infant and child is the most common orthopedic complaint parents have for the primary care physician during the course of well-child care. The most prevalent causes of intoeing are (1) metatarsus adductus in the young infant, (2) internal tibial torsion in the toddler, and (3) femoral anteversion in the preschool and school-age child. Although all of these tend to resolve with growth of the child, they should be quantitated at each visit to document that resolution. A minority of patients with each of these deformities may require special exercises or orthopedic referral for excessive degrees of the deformity or failure to resolve.

I. **Physical examination** is best performed with the child in the prone position, thighs extended, legs flexed to 90 degrees, and the examiner at the foot of the examining table (Fig. 42-1). In this position, the three causes of intoeing can be differentiated. As the examiner looks down on the bottoms of the feet, the C-shaped foot of metatarsus adductus is apparent (Fig. 42-2).

   If the foot is straight, but there is internal rotation of the long axis of the foot relative to the femur, internal tibial torsion is present (Fig. 42-3).

   If metatarsus adductus and internal tibial torsion are both absent and there is increased internal rotation at the hips (usually to 90 degrees), femoral anteversion is present (Fig. 42-4).

II. **Metatarsus adductus.** The treatment of metatarsus adductus depends on the degree of the deformity.

   A. **Grade I.** Stroking the lateral margin of the foot causes it to straighten out. No treatment is necessary, and the condition resolves spontaneously.

   B. **Grade II.** Stroking does not straighten the foot, but the forefoot can be stretched passively past neutral. The physician should demonstrate stretching exercises for the caregiver and recommend them at each diaper change. Metatarsus adductus should be checked for resolution at each visit. If it does not resolve by age 5–6 months, orthopedic referral is indicated.

   C. **Grade III.** The forefoot cannot be moved passively past the neutral position. This requires immediate orthopedic referral for serial casting (preferably by 2 months of age).

III. **Internal tibial torsion** usually requires no specific treatment and resolves spontaneously. When diagnosed, the degree of torsion should be quantitated with a goniometer by measuring the angle formed by the intersection of a line drawn through the long axis of the foot and one drawn through the long axis of the femur with the child in the prone position as above. At subsequent well-child examinations, the angle should be remeasured. If there is a significant decrease in the angle after the

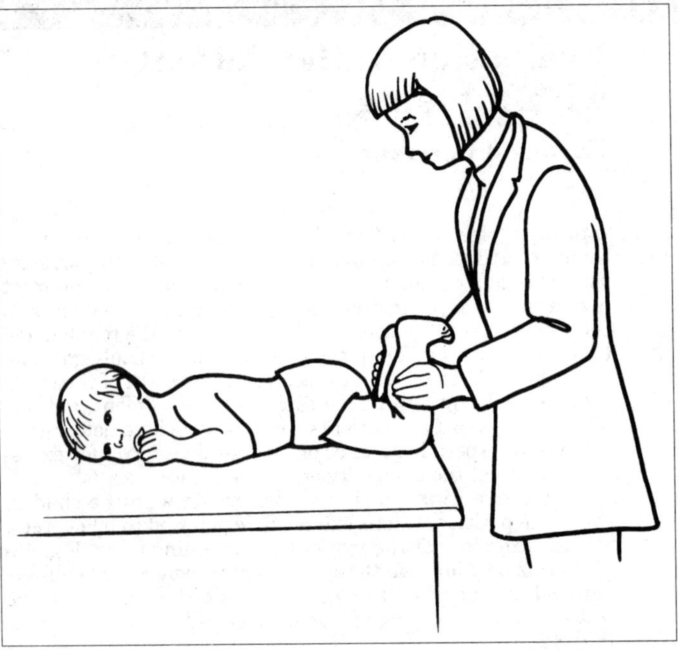

**Fig. 42-1. Best position for performing the physical examination for intoeing.**

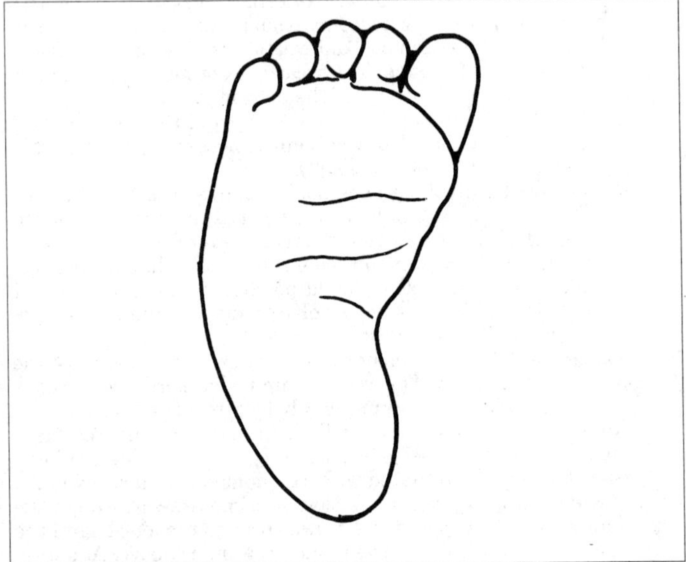

**Fig. 42-2. Metatarsus adductus.**

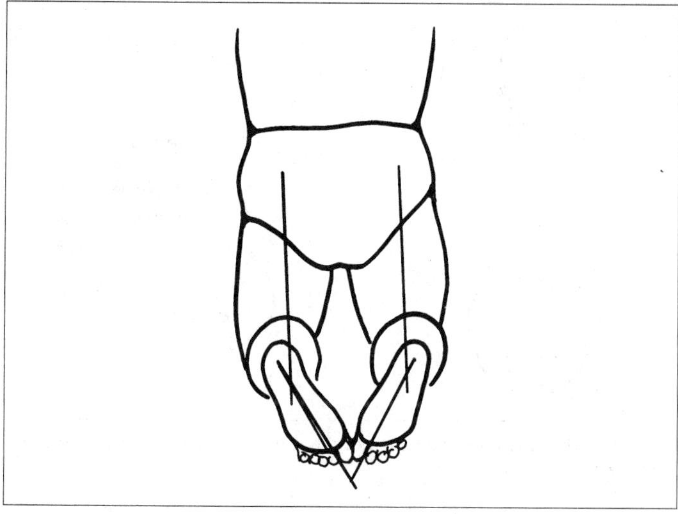

**Fig. 42-3. Internal tibial torsion.**

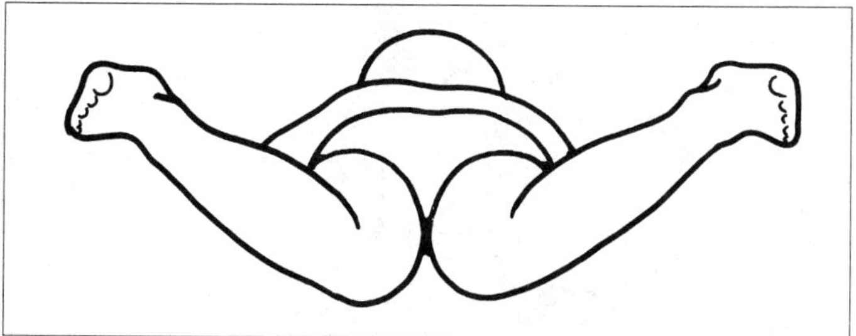

**Fig. 42-4. Femoral anteversion.**

child has been walking for 1 year, the problem usually resolves without further treatment. If there is no significant resolution, orthopedic referral is appropriate (for night splints). The habit of sitting or lying on the feet with the hips and legs flexed and feet internally rotated underneath (Fig. 42-5) exacerbates this problem and should be discouraged.

**IV. Femoral anteversion** is seen usually in females and is the most common cause of intoeing in preschool and school-age children. In femoral anteversion, the hips usually can be internally rotated 90 degrees easily while external rotation is decreased or normal. The habit of sitting in the "W," or "TV," position (thighs flexed and internally rotated, legs flexed 90–120 degrees; Fig. 42-6), tends to exacerbate this condition and should be discouraged. The child should be encouraged to sit Indian-style. If the hips can be externally rotated more than 25 degrees, the deformity can be compensated for by age 12 years, usually consciously by the child. Orthopedic referral

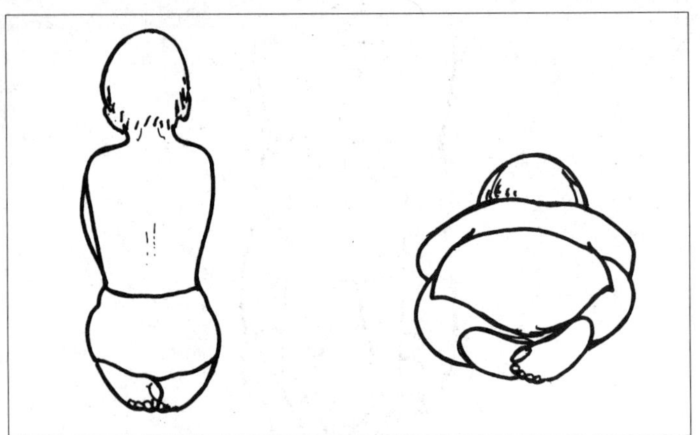

**Fig. 42-5. These two positions exacerbate internal torsion and should be discouraged.**

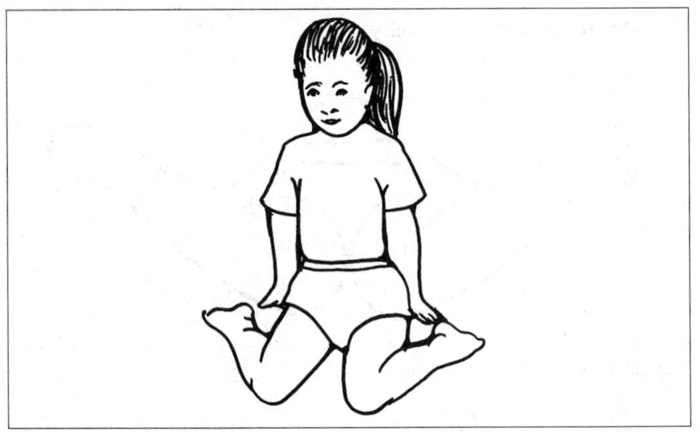

**Fig. 42-6. The "W," or "TV," position exacerbates femoral anteversion and should be discouraged.**

is rarely necessary for this condition; however, if the child's gait is affected enough to cause frequent falls, referral to an orthopedist is appropriate.

## Selected Readings

Bunnell WP, Shook JE. Orthopedics in the pediatric office. *Curr Prob Pediatr* 22:13, 1992.

Scoles PV. *Pediatric Orthopedics in Clinical Practice* (2nd ed). Chicago: Year Book, 1988.

Staheli LT. Torsional deformity. *Pediatr Clin North Am* 33:1373, 1986.

# Evaluation and Management of Headaches in Children

David N. Franz

Headache is the most common neurologic complaint to face the primary care physician. A straightforward diagnostic strategy and therapeutic intervention are successful in the majority of cases. Primary diagnostic concerns are to differentiate neurologic from non-neurologic causes and differentiate neurologic causes associated with significant morbidity (e.g., malignancy, pseudotumor cerebri) from those that are less serious (e.g., migraine). Most pediatric patients with headache do not have a serious neurologic disorder; however, it is the clinician's responsibility to identify children whose headaches result from a serious cause and to do so in a cost-effective manner.

I. **History** is the crucial element in the categorization of headache and should be an active process—with questioning designed to include or exclude specific entities—rather than just a rote interrogation. Headache episodes first should be characterized as accurately as possible with respect to frequency, duration, and quality of pain. The physician should ask the patient and parents questions that may help determine the source of the headaches. Are there any provoking factors or patterns to the attacks, such as ingestion of certain foods, particular activities, or times of day? Are they of recent onset and increasing in severity or frequency, or chronic and nonprogressive? Is there an aura, visual or sensory changes, fever, or stiff neck?

Complex neurologic symptoms such as diplopia, hemiparesis, or aphasia can indicate structural CNS disease. Children who experience syncope or presyncope may have residual headache following a syncopal event, which can lead to an erroneous diagnosis of complicated migraine. Neurocardiogenic syncope or arrhythmia should be considered in patients with an altered level of consciousness.

Patients with headache from non-neurologic causes, such as sinusitis or temporomandibular joint (TMJ) dysfunction, often have pain involving the face, maxillae, or temporal regions as opposed to having hemicrania or holocephalgia. Associated fever, meningismus, or both raises the possibility of subarachnoid hemorrhage or infection. These conditions need not be fulminant, as with aneurysmal rupture or bacterial meningitis. Venous angiomas and other types of vascular malformations may intermittently leak small amounts of blood (sentinel hemorrhage), producing episodic symptoms and focal neurologic deficits. Affected children may appear normal between events. The headache of subarachnoid hemorrhage is described classically as acute and severe ("the worst headache I've ever had").

Subacute and chronic infectious processes (e.g., Lyme disease; fungal, mycobacterial, viral meningoencephalitis) should

**Table 43-1. Characteristics of headache pain in children**

| Serious | Migraine |
|---|---|
| Always in morning | Any time of day |
| Awakens from sleep | Better with recumbency, emesis |
| Worse with recumbency | Obvious precipitants |
| Early morning vomiting | Family history of migraine |
| Persistent neurologic deficit | Transient neurologic deficit |
| Chronic progressive (increased severity or frequency) | Facial pain |
| Polydipsia | Stress |
| Short stature | Complaints of tightness, aching |
| Personality change | Bilateral band |
| Immunosuppression | |
| Valvular heart disease | |
| "Worst headache I've ever had!" | |
| Excessively stereotyped | |
| Bruits | |

be considered, particularly in the immunosuppressed host or one who has recently had a course of steroid therapy. Headaches that awaken the patient from sleep or are relieved by upright posture can be related to increased intracranial pressure. Migraine sufferers usually prefer to lie down in a dark room during an attack. Sleep disturbances such as bruxism, snoring, enuresis, night terrors, and insomnia can be clues to underlying causes, such as TMJ dysfunction, sleep apnea, epilepsy, or a psychological disorder.

The physician should ask what has been tried for relief and how the headaches have affected the child's daily activities. (Some patients with "severe" headaches have never missed school or favorite activities as a result.) Changes in personality, school performance, or emotional state may indicate an ongoing encephalopathy. Issues of secondary gain, personal stressors, potential drug abuse, and pregnancy should be considered when appropriate. Cocaine and amphetamine abuse can produce headache, subarachnoid hemorrhage, toxic vasculitis, and stroke even when not taken intravenously (IV). Refractive error (eyestrain) is rarely a source of significant head pain. Likewise, allergies in the absence of rhinorrhea, nasal congestion, and tenderness over the affected sinus(es) are not commonly a source of headache pain.

Table 43-1 classifies headache symptoms as serious (i.e., potentially associated with serious neurologic pathology) and migraine.

**II. Past medical history** is important particularly to identify conditions that may indicate an increased risk of neurologic pathology or direct therapy, such as seizures, asthma, or renal or cardiac disease. A positive family history of migraine or severe episodic headache usually supports this diagnosis; however, such a history can be obtained in up to 60% of the general population. Head pain can be associated with certain types of inherited epilepsy, which may not always produce major motor seizures. Certain cerebrovascular malformations may be familial as well.

Many prescription and proprietary medications have headache as a side effect; examples are psychostimulants, beta-agonists, theophylline, caffeine, oral contraceptives, and sympathomimetic decongestants (ephedrine and pseudoephedrine). Migraine sufferers, particularly those who smoke cigarettes, are at increased risk for stroke, which is increased further by oral contraceptive use. Tetracyclines and chronic steroid use, especially when being tapered, have been associated with pseudotumor cerebri.

III. **Physical examination** supplements the history in determining specific causes of headache pain. Blood pressure, heart rate, height, and weight always should be recorded. These may indicate the presence of systemic illnesses that may be causing headache, such as hypertension, renal disease, or cardiac arrhythmia. Children with a postural component to their headache should have orthostatic blood pressure and heart rate determinations. Obese individuals are at increased risk for pseudotumor cerebri. Poor weight gain can indicate a malabsorptive or chronic inflammatory process. Failure to thrive with preservation of linear growth can be a sign of a diencephalic lesion or tumor (diencephalic syndrome). Short stature and/or dwarfism can be associated with malformations of the posterior fossa or craniocervical junction.

Examination of the nasopharynx may reveal signs of sinusitis; dental caries, abscess, or both; or tonsillar hypertrophy. Otoscopic assessment rules out chronic or acute otitis media. Cervical and temporal muscle spasm or tenderness may indicate trauma or an overuse syndrome.

IV. **Neurologic examination.** It is important for the physician to take time to perform a careful ophthalmologic examination, including visualization of the optic disc and fundus. Besides papilledema, the fundus should be examined for spontaneous pulsations of the retinal vessels as they cross the disc margin. When present, spontaneous venous pulsations rule out increased intracranial pressure. Their absence, however, does not necessarily mean the reverse is true. Cranial nerves, deep tendon reflexes, and cerebellar function, including tandem walking, should be checked. Brisk but symmetric tendon reflexes in the absence of extensor plantar responses (positive Babinski sign) or other abnormal signs generally do not indicate neurologic pathology. Weakness should be screened for by checking upper extremity drift. Despite a careful neurologic examination, most children with headache have a normal neurologic exam when symptom-free. It is advantageous to examine the patient when he or she is experiencing a headache to increase the likelihood of uncovering abnormal signs.

V. **Laboratory studies.** Neuroimaging studies are the primary consideration in evaluating a patient with headache, particularly to exclude structural CNS disease. CT scans and MRI are of low yield when performed indiscriminately in children with uncomplicated headache. Conversely, head pain caused by potentially serious lesions may be clinically indistinguishable on rare occasions from migraine or other more benign

**Table 43-2. Indications for neuroimaging in headache patients**

| |
|---|
| Focal neurologic deficit |
| Alteration in mental status |
| Fever, stiff neck |
| Recent trauma |
| Prior history of neurologic disorder |
| Complicated migraine |
| Postural headache (i.e., worse with recumbency) |
| Acute progressive symptoms |
| Age less than 5 yrs |

types of headache. There is no "cookbook" recipe to define precisely which patients need neuroimaging; this judgment is made on clinical grounds and will continue to be for the foreseeable future.

Table 43-2 lists factors that mandate neuroimaging in a headache patient. It is also appropriate to consider imaging in patients whose headaches seem atypical, have the potentially serious symptoms listed in Table 43-1, or who have concurrent systemic illnesses, such as congenital heart disease. A CT scan, with and without contrast, is sufficient in most patients to screen for structural lesions. CT is quicker, less expensive, and superior to MRI in the acute detection of subarachnoid blood. MRI is preferable for visualization of the brain stem, craniocervical junction, and cerebral white matter. Small vascular malformations may be better visualized on MRI, and concurrent magnetic resonance angiography can further define larger vascular lesions. Small malformations still can be missed on magnetic resonance angiography and require traditional angiographic techniques.

EEG often is requested in evaluating headache patients, but its usefulness is limited to identifying headaches that are part of an underlying epileptic syndrome. EEG has no role in the routine screening of children with headache. It has poor sensitivity for intracranial mass lesions, and a normal EEG does not exclude a structural lesion. Conversely, focal findings on EEG (either epileptiform discharges or background slowing) are an absolute indication for neuroimaging. Lumbar puncture (LP) should be performed in children suspected of having meningoencephalitis, pseudotumor cerebri, or subarachnoid hemorrhage if clinically suspected even if not apparent on neuroimaging. Prior to a LP, a mass lesion first should be excluded using a CT scan or MRI. Performance of the LP should include opening and closing pressures. Normal CSF pressure in the lateral decubitus position is less than 200 mm of water, up to 250 mm of water in obese persons. Additional studies may be indicated if there is evidence of a coexistent systemic illness.

**VI. Migraine.** Most children with headache have migraine; estimates of the incidence vary widely. Recurrent, severe headaches have been reported to occur in 33–77% of children. Certainly, most migraine sufferers have their first attacks in childhood, which may be followed by a long period of quiescence stretching well into adulthood. The relapsing and remitting character of migraine (plus the significant placebo effect reported in migraine) not only confounds estimates of its prevalence but also hampers the evaluation of therapies. A variety of classifications have been used for migraine. Functionally, it is usually adequate to consider three types: classic, common, and complicated. Tension-type headaches are now thought to be similar in pathogenesis to migraine; therefore, treatment strategies should be similar.

A. **Classic migraine** consists of a stereotypic, usually visual aura followed by throbbing hemicranial pain, nausea, and vomiting.

B. **Common migraine** generally is less severe, has no aura, and may be described as a tight, bandlike holocephalgic pain.

C. **Complicated migraine** refers to headache associated with complex neurologic symptoms, such as hemiparesis, ophthalmoplegia, torticollis, visual loss, or unconsciousness, provided that these symptoms are not attributable to another neurologic disorder.

Current thinking on the pathogenesis of migraine suggests a disturbance of central serotonergic neurotransmission. Many, if not most, of the seemingly disparate medications for migraine can be found to have direct or indirect effects on central serotonin receptors.

D. **Management.** In addition to the "active" interventions of pharmacotherapy, there are several "passive" aspects essential to successful management of headache.

It is extremely useful for patients to keep a "headache diary." Patients note on a calendar the dates and times that headaches occur and document intensity of symptoms according to an arbitrary scale. (A sample scale is one numbered 1–10; 1 = least severe, and 10 = most severe.) Patients should be asked to note any associated or precipitating factors. If such factors can be identified, avoidance of them in combination with the occasional use of simple analgesics (e.g., acetaminophen) may be sufficient. Migraine precipitants include exertion, emotional stress, bright lights, pungent odors such as certain perfumes or cigarette smoke, and a variety of foods. Common food offenders are chocolate, cheese, caffeine, nitrates (as in processed meats), and alcoholic beverages. Patients are counseled on potential migraine precipitants and then asked to note if any of these factors are associated with their headaches. These factors then are avoided and any change in headache frequency noted. In this way, a few culprits often can be implicated. Stress reduction and biofeedback also may be useful. Success with this method requires an ongoing commitment by the patient and family and access to a qualified practitioner (usually a clinical psychologist).

VII. **Pharmacotherapy** of migraine is divided into abortive and prophylactic measures. Tables 43-3 and 43-4 summarize the various agents useful in pediatrics.

A. **Abortive treatment** (see Table 43-3) should be administered as early in the attack as possible. Simple analgesics such as acetaminophen or ibuprofen should be tried first. The nonsteroidal anti-inflammatory drug

**Table 43-3. Commonly used drugs for migraine treatment: Abortive therapy**

| Agent | Dosage* | Side effects |
|---|---|---|
| Ibuprofen (e.g., Motrin) | 10 mg/kg PO q4–6h (maximum 800 mg/dose) | Gastritis, renal injury, inhibition of platelet function |
| Naproxen (e.g., Naprosyn) | 5 mg/kg PO bid (maximum 375 mg PO bid) | Same as ibuprofen |
| Diphenhydramine (e.g., Benadryl) | 1.5 mg/kg PO qid prn for sleep (max. 50 mg/dose) | Anticholinergic toxicity, exacerbation of seizures, sedation |
| Promethazine (e.g., Phenergan) | 0.5 mg/kg IV or PR q4–6h prn (maximum 50 mg/dose) | Extrapyramidal movements, anticholinergic toxicity, exacerbation of seizures, sedation |
| Prochlorperazine (e.g., Compazine) | 0.10–0.15 mg/kg IM q6h (can be given IV in children >2 yrs of age) (maximum 10 mg/dose) | Same as promethazine |
| Chlorpromazine (e.g., Thorazine) | 1 mg/kg IM or IV | Same as promethazine |

*Per dose unless otherwise indicated.

**Table 43-4. Commonly used drugs for migraine treatment: Prophylactic therapy**

| Agent | Dosage* | Side effects |
|---|---|---|
| Amitriptyline | 10 mg PO qhs<br>Increase by 10 mg at weekly intervals until headache controlled, side effects intolerable, or maximum dose 3 mg/kg/day | Sedation, dry mouth, urinary retention, constipation |
| Cyproheptadine | 0.12–0.25 mg/kg PO bid | Sedation, increased appetite |
| Propranolol | 10 mg PO bid or 0.5 mg/kg bid (whichever is less)<br>Increase at weekly intervals until headache controlled, side effects intolerable, or maximum dose 4 mg/kg/day | Lethargy, syncope, hypotension, exacerbation of bronchospasm |

*Per dose unless otherwise indicated.

naproxen (Naprosyn, Anaprox, Aleve) is also effective. Patients with migraine who suffer vomiting with their attacks may try promethazine (Phenergan) suppositories. Sleep can be helpful in aborting more severe attacks; diphenhydramine (Benadryl), which has sedative properties, is readily available and can be given at home.

Intravenous ( if >2 year of age) or intramuscular (at any age) prochlorperazine (Compazine) can be given in the hospital setting. Chlorpromazine (Thorazine) given IM also has been advocated for abortive therapy. Patients should be monitored closely for side effects of hypotension and extrapyramidal reactions, such as oculogyric crisis and other dystonic symptoms and signs. Drugs with sedative properties should not be given to patients in whom an intracranial mass, hemorrhage, or infection have not been excluded. Phenothiazine and antihistamine drugs also should be used cautiously in patients with epilepsy because these agents can lower the seizure threshold.

**B. Prophylactic therapy** (see Table 43-4) should be considered in children with one or more migraines a week. The goal is not to continue prophylaxis indefinitely but to attain headache control for 6–8 weeks and then discontinue medication. A daily dose of ibuprofen 10 mg/kg can be given as prophylaxis and additional doses taken as needed for acute headache, up to 40 mg/kg/day or 800 mg/dose. Amitriptyline is inexpensive, effective, given in a single daily dose, and generally well tolerated. Cyproheptadine (Periactin) is preferred for very young children (<5 years) with migraine, those with concomitant allergic symptoms, and those intolerant of amitriptyline. Propranolol is effective but can cause lethargy and exacerbation of reactive airways disease. Prophylaxis always should be tapered rather than abruptly discontinued to avoid precipitating a rebound headache. Beta-blockers must always be tapered to avoid rebound hypertension or tachycardia.

**VIII.** In **pseudotumor cerebri**, there is increased intracranial pressure, presumably from an excessive volume of cerebrospinal fluid (CSF). Patients with pseudotumor cerebri have postural headache, vomiting, and papilledema without obstructive hydrocephalus or an intracranial mass. Risk factors include obesity, tetracycline use, cachexia, excessive intake of fat-soluble vitamins, and chronic corticosteroid treatment, especially if tapered too rapidly. Affected individuals may have associated cranial neuropathies, most commonly of the sixth (abducens) or seventh (facial) nerves. LP after appropriate neuroimaging is both diagnostic and therapeutic. Sufficient CSF is drained to bring the CSF pressure to a normal level (<200 mm of water). Untreated patients with pseudotumor cerebri may suffer permanent visual loss or blindness. When symptoms recur after an initial LP, treatment options include agents to decrease CSF production, such as acetazolamide (Diamox) or furosemide (Lasix), or surgical intervention to enhance CSF drainage. Optic nerve fenestration usually is tried first; refractory cases may require lumboperitoneal shunting.

**IX. Referral.** Neurological or neurosurgical consultation should be sought for any child who has headache associated with focal deficits, is under 5 years of age, does not respond to abortive or prophylactic interventions described above, or who has head pain thought to be related to a nonmigrainous etiology, such as pseudotumor, infection, or hemorrhage. Consultation also should be considered in any patient with one or more of the serious symptoms noted in Table 43-1 or with a history of antecedent trauma or neurologic disorder such as seizures.

## Selected Readings

Fenichel GM. *Clinical Pediatric Neurology* (2nd ed). Philadelphia: Saunders, 1992.

Hanson R. Headaches in childhood. *Semin Neurol* 8:1, 1988.

Raskin NH. *Headache*. New York: Churchill Livingstone, 1988.

Singer H. Migraine headaches in childhood. *Pediatr Ann* 21:369, 1992.

# 44

# Febrile Seizures

**Julie Jaskiewicz**

Febrile seizures are defined broadly as seizures caused by or associated with fever. From a clinical perspective, febrile seizures must be subdivided based on their pathogenesis, etiology, and prognosis to manage the patient and educate parents.

**I. Classification.** Febrile seizures are subdivided into three types: complicated febrile seizures (secondary febrile seizures), idiopathic epilepsy triggered by fever, and simple febrile seizures (which constitute the majority). Complicated febrile seizures, or secondary febrile seizures, are those with a recognizable cause, including intracranial infection, exogenous toxins (e.g., *Shigella* or metabolites), and intracranial structural abnormalities (e.g., vascular malformation or tumor).

The most common type of febrile seizure in the pediatric population is simple febrile seizure, which occurs in an otherwise healthy and neurologically normal child between 6 months and 5 years of age. The seizure is generalized, usually lasts less than 15 minutes, and is associated with a febrile illness. Shortly after the seizure, the child is neurologically normal and appears well. Because simple febrile seizures are benign in childhood, making an accurate diagnosis and providing information and reassurance for parents are important.

**II. Evaluation**

**A. EEG and imaging.** No single laboratory test, including an EEG, is able to confirm a seizure's occurrence or prove that a particular seizure was the result of fever. The diagnosis of a seizure is made solely by interpreting the description of the event. An EEG performed immediately after a seizure may be normal, and unless the EEG is extremely abnormal, its usefulness following a single febrile event is limited. Since an EEG does not help distinguish between a first simple febrile seizure and the onset of epilepsy brought about by fever, most neurologists do not recommend an EEG following the first febrile seizure. Likewise, because tumors are an unusual cause of seizures in children, a CT scan or cranial MRI is not indicated in a child with a normal neurologic exam following the first typical simple febrile seizure.

**B. Laboratory.** Searching for the fever's cause with appropriate laboratory tests is warranted and varies according to the child's age and clinical presentation. A CBC, blood culture, urinalysis, and urine culture should be obtained in most children less than 2 years of age. A lumbar puncture should be considered in all children with a febrile seizure, especially in infants (<18 months), if meningitis is suspected. Other laboratory tests, including serum electrolytes, calcium, phosphorus, and magnesium, should be obtained only if an underlying metabolic disorder is suspected.

**III. Natural history.** Simple febrile seizures occur in 3–4% of all children before school entry. The risk is three to four times greater if one parent had febrile seizures. Both the height of fever and the intercurrent illness have an impact on a child's likelihood of having a febrile seizure. In some children with a very low threshold for seizures, even a low-grade fever may trigger a simple febrile seizure. Most children "outgrow" their tendency to have febrile seizures, and the frequency of febrile infections and the height of fever with those infections diminishes with increasing age.

A. **Risk of subsequent simple febrile seizures.** While the risk of a second febrile seizure during the same febrile illness is low, up to 30% of children who have one febrile seizure will have a second one with a subsequent febrile illness. This risk is somewhat greater for children with a family history of seizures if the first febrile seizure occurred before 12 months of age or the seizure was prolonged or complex. Most febrile seizures recur within 6 months of the first seizure. If there is no recurrence within 1 year of the first seizure, the child's risk of a subsequent febrile seizure drops to only 10–15%.

B. **Risk of status epilepticus with febrile seizures.** Status epilepticus associated with fever makes up about one-fourth of all status epilepticus in children. There is no evidence that brain damage is associated with febrile status epilepticus. A neurologically normal child has only a 3% risk of a recurrence of febrile status epilepticus.

C. **Risk of subsequent afebrile seizure disorder (epilepsy).** The child who has a simple febrile seizure has only a slightly increased risk for developing epilepsy (in contrast to the complicated febrile seizure, for which the risk of developing epilepsy is significant). There is also no link between the number of simple febrile seizures a child has and his or her risk of developing epilepsy. Risk factors associated with a higher risk of epilepsy in a child with a febrile seizure are a prolonged (>15 minutes) febrile seizure; atypical or focal seizure; two or more seizures in 1 day; a parent or sibling with epilepsy; and underlying neurologic problems, developmental delay, or both. All of these factors exclude the diagnosis of simple febrile seizure and change the category of febrile seizure to complicated seizures (secondary seizures), which have an increased risk for subsequent epilepsy.

IV. **Management.** The mainstay of managing febrile seizures is to differentiate the type of febrile seizure, determine the cause of fever, promptly treat any specific inciting event, and educate parents.

A. **Reassurance.** With simple febrile seizures, the benign nature of the event and the lack of progression to epilepsy should be emphasized. In most cases, primary care physicians are well-suited to manage simple febrile seizures in the office. Some parents may be particularly anxious and frightened by the seizure, especially recurrent febrile seizures, and referral to a neurologist may be warranted on occasion primarily to ease parental concerns.

B. **Medication.** Treatment of simple febrile seizures with anticonvulsant medication is not appropriate because the side effects of medication often outweigh the benefits. Only two anticonvulsant medications—phenobarbital and sodium valproate—have been effective in preventing the recurrence of febrile seizures. Phenobarbital has significant side effects in up to 40% of children, including irritability, sleep disturbance, hyperactivity, and learning and concentration problems. Sodium valproate is not recommended for any child less than 2 years of age, given the significant incidence of fatal liver failure associated with its use in this age group (up to 1 out of 800).

Parents vary in their ability to tolerate repeated episodes of febrile seizures in their children. Occasionally, rectal diazepam (0.5 mg/kg q8h) during a febrile illness for temperature higher than 38.5°C may be recommended. Some physicians prescribe prophylaxis to children who had neurologic abnormalities before their first febrile seizure, especially to children at risk for febrile status epilepticus.

V. **Outcome.** Simple febrile seizures in young children are usually benign. The greatest risk from a first simple febrile seizure is an increased chance of having a second simple febrile seizure, and even then, the consequences of a second or multiple febrile seizures are minimal. Children with a simple febrile seizure do not have an increased likelihood of death, brain damage, or learning or behavior disorders. One of the greatest morbidities may be the family's fear and anxiety about dangerous effects on the child. Education and reassurance are therefore critical.

## Selected Readings

Freeman JM, Vining EPG. Decision-making and the child with febrile seizures. *Pediatr Rev* 13:298, 1992.

Gerber MA, Berliner BC. The child with a "simple" febrile seizure. *Am J Dis Child* 135:431, 1981.

Wallace SJ. *The Child with Febrile Seizures*. London: Wright, 1988.

Weiner HL, Bresnan MJ, Levitt LP. *Pediatric Neurology for the Houseofficer* (2nd ed). Baltimore: Williams & Wilkins, 1982.

H

# Hematologic Disorders

# 45

# Iron Deficiency


## Omer G. Berger


Iron deficiency occurs when the amount of iron in the body is less than required for the normal formation of hemoglobin, iron enzymes, and other functioning iron compounds. Iron deficiency remains the most prevalent nutritional disease worldwide. Although iron status in children has been improving, iron deficiency is the most common nutritional deficiency state in the age group 9 months to 3 years.

I. **Pathogenesis.** Iron deficiency in infants is due to rapid growth and a low-iron diet. Iron stores are depleted by 4–6 months in full-term infants and by 2–3 months in premature infants. Perinatal blood loss and exchange transfusions increase the risk of iron deficiency. The typical iron-deficient child is 12–24 months old and consumes cow's milk or juice for the majority of his or her calories. Iron deficiency is rare in a term infant taking iron-fortified formula.

II. **Signs and symptoms of iron deficiency.** Severe iron deficiency may result in anemia with pallor, fatigue, and anorexia. Most children have iron deficiency without anemia, which may result in irritability, decreased attention span, and other developmental disturbances presumably due to depleted iron-containing enzymes and dopamine receptors.

III. **Diagnosis.** Hemoglobin and hematocrit measurements are the usual screening methods for iron-deficiency anemia. Electronic measurement of RBC indices has improved the CBC's sensitivity in detecting iron deficiency without anemia. In the office or clinic, diagnosis can be made using the CBC, RBC indices, and the red blood cell distribution width (RDW), followed by a therapeutic trial of iron. The most sensitive and specific test is serum ferritin.

IV. **Stages of iron deficiency.** Iron deficiency is staged based on the following laboratory test values (Table 45-1): ferritin, percent transferrin saturation, zinc protoporphyrin, hemoglobin, and RDW.

V. **Prevention and treatment.** In full-term infants, preventing iron deficiency is ensured by feeding children human milk or iron-supplemented formula for the first year, with intake of iron-containing solid foods at appropriate times. After age 6 months, breast-fed infants should receive supplemental iron, 1 mg/kg/day. Iron-enriched cereal should be a child's first solid food.

In premature infants, iron stores may be depleted by 2 months. Iron sulfate drops, 2 mg/kg/day of elemental iron divided bid, should be added until adequate dietary iron intake is established.

For infants and toddlers with confirmed iron deficiency, treatment with iron sulfate drops should be started at 3–4 mg/kg/day of elemental iron divided bid. A full dropper (0.6 ml) of iron sulfate drops contains 15 mg of elemental iron; therefore, a 10-kg child should receive 0.6 ml of iron sulfate drops

**Table 45-1. Stages of iron deficiency**

| | Normal | Iron depletion | Iron-deficiency anemia |
|---|---|---|---|
| Ferritin (ng/ml) | >12 | <12 | <12 |
| Transferrin saturation (%) | >12 | >12 | <12 |
| Zinc protoporphyrin (μg/dl whole blood) | 60 | 60 | >85 |
| Hemoglobin (g/dl) | 11.5 | 11.5 | <11 |
| Red blood cell distribution width (%) | <14.5 | >14.5 | >14.5 |

(one full dropper) twice daily. After 5 days, hemoglobin increases 0.25 g/day until a normal level is attained. Treatment should continue 2–3 months to allow iron stores to reaccumulate.

## Selected Readings

Beutler E. The common anemias. *JAMA* 259:2433, 1987.

Lozoff B, Jimenez E, Wolf AW. Long term developmental outcome of infants with iron deficiency. *N Engl J Med* 325:687, 1991.

Oski FA. Iron deficiency in infancy and childhood. *N Engl J Med* 329:190, 1993.

Yip R, Binkin JJ, Fleshood L et al. Declining prevalence of anemia among low-income children in the United States. *JAMA* 258:1619, 1987.

# Lead Poisoning in Childhood: Screening and Evaluation

## Omer G. Berger

In 1991, the Centers for Disease Control (CDC) defined an elevated blood lead level (PbB) as a confirmed concentration of lead in whole blood of 10 μg/dl or more. Older buildings and houses in poor condition with interior and exterior lead-based paint represent a significant hazard to children, especially children with compulsive hand-to-mouth behavior. Those at highest risk for lead poisoning are children age 6–36 months who live in or frequent old (pre-1960), dilapidated housing and children living in older housing undergoing renovation. Also at risk are children with parents or household members who work in lead-related industries who may bring lead home on their clothing and children with siblings with known lead toxicity.

**I. Screening**

**A.** All children need a lead risk assessment at age 6 months based on the above risk factors. If they are at high risk, a PbB should be obtained. If the PbB is less than 10 μg/dl, the infant is retested in 6 months; if the PbB is greater than 10 μg/dl, the infant should be retested every 3 months until the PbB declines.

**B.** If at low risk by history, lead testing should begin at 12 months of age. If the PbB is less than 10 μg/dl, the child is retested at age 24 months.

**C.** For children older than 36 months, the PbB is rechecked annually if elevated or if previous PbBs have exceeded 15 μg/dl.

**II. Classification and recommended action.** Lead intoxication is classified according to PbBs and divided into management stages (Table 46-1).

**III. Management**

**A. Class IIB**. Retest the child within 1 month (venous blood is preferred). Finding the lead source is key; contact the local health department for advice and action. Advise a low-fat diet high in calcium, iron, and zinc. Advise vitamins with iron and weaning the child from the bottle. Discuss pica and hazard reduction (e.g., reducing exposure to lead paint and lead-contaminated dust).

**B. Class III**. Retest the child with a venous sample within 1 week. Contact the health department and consider consultation with or referral to a lead clinic. Assess the child for signs and symptoms of lead toxicity (e.g., periodic vomiting, frequent falling, and ataxia). Symptomatic children should be removed from their environment and chelation therapy considered.

**C. Class IV**. Retest the child immediately. If he or she is symptomatic, refer for immediate consultation and chelation therapy.

**Table 46-1. Blood lead classification and management**

| Class | Blood lead (μg/dl) | Action |
|---|---|---|
| I | ≤9 | None |
| IIA | 10–14 | Retest the child according to risk assessment. |
| IIB | 15–19 | Take child's history to assess lead source; educate parents and patient regarding diet, cleaning, etc.; consider iron deficiency. |
| III | 20–44* | Complete medical evaluation; initiate nursing and environmental assessment. |
| IV | 45–69* | Begin medical treatment and environmental assessment within 48 hrs. |
| V | >70 | Admit the child for chelation therapy. |

*Confirmed (venous sample preferred).

**D. Class V.** Admit the child for chelation therapy immediately; an assessment of the child's environment and remediation should be performed.

IV. **Prevention** is clearly the best treatment for lead poisoning. The physician should ask about pica behavior and note excessive hand-to-mouth activity, such as thumb- or finger-sucking and fingernail biting. It is important for the physician to be certain that patients and parents are aware of the danger of lead toxicity and screened if at risk.

## Selected Readings

Centers for Disease Control. Preventing lead poisoning in young children. Atlanta: Centers for Disease Control, October 1991.

Committee on Environmental Health, American Academy of Pediatrics. Lead poisoning: From screening to primary prevention. *Pediatrics* 92:176, 1993.

Schonfeld D. New developments in pediatric lead poisoning. *Curr Opin Pediatr* 5:537, 1993.

47

# Sickle Cell Disease Episodes and Infections

Paul S. Bellet

I. **Sickle episodes** are classified as vaso-occlusive, sequestration, and aplastic.

A. **Vaso-occlusive sickle episodes** are due to intravascular sickling and commonly involve the bones, lungs, brain, and penis.

1. **Bone pain.** The most common vaso-occlusive sickle episode is acute bone pain. Usually, there are no physical findings, but local tenderness, swelling, and warmth may occur. In children less than 5 years of age, painful swelling of the small bones of the hands, feet, or both (dactylitis) is common. If the bone is involved near a joint, a joint effusion may occur; however, septic arthritis also should be considered. If fever occurs with bone tenderness, bone infarction is mostly likely, but osteomyelitis also should be considered.

Pain management must be individualized. Many painful episodes can be managed at home with oral analgesics. Doses described are initial starting doses; subsequent doses can be titrated up or down as needed. Mild pain may be managed with acetaminophen, 15 mg/kg PO q4h. Mild to moderate pain may be managed with acetaminophen and codeine (1 mg/kg PO q4h); a nonsteroidal anti-inflammatory drug (NSAID), such as naproxen (5 mg/kg PO tid or 250 mg PO q6–8h) or ibuprofen (10 mg/kg PO q4–6h or 400–600 mg PO q4–6h); or a combination of acetaminophen, codeine, and a NSAID.

For moderate to severe pain, oxycodone and acetaminophen (Tylox), ketorolac, oral morphine, sustained-release oral morphine (MS Contin), or oral hydromorphone hydrochloride (Dilaudid) may be used. The dose of Tylox is one capsule PO q6h for children 8–12 years of age, and 1–2 capsules PO q6h for those older than 12 years of age. Ketorolac may be given 30–60 mg IV as a loading dose and then 30 mg IV q6h in the hospital. It can be used with around-the-clock morphine or with prn rescue doses of morphine or patient-controlled analgesia (PCA). It also can be given 10 mg PO q6h; morphine, 0.2 mg/kg PO q3h, can be used as a rescue dose if needed. MS Contin can be used in patients with prolonged pain episodes and should be given around-the-clock q8–12h; the usual dose is 30 mg PO q8h. In a child less than 12 years of age, a lower dose may be given, such as 15 mg PO q8h, depending on his or her tolerance and experience with morphine sulfate. Oral Dilaudid may be given in a dose of 0.05-0.10 mg/kg PO q3h.

For severe pain, the episode may be treated in the emergency department with morphine sulfate (0.15 mg/kg IV or IM q3h). If morphine is not well-tolerated, Dilaudid (0.05 mg/kg IV or IM q3h) is an alternative; in an adolescent, this dose is usually 2–3 mg/dose. Demerol (1.0-1.5 mg/kg IM or IV q3–4h) is only used if the patient cannot tolerate morphine or Dilaudid. The usual IV fluid is D5 1/2 normal saline at 1.0–1.5 times maintenance as cardiopulmonary and renal status allow. The importance and necessity of IV hydration in an older sickle cell patient with an uncomplicated pain episode who is not dehydrated and able to take oral fluids are not well established. It is acceptable to hydrate orally and give parenteral narcotics while determining whether hospitalization is necessary. If the pain is not relieved sufficiently following one or two doses of parenteral morphine, the patient usually requires hospital admission.

2. **Acute chest syndrome.** An acute illness characterized by chest pain and pulmonary infiltrate on the chest radiograph is referred to as acute chest syndrome. Fever is a variable finding. This syndrome has been attributed to pneumonia, pulmonary infarction, pulmonary thromboembolism, fat emboli from necrotic bone marrow, and rib infarction. Children with acute chest syndrome may become hypoxic and extremely ill. In general, a CBC, reticulocyte count, blood culture, chest radiograph, and measurement of oxygen saturation by pulse oximeter should be performed. Management consists of IV fluids; effective analgesia; antibiotics if febrile; and close monitoring of vital signs, pulmonary status, and oxygenation. A patient with suspected acute chest syndrome should be admitted to the hospital.
3. **Acute CNS event.** Acute vaso-occlusion in the brain can result in a potentially fatal cerebrovascular accident, which may occur spontaneously or accompanying a painful episode, viral infection, pneumonia, dehydration, aplastic episode, or priapism. Common neurologic signs are hemiplegia, seizures, speech defects, visual disturbances, and coma. The management of a CNS event in sickle cell disease involves the following: (1) CT scan to diagnose a ruptured cerebral aneurysm or other intracranial hemorrhage, (2) exchange transfusion or RBC apheresis on the ward as quickly as possible to reduce hemoglobin S (Hb S) below 30% of total hemoglobin, (3) an MRI and magnetic resonance angiography when the patient is stable for further characterization of the lesions, and (4) possible cerebral angiography. Chronic transfusion therapy given once a month to keep the Hb S level below 30% has been successful in reducing the risk of recurrent stroke.
4. **Priapism** can occur in males of all ages. The penis becomes swollen, edematous, and tender, and urination may be difficult. Management for the first 24 hours includes pain control, IV hydration, and a urinary catheter placed for inability to void. If there is no

improvement, nifedipine, 10 mg PO q8h for 1–2 days, may be given. If this fails, a packed RBC transfusion to raise the hemoglobin level to 9–10 g/dl should be given. If no improvement occurs, an exchange transfusion should be performed to reduce Hb S to less than 30% of total hemoglobin.

B. **Acute splenic sequestration** may be a fatal complication in children with homozygous sickle cell disease (Hb SS), sickle cell-hemoglobin C disease (Hb SC), or sickle-beta zero thalassemia disease (Hb S-$B^0$). The usual age of presentation in a child with Hb SS or Hb S-$B^0$ is 1–3 years. In a child with Hb SC, acute sequestration may develop at 4–7 years of age or as late as 12–13 years of age. The spleen massively enlarges, trapping a considerable portion of the RBC mass and possibly leading rapidly to hypotension and shock. The hematocrit level is low, and there is thrombocytopenia and reticulocytosis with an increase in nucleated RBCs. The immediate goal of treatment is to expand intravascular volume with crystalloid and then transfuse with packed RBCs. If available, whole blood may be given to expand intravascular volume and increase the blood's oxygen-carrying capacity. Usually, the spleen becomes smaller in a few days, and thrombocytopenia resolves. Monthly transfusions may be given for 6–12 months following the first episode to prevent subsequent episodes.

Sequestration may also occur in the liver. The usual clinical features are liver enlargement, hyperbilirubinemia, severe anemia, and marked reticulocytosis. Because the liver is not as distensible as the spleen, there is rarely pooling of RBCs significant enough to cause cardiovascular collapse.

C. **Aplastic episodes** are usually due to intercurrent viral or bacterial infections. Human parvovirus infection has been associated with aplastic episodes. Fatigue or dyspnea may occur due to a progressive fall in the hematocrit level without compensatory reticulocytosis. Most of these crises are mild and short and require no therapy. When the reticulocyte count is 0, the hemoglobin level can decrease 0.5-1.0 g/dl/day. Close follow-up is essential if the patient does not receive a transfusion, which may be required if anemia becomes severe (Hb $<5$ g/dl).

II. **Infection** is the most common cause of death in children with sickle cell anemia. This is due to increased susceptibility to infection secondary to abnormal opsonic activity, which results from functional asplenia. Functional asplenia regularly occurs in children with sickle anemia during the first year of life. Common infections in sickle cell disease include septicemia (*Streptococcus pneumoniae*, *Haemophilus influenzae* type b, *Escherichia coli*), meningitis (*S. pneumoniae* and *H. influenzae*), pneumonia (*S. pneumoniae, H. influenzae, Mycoplasma pneumoniae*), urinary tract infection (*E. coli*, *Klebsiella*), osteomyelitis and septic arthritis (*Staphylococcus aureus*, *S. pneumoniae*, *Salmonella* species), and dysentery (*Salmonella* and *Shigella* species). Sickle cell patients who present with a known infection or fever should be seen promptly by a physician because their risk of septicemia is 300 times higher than that of the normal population. The common occurrence of fever with no obvious source in young children with sickle cell disease makes the distinction between serious bacterial infections and benign, self-limited viral infections a difficult problem.

On presentation with significant fever (>101° F), the child with Hb SS or Hb S-B thalassemia ($B^0$ or $B^+$) should have a CBC, reticulocyte count, and blood culture performed. In most cases, ceftriaxone, 50 mg/kg IV or IM, should be given even before any test results are available or other studies performed (e.g., urinalysis, urine culture, x-ray). The decision to hospitalize a child is based on the child's age, clinical appearance, height of fever, change in hematologic values from their steady state, recent compliance with prophylaxis vaccines and penicillin therapy, and the parents' ability to return promptly if the child's condition deteriorates. Most patients without a known source of infection managed as outpatients are given amoxicillin, 40 mg/kg/day PO tid, for at least 3 days until blood culture results are known. Every child should be reexamined the following day. Prophylactic penicillin should be begun when the antibiotic is finished.

Children with Hb SC are at increased risk for septicemia, although not as much as those with Hb SS. (One reason is that the spleen remains functional for a longer period of time [the first 3–4 years of age] in patients with Hb SC.) It is controversial whether Hb SC patients should be on daily penicillin.

Patients with Hb S-$B^+$ thalassemia probably have only a slightly increased predisposition to infection with *S. pneumoniae*. The indications for hospitalization are the same as those for children without hemoglobin abnormality (e.g., meningitis, significant pneumonia).

## Selected Readings

Gill FM. Sickle Cell Disease. In MW Schwartz (ed), *Principles and Practice of Clinical Pediatrics*. Chicago: Year Book, 1987.

Lampkin BC, Gruppo RA, Lobel JS et al. Pediatric and oncologic emergencies. *Emerg Med Clin North Am* 1:63, 1983.

Platt OS, Dover DJ. Sickle Cell Disease. In DG Nathan, FA Oski (eds), *Hematology of Infancy and Childhood* (4th ed). Philadelphia: Saunders, 1993.

Rogers ZR, Morrison RA, Vedro DA et al. Outpatient management of febrile illness in infants and young children with sickle cell anemia. *J Pediatr* 117:736, 1990.

# I

# Medicolegal Issues

# Physical Abuse

Robert A. Shapiro

Child abuse is a problem virtually all primary care physicians encounter in their practice. Physicians are required by state laws to report suspected physical abuse or neglect to the legally mandated agency in their community. Although the legal definition of child abuse varies from state to state, the accepted medical meaning of physical abuse includes any injury to or death of a child less than 18 years of age resulting from the intentional commission of an act(s) by the child's caretaker. The commonly accepted medical meaning of neglect includes any injury to, suffering of, or death of a child younger than 18 years old resulting from the omission of an act(s) by the child's caretaker.

I. **Statistics.** In 1993, there were nearly 3 million reports of alleged child abuse—that is, 45 reports for each 1,000 children in the United States. More than 1 million of those reports were verified as abuse by children's protective agencies. Twenty-five percent of the reports were for physical abuse; 47% were for neglect. There were 1,299 documented deaths in the United States due to child abuse in 1993.

II. **Risk factors for abuse and neglect.** Young children are the most frequent victims of physical abuse and neglect because of their greater dependence on adults compared to older children. The likelihood of abuse increases for children born prematurely, with mental or physical handicaps, with temperamental or needy behavior, or living in dysfunctional families. Caretakers are more likely to abuse children if they were abused or neglected as children, are isolated, are impulsive, have poor parenting skills, have unrealistic expectations for their children, are substance abusers, or suffer from mental illness. Awareness of risk factors for abuse in families can enable the physician to maintain increased vigilance. Abuse is often diagnosed, however, in families in which specific risk factors are absent.

III. **History.** The history should document the circumstances surrounding any suspicious injury, including how, when, where, and with whom the injury occurred. Abuse should be suspected whenever the history (1) is inconsistent with the degree or mechanism of trauma, (2) is incompatible with the child's developmental abilities, or (3) changes by the historian, who is "fishing" for a valid explanation. Fictitious histories are likely to be incomplete and may contain conflicting details. Abuse should be considered when a caretaker claims no knowledge of how an infant's injuries occurred.

IV. **Specific injuries.** The physician must be aware of unusual injuries that are the hallmarks of physical abuse, including the following:

A. **Bruises** are the most common type of injury resulting from physical abuse. There are distinguishing differences between accidental and inflicted bruises. Accidental bruises most commonly occur over body areas that lack "padding," such as the forehead, elbows, iliac crests, knees, and shins. Inflicted bruises are often found on the more "fleshy" parts of the body, such as the cheeks, abdomen, flanks, buttocks, and thighs. The physician should suspect abuse if the child has a large number of bruises over different areas of the body of different ages. Young, nonambulatory children should not have bruises without a reasonable explanation. Loop marks, indicating beating with a belt or cord, hand imprints, bite marks, and trauma from other recognizable objects all strongly suggest abuse.

Color photographs of the injuries should be obtained if abuse is suspected; parental consent is not required. Sketches should be made in the chart documenting the bruises' locations, sizes, shapes, and colors. It is not possible to determine the exact age of a bruise by its appearance, but its color provides a general guide to its degree of healing (Table 48-1).

**B. Fractures**. In the nonambulatory infant, any fracture should alert the physician to the possibility of abuse. The physician should suspect child abuse in children who present with rib, metaphyseal, and scapular fractures. Fractures resulting from allegedly minor trauma and multiple fractures of various ages are typical findings in the abused child. The presence and degree of callous about the fracture site dates a fracture.

**C. Burns.** The burn's appearance usually provides clues as to its cause (e.g., hot water, grease, cigarettes). Water burns from immersion cause a "glove and stocking" distribution on an extremity, and scalds (as from dipping in hot water) on other parts of the body (e.g., buttocks) are clearly demarcated with sharp borders. Grease burns show a "dripping" or "running" pattern down the skin and often are accompanied by smaller "splatter" burns around the burn site. Cigarette burns are round and have the same diameter as a cigarette. Table 48-2 lists the time required to cause a third-degree burn in adults exposed to water at different temperatures.

**D. Abdominal trauma** results from direct blows to the abdomen. Initially, signs of injury may be minimal. Specific injuries include liver lacerations, splenic rupture, traumatic pancreatitis and pseudocyst, and duodenal hematomas.

**E. Human bites** must be distinguished from animal bites, which are usually smaller. The trauma from animal teeth will be deeper and narrower compared to that of a human and often causes a ripping type of injury. Bites from adult humans are oval in shape, whereas bites from children are circular. If impressions from the upper canines are present, the distance between them should be measured. A distance of greater than 3 cm indicates that the bite was caused by someone older than 8 years old. Bites should be photographed using a high-quality 35-mm camera, and a tape measure should be included in the camera field so that accurate measurements can be made at a later time. If the bite is fresh and the skin has not yet been washed, saliva from the perpetrator may be present. The skin around the bite should be swabbed with a moistened sterile swab,

**Table 48-1. Color of healing bruises**

| Color | Approximate age of bruise |
|---|---|
| Red or blue | 0–5 days |
| Green | 5–7 days |
| Yellow | 7–10 days |
| Brown | 10–14 days |
| Resolved | 14–28 days |

**Table 48-2. Length of time to cause third-degree burns from water in adults**

| Water temperature (°F) | Time to cause third-degree burn |
|---|---|
| 120 | 10 min |
| 122 | 5 min |
| 127 | 1 min |
| 130 | 30 sec |
| 140 | 5 sec |
| 150 | 2 sec |

Source: Adapted from M Katcher. Scald burns from hot tap water. *JAMA* 246:1219, 1981.

which should be placed into a paper envelope (not plastic) and labeled with the patient's name and description of the specimen's source. The envelope must be locked in a secure location until it is given to the police.

F. **Head injury.** The greatest cause of morbidity and mortality from child abuse is inflicted head injury, which may occur after blunt trauma or as the result of severe shaking ("shaken baby syndrome"). Presenting signs include altered mental status, irritability, seizures, or respiratory arrest. Signs of external injury are frequently absent in shaken baby syndrome, but 80% of shaken children have retinal hemorrhages. A CT scan of the head or MRI is diagnostic. Head ultrasound is inadequate for the diagnosis.

V. **Evaluation.** A platelet count, prothrombin time, partial thromboplastin time, and bleeding time should be determined in children with significant bruising to rule out a bleeding diathesis. Abused children younger than 2 years old also should have a skeletal survey to look for occult fractures, which should include at least two views of each long bone, the skull, and the spine. A so-called babygram is inadequate. A bone scan can augment information obtained by the skeletal survey and is particularly good for diagnosing rib fractures. Young children with any neurologic abnormalities or retinal hemorrhages in whom shaken baby syndrome is being considered require a MRI or CT scan of the head. If there is any abdominal tenderness or bruising, SGOT, SGPT, and amylase levels should be obtained in addition to appropriate imaging. The physician also must consider diagnoses other than abuse and perform the appropriate work-up to exclude a medical explanation for the injuries found.

**VI. Reporting.** Physicians are required to report all cases of suspected child abuse to the local child protective services (CPS) or the police. The physician need not accuse the family of abuse but should notify them of his or her concerns and that he or she is required by law to make a report. The physician should inform the family using statements such as the following: *"Your child's injuries seem too severe to have been caused by the incident you are describing. I am concerned that someone may be hurting your child. Do you have any of these same concerns?"*

If the examining physician believes that by notifying the family the child's safety may be jeopardized, the CPS social worker should be informed first. In all cases, the initial report is phoned to the CPS social worker and followed by a complete written report. The report should describe the injuries observed, the history given, and the reason for the report. Nonmedical terminology should be used throughout the report so that social workers, police officers, and lawyers can understand the findings and concerns. Physicians are immune from civil or criminal law suits brought by the family for making reports of alleged child abuse if the report is made in good faith.

**VII. Follow-up**. The physician must maintain objectivity throughout the investigation and be available to social workers and police for questions. Court testimony also may be necessary.

**VIII. Disposition.** Once abuse is suspected, the child must be protected from further harm. The CPS social worker is responsible for the child's safety and must secure safe placement. If the child's home is unsafe and no other arrangements can be made by the CPS social worker, the child can be admitted to the hospital. Some states allow the physician to place a temporary "medical hold" on a child's discharge; other states require an order by a juvenile court judge.

## Selected Readings

Kleinman P. *Diagnostic Imaging of Child Abuse*. Baltimore: Williams & Wilkins, 1987.

Ludwig S, Kornbert A. *Child Abuse: A Medical Reference* (2nd ed). New York: Churchill Livingstone, 1992.

Reece R. *Child Abuse: Medical Diagnosis and Management*. Philadelphia: Lea & Febiger, 1994.

# Sexual Abuse

Robert A. Shapiro

Sexual abuse is the exploitation or involvement of a child in sexual activities. Sexual activities include but are not limited to exposure, fondling, and genital contact. Statutory rape in Ohio is defined as sexual intercourse with a child younger than 14 years old by a person 18 years old or older, but the definition varies somewhat from state to state.

I. **Statistics.** The prevalence of sexual abuse is difficult to determine because much remains undiagnosed. In 1994, there were 750,000 reports of sexual abuse filed in the United States. Sexual abuse has been diagnosed in children of all ages, races, and socioeconomic groups. The perpetrator is often a male family member, family friend, or neighbor who has access to or authority over the child.

II. **Presentation**. Children who have been sexually abused may act out sexual behaviors, experience sleep disturbances, develop phobias, perform poorly in school, or regress in their behavior. They may complain of genital-rectal symptoms, such as pain, itching, redness, discharge, bleeding, enuresis, or encopresis. Even though sexual abuse may have been ongoing for months or years before diagnosis, however, many children have no behavior changes or physical complaints. Children may be brought to the physician for evaluation of sexual abuse because of nonspecific family concerns or recent disclosure by the child of abuse. If a report has been made to the children's protective services (CPS), a CPS social worker may ask that the child be examined as part of an investigation.

III. **History**. The purpose of the interview is to collect information that validates the history of abuse, determine what testing needs to be done, and begin the healing process for the child. Children who previously have been interviewed by a CPS social worker will not need as complete an interview as children being seen for the first time. The history should be obtained in a calm, relaxed, and accepting manner. Before referring to body parts, the physician should ask the child or caregiver what words he or she uses when referring to the genitalia and rectum. The physician should encourage the child to tell the story himself or herself without asking prompting or leading questions. During the interview, it is important to tell the child that disclosing the abuse is the right thing to do and that you will work to prevent the abuse from happening again. If the perpetrator is a family member or a close friend, the physician should be aware that the child's parents may not want to believe that the abuse has occurred. If parental support is lacking, the child may recant because of family pressures. The history should be documented thoroughly in the child's chart, and statements made by the child should be delineated with quotation marks.

**IV. Forensic evidence**

**A.** If the sexual assault occurred less than 72 hours ago *and* the history suggests that seminal fluid, pubic hair, saliva, or blood belonging to the perpetrator might be recovered from the patient's body, forensic specimen collection is required. The physician should refer the patient immediately to an emergency facility or similar site capable of forensic evidence collection. It is important to instruct the patient not to bathe or change clothes prior to the examination.

**B.** If there is no possibility of forensic material being present and no acute injury is present, the physical examination can be scheduled at a convenient time and place. Children with acute injuries should be evaluated as soon as possible to assess and document the degree of injury and need for treatment.

**V. Examination.** The purpose of the examination is to look for supporting evidence of sexual abuse, screen for sexually transmitted diseases (STDs), and reassure the child and his or her parents or other care providers.

**A. Examining the genitalia**

**1. Prepubertal female.** Examine the external genitalia for signs of injury and infection. Assure the child that nothing will be placed inside her vagina and that the examination will not hurt. Position the girl in a supine position with her knees out and soles together (frog leg position) or in a knee-chest position. The child can lie on an examination table or sit on the caregiver's lap, whichever makes her most comfortable. Examine the perineum for injuries, condylomata, herpetic lesions, bruises, tears, or discharge. Visualize the hymen by holding onto the labia majora with the thumb and forefinger of each hand and retracting them laterally and outward (toward the examiner). When done properly, the introitis will open, and the inner hymeneal ring will be visible. A vaginal speculum is contraindicated in most prepubertal examinations. Examine the hymen for indications of trauma. The inner hymeneal ring should be smooth and uninterrupted, although there may be congenital clefts at the 3 and 9 o'clock positions. Many girls have a crescent-shaped hymen with little or no hymen between 10 and 2 o'clock. Look for injuries, such as tears and scars, or absence of the hymeneal tissue. If the horizontal opening through the hymen appears to be large for age, look carefully for signs of injury to the lateral hymeneal edges. An enlarged hymeneal opening without signs of trauma should not be considered indicative of vaginal penetration.

Less than 10% of prepubertal girls have genital findings that are clear evidence for sexual abuse, 15% have findings that are suggestive but not diagnostic of abuse, 50% have nonspecific findings, and 30% have normal genital examination findings.

**2. Pubertal female.** Inspect the external genitalia for acute injury, condylomata, herpes, and lice. If possible, perform an internal speculum and bimanual examina-

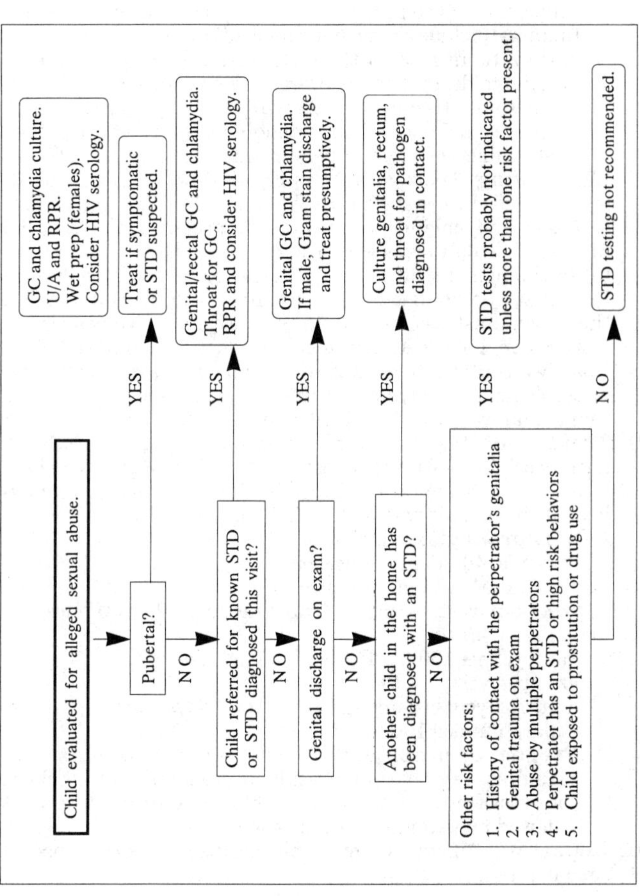


**Fig. 49-1. Algorithm for testing for sexually transmitted diseases.**

tion and obtain routine cultures for STDs. Findings suggestive of hymeneal injury can be confused easily with normal adolescent anatomy, as virginal adolescents can have redundant folds and notching of the hymen.

3. **Male.** Inspect the genitalia for infection or injury.

B. **Examining the rectum**. Examine the rectum for trauma, including scars, bruising, or tears. Normal or nonspecific findings include anal tags, thick or smooth skin in the midline, anal gaping with stool in the rectal vault, flattened or thickened anal folds, fissures, and delayed venous congestion of the perianal tissues. Suspicious or suggestive findings include immediate anal dilatation of 15 mm or more without stool in the rectal vault, distorted or irregular anal folds, immediate or extensive venous congestion of the perianal tissues, and scarring in the perianal area. A deep perianal laceration extending beyond the external anal sphincter indicates penetrating trauma.

VI. **STD testing.** The algorithm in Fig. 49-1 will assist in deciding when to culture for STDs. When obtaining *Neisseria gonorrhoeae* and chlamydia cultures in prepubertal girls, the highest yield culture is from the mucosa just proximal or distal to the hymen with type I Calgiswabs (moisten the swabs first in sterile nonbacteriostatic saline). In pubertal females, the cervix must be cultured. Presumptive positive gonococcal cultures on Thayer-Martin medium must be confirmed by at least two confirmatory tests (biochemical, enzyme substrate, or serologic). Chlamydia cultures should be obtained because rapid chlamydia tests are inadequate for legal evidence.

VII. **Treatment.** Prepubertal children do not require prophylactic antimicrobial treatment unless infection is thought to be likely. Adolescents should be offered STD and pregnancy prophylaxis if the assault was within 72 hours of treatment.

A. **STD prophylaxis** includes:
cefixime, 400 mg PO once, *or*
ceftriaxone, 125 mg IM once, *or*
spectinomycin, 40 mg/kg (maximum dose 2 g) IM once
*plus*
doxycycline, 100 mg PO bid for 7 days, *or*
azithromycin, 1 g PO once, *or*
erythromycin, 10 mg/kg PO qid for 7 days (for prepubertal children under 100 lb).

B. **Pregnancy prophylaxis** should be offered in all cases of sexual assault that may result in pregnancy. Prophylaxis consists of two Ovral tablets within 72 hours of the assault followed by two more 12 hours later.

VIII. **Reporting.** All states require physicians to report suspected sexual abuse.

## Selected Readings

Heger A, Emans S. *Evaluation of the Sexually Abused Child. A Medical Textbook and Photographic Atlas*. New York: Oxford University Press, 1992.

# 50

# Ethical Issues in the Outpatient Setting

Christine L. McHenry

Ethics is a systematic reflection about right character, right conduct, or both in a given situation. Ethics uses principles, rules, virtues, and values as guides in this systematic reflection. When these principles, rules, virtues, or values conflict, an ethical dilemma results.

It is fairly easy to recognize ethical dilemmas in areas where medical technology is used, such in as the newborn intensive care unit or the pediatric intensive care unit, and where questions about withholding or withdrawing life-sustaining treatment arise. Health care providers tend not to recognize ethical dilemmas as frequently on a general pediatric ward or in the outpatient department, however. Nevertheless, ethical dilemmas do exist in these areas, and health care providers must be sensitive to their possibilities. This chapter addresses several issues that pertain both to the inpatient and outpatient arenas.

I. **Informed consent** is based on the ethical principles of respect for autonomy, beneficence, and nonmaleficence. Everyone has the right to informed consent.
   A. **The process of informed consent** consists of the following components:
      1. A competent individual as the decision maker (either patient or surrogate decision-maker)
      2. Disclosure of information to the competent individual, including the following examples:
         a. The patient's condition, including diagnosis and prognosis
         b. The nature and purpose of the proposed treatment
         c. The risks and benefits of the proposed treatment
         d. Alternative treatments
         e. Consequences if the proposed treatment is not accepted
         f. Names of the health professionals who are to perform any procedure
      3. Understanding of the information by the decision maker
      4. Voluntary agreement by the decision maker
      5. Authorization by the decision maker
   B. **Exemptions to informed consent**. The following are exemptions to informed consent.
      1. **Emergencies** (e.g., an unconscious person in need of medical treatment brought to the emergency department)
      2. **Waivers** (e.g., a competent patient or surrogate decision-maker who specifically says he or she does not want to know)
      3. **Therapeutic privilege** (e.g., a physician who intentionally withholds information from a patient with cancer because the physician thinks the information may harm the patient. This exception is *very controversial* and should not be used frivolously.)

**II. Religious exemptions**. The First Amendment of the Constitution grants religious freedom. This religious freedom is freedom of belief and practice as long as the practice does not infringe on the rights of or potentially harm an innocent third party. In general, competent adult patients have the right to reject recommended treatment based on religious or other convictions. A dilemma arises, however, when parents reject recommended treatment for their child based on their own religious convictions. Parents are required to provide "adequate" medical care for their children or face potential criminal charges under state child abuse and neglect statutes. The definition of "adequate" varies from situation to situation.

**A. Religious exemptions for treatment**. When parents refuse medical treatment for their child based on religious conviction, a conflict arises between wanting to respect the parents' wishes to raise their child according to their religious beliefs and doing what the health care provider believes is in the best medical interest of the child. How this conflict is resolved depends on the nature of the illness (minor versus life-threatening), prognosis with and without recommended treatment, and the nature of the recommended treatment (conventional versus experimental).

**B. Religious exemptions for immunizations**. When parents bring their healthy child to a physician for a well-child visit and refuse immunizations based on religious convictions, preserving the physician's relationship with the parents should take precedence over trying to coerce them into agreeing to the immunizations. The physician should use this time to educate parents about the recommended immunizations. If this is done in a nonthreatening manner, parents are more likely to bring their child back to the physician for medical care. If, on the other hand, there is an epidemic of a preventable childhood disease from which children have become seriously ill or have died and the patient has not been immunized, it may be in the best interest of the child for the physician to obtain a court order to immunize the child. In addition, the physician must be familiar with the state's statute regarding religious exemptions for immunizations and admission to public school.

**III. Confidentiality** is based on the ethical principle and rule of respect for autonomy and fidelity. It can be violated by deliberately disclosing confidential information without the person's permission or carelessly handling information.

**A. Justified infringements to confidentiality.** The following areas are justified infringements to confidentiality:

1. **Obligation to obey the law**
   - **a.** Reporting child abuse, elder abuse, gunshot wounds, stab wounds, sexually transmitted diseases
   - **b.** Certain legal proceedings such as a malpractice claim
2. **Obligation to protect the welfare of the community.** Confidentiality may be breached to protect an innocent third party if the individual who may be harmed is identifiable, the harm to be averted is serious, and disclosure is the minimum required to protect the third party.
3. **Obligation to protect the patient** if the patient presents a clear danger to himself or herself.

B. **Areas of heightened confidentiality** (usually specified by state statute)
   1. Drug and alcohol rehabilitation
   2. Psychiatric treatment
   3. Minors seeking birth control and abortion (in some states)
   4. HIV infection

IV. **Mature minors and emancipated minors**

A. **Mature minors** are individuals 14 years of age or older who have decision-making capacity—that is, they are capable of understanding their diagnosis and prognosis, the risks and benefits of proposed treatment, and consequences if they refuse treatment. Mature minors are capable of giving informed consent to the same degree as an adult. If the treatment does not involve serious risk, such as treatment for a *Streptococcal* pharyngitis or acne, the mature minor has the right to consent to such treatment without parental consent. A mature minor would not, however, have the right to consent to treatment that involves serious risk, such as organ transplantation, without the consent of the minor's parent or guardian.

B. **Emancipated minors** are individuals under the age of 18 years living on their own without parental support and not subject to parental control. Historically, certain groups of individuals have been considered emancipated, including minors in the military, married minors, and in some states, minors who are pregnant or have a child. In addition, college students living on their own may be considered emancipated even if they depend on their parents to pay the bills. Emancipated minors are considered adults in the medical arena, and therefore, parental permission is not required for treatment. The physician should be familiar with the specifics of the "mature minor" and "emancipated minor" statutes in his or her state.

## Selected Readings

Alderman EM, Fleischman AR. Should adolescents make their own health care choices? *Contemp Pediatr* January 1993, P 65.

Beauchamp TL, Childress JF. *Principles of Biomedical Ethics* (3rd ed). New York: Oxford University Press, 1989.

Etkind P, Lett SM, Macdonald PD et al. Pertussis outbreaks in groups claiming religious exemptions to vaccinations. *Am J Dis Child* 146:173, 1992.

Holder AR. Minors' rights to consent to medical care. *JAMA* 257:3400, 1987.

Holder AR. *Legal Issues in Pediatrics and Adolescent Medicine* (2nd ed). New Haven, CT: Yale University Press, 1985.

Landwirth J. Religious exemptions in child abuse law. *Infect Dis Child* December 1989, P 14.

Religion and medicine clash over deadly measles epidemic. *Med Ethics Adv* 7:41, 1991.

Sigman GS, O'Connor C. Exploration for physicians of the mature minor doctrine. *J Pediatr* 119:520, 1991.

J

# Miscellaneous Topics

51

# The Evaluation of Fever in Infancy

**Sherman J. Alter**

Children from birth to 36 months with fever of unknown source comprise a large fraction of ambulatory pediatric ill visits. While fever is frequently self-limited and the incidence of serious bacterial infections (SBIs) in febrile children is relatively low, serious infections may be present. The most common SBIs are bacterial meningitis, bacteremia, and urinary tract infection (UTI).

Proposed management strategies seek to identify infants at low risk for SBI. It is assumed that the ability of very young infants' immune systems to defend against pathogens is limited and that this ability matures during the early months of life. Such young infants, therefore, are at higher risk for serious infections than are older children. Because of this higher risk, it is standard practice in many areas to admit febrile neonates, perform a complete diagnostic evaluation for SBI, and administer parenteral antibiotics until results of blood, urine, and cerebrospinal fluid (CSF) cultures are negative. Recent investigations, however, have attempted to evaluate the efficacy of managing fever even in young infants in an ambulatory setting with or without empirical antibiotics.

Infants and young children usually are divided into two groups based on age and the ability to clinically assess severity of illness: birth to 2 months and 3–36 months.

I. **Epidemiology.** SBIs include meningitis, bacteremia, UTI, pneumonia, enteritis, and bone or joint infections. Depending on clinical screening criteria and the definition of toxicity used, febrile infants less than 60–90 days of age with temperatures of 38°C or higher rectally have a 1.4–17.3% probability of having a SBI, including a 1.1–10.7% probability of bacteremia and a 0.5–3.9% probability of meningitis. The risk of occult bacteremia in children 3–36 months of age is less, reported to be from 3% to 11% with a mean probability of 4.3% in children with a temperature of 39°C or higher.

II. **Etiology.** Etiologic agents of bacteremia in infants 2 months of age and younger include group B streptococci, *Streptococcus pneumoniae, Salmonella* sp., *Escherichia coli, Neisseria meningitidis,* and *Haemophilus influenzae* type B. The bacteria most commonly isolated from the blood of children age 3–36 months with fever without a source are *S. pneumoniae, H. influenzae* type B, and *N. meningitidis*, accounting for approximately 85%, 10%, and 3% of positive blood cultures, respectively. Other pathogens associated with bacteremia include *Staphylococcus aureus*, *Streptococcus pyogenes*, and *Salmonella* species.

Pathogens associated with bacterial meningitis in infants in the first 2 months of life include group B streptococci, *E. coli* and other enteric gram-negative bacilli, and *Listeria monocy-*

*togenes*. Pathogens typically causing community-acquired meningitis in older children—*S. pneumoniae*, *N. meningitidis*, and *H. influenzae* type B—also may be found in younger infants. The proportion of children with invasive disease caused by *H. influenzae* type B has decreased significantly due to widespread use of the vaccine against this organism.

**III. Clinical assessment and management.** No reliable method of identifying all children with SBIs has been developed. Screening criteria to identify infants and young children at low or high risk for SBIs, however, have been used by a number of investigators. These criteria most commonly involve history, physical examination, and specific laboratory parameters that then are used to identify patients who require no antibiotics and can be managed as outpatients and patients who require antibiotics either as an outpatient or an inpatient.

**A. Young infants less than 3 months of age.** Traditionally, young infants with fever have been managed very conservatively because they are notoriously difficult to assess clinically and more prone to SBIs because of their immature immune systems. Febrile neonates (0–28 days old) are considered high-risk patients. A sepsis evaluation should be performed, including CBC and differential, blood culture, cytology and culture of CSF, urinalysis and culture of urine obtained by catheterization or bladder tap, stool culture, and chest radiographs if indicated. Antimicrobial therapy should be instituted in the hospital.

Febrile infants 28–60 days old should have an assessment of toxicity, careful physical examination, and laboratory testing performed as above. Low-risk, non–toxic-appearing infants with normal CSF may be managed as outpatients and receive therapy with an antibiotic that will empirically treat the presumed agents of bacteremia. The third-generation cephalosporin, ceftriaxone, at a dose of 50 mg/kg IM is a particularly suitable antibiotic due to its long half-life. The child should return for re-evaluation within 24 hours. Any child who cannot return for repeat evaluation should be admitted to the hospital. At the return evaluation, results of cultures should be reviewed. Ill-appearing infants or those with positive blood or CSF cultures must be admitted for therapy. A second intramuscular injection of ceftriaxone may be an option. Continued close observation and immediate return to the hospital if needed must always be ensured.

Alternatively, some investigators have advocated selecting a subgroup of infants at low risk for SBI based on certain criteria and managing them without antibiotics as outpatients. These low-risk criteria have been studied by the Rochester group and include the following:

1. The infant appears generally well.
2. The infant has been previously healthy and has the following characteristics:
   - **a.** Was born at term ($\geq$ 37 weeks gestation)
   - **b.** Did not receive parenteral antibiotics
   - **c.** Was not treated for unexplained hyperbilirubinemia
   - **d.** Has not received and was not receiving antimicrobial agents

   e. Has not been previously hospitalized
   f. Has no chronic or underlying illness
   g. Was not hospitalized longer than the mother
3. Physical examination of the infants reveals no evidence of skin, soft tissue, bone, joint, or ear infection.
4. Laboratory values
   a. Peripheral blood WBC count 5,000–15,000/μl
   b. Absolute band form count <1,500/μl
   c. <10 WBC per high-power field (40× magnification) on microscopic examination of a spun urine sediment
   d. <5 WBC per high-power field (40× magnification) on microscopic examination of a stool smear (for infants with diarrhea)

Patients must be evaluated by a physician who is thoroughly familiar with caring for young children. Infants who meet such clinical criteria appear to be at low risk for SBI and may be candidates for outpatient management with follow-up examination in 24 hours.

B. **3–36 months**. Well-appearing older children who are 3–36 months of age with a fever of less than 39°C without a source need neither laboratory testing nor antibiotics. Parents, however, must be instructed to return if fever persists for more than 48–72 hours or if the child's condition deteriorates.

The appropriate and cost-effective evaluation and management of children with fever of 39°C or higher vary both in the pediatric literature and in practice. Conservative management consists of attempting to identify a subgroup of febrile children at increased risk for SBI, specifically occult bacteremia (OB), by obtaining a CBC, blood culture, and urinalysis and culture (the latter on all females; males less than 6 months of age). Chest radiographs and cultures of stool are performed if indicated by the history. A child with a WBC count ≥ 15,000/μl is at increased risk for OB and should receive expectant antibiotic therapy pending culture results. Before penicillinase-producing *H. influenzae* became significant (and before *Haemophilus* immunization), oral amoxicillin alone or procaine penicillin and amoxicillin was commonly used. Currently, ceftriaxone, 50 mg/kg IM, is popular because of its long half-life and extended coverage. Patients should be re-evaluated within 24 hours. Ill-appearing children or those with positive blood cultures should be admitted for further treatment.

Alternatively, concerns about cost containment, the dramatically decreased incidence of OB due to *H. influenzae* since the vaccine, and increased knowledge and experience with OB have prompted practitioners to practice other treatment options. The site of care and the relationship between the physician and patient affect treatment decisions. In a primary care setting with patients who are followed on a regular basis, the practitioner may elect to follow the patient clinically with no laboratory evaluation (or blood culture only) in the non–toxic-appearing infant. If the fever persists beyond 24–48 hours or the patient does not respond to antipyretics with improved clinical appearance, further work-up may be appropriate. On the other hand, a physician evaluating a febrile infant unknown to him or her in an emergency room or urgent care setting is more likely to obtain a CBC and blood culture and treat expectantly using the above criteria.

Any ill- or toxic-appearing child in this age range must be admitted to the hospital following appropriate laboratory evaluation, usually including a CBC, blood culture, and CSF evaluation. Toxicity generally is defined as a clinical appearance consistent with sepsis (e.g., inconsolable irritability, lethargy, signs of poor perfusion, hypoventilation, cyanosis). Unfortunately, clinical assessment of toxicity is the least objective screening criterion available to the primary care physician and requires the most clinical experience. McCarthy attempted to quantitate clinical toxicity by developing the Infant Observation Scale, but the appearance of toxicity is affected by the presence of fever. Some children may appear toxic while their temperature is elevated, but become less ill-appearing, even playful and well-appearing, after defervescence, leading to the common practice of giving antipyretics to febrile children on arrival in a care facility even before evaluation. Improved clinical appearance with defervescence may obviate the need for lumbar puncture and hospital admission in some children.

No management strategy will identify all patients at risk for SBI. Meticulous clinical assessment, judicious use of laboratory testing, and close follow-up are warranted when caring for the febrile infant or young child.

## Selected Readings

Baker MD, Bell LM, Avner JR. Outpatient management without antibiotics of fever in selected infants. *N Engl J Med* 329:1437, 1993.

Baker RC, Tiller T, Bausher JC et al. Severity of disease correlated with fever reduction in febrile infants. *Pediatrics* 83:1016, 1989.

Baraff LJ, Bass JW, Fleisher GR et al. Practice guideline for the management of infants and children 0 to 36 months of age with fever without source. *Ann Emerg Med* 22:1198, 1993.

Baskin MN, O'Rourke EJ, Fleisher GR. Outpatient treatment of febrile infants 28 to 89 days of age with intramuscular administration of ceftriaxone. *J Pediatr* 120:22, 1992.

Dagan R, Powell KR, Hall CB et al. Identification of infants unlikely to have serious bacterial infection although hospitalized for suspected sepsis. *J Pediatr* 107:855, 1985.

Jaskiewicz JA, McCarthy CA, Richardson CA et al. Febrile infants at low risk for serious bacterial infection—an appraisal of the Rochester criteria and implications for management. *Pediatrics* 94:390, 1994.

McCarthy PL, Sharpe MR, Spiesel SZ et al. Observation scales to identify serious illness in febrile children. *Pediatrics* 70:802, 1982.

Wilson CB. Immunologic basis for increased susceptibility of the neonate to infection. *J Pediatr* 108:1, 1986.

# 52

# Antibiotic Selection and Compliance

Raymond C. Baker

Many effective oral antibiotics with a broad spectrum of activity against organisms causing the common infections in pediatric outpatients are available. The choice of antibiotic depends on many factors, the most important being the sensitivity of the probable etiologic organism; however, many subjective factors also must be considered. Acute otitis media and skin infections are examples of common diseases in outpatients for which several choices of oral antibiotics are possible. For acute otitis media, *Streptococcus pneumoniae,* nontypeable *Haemophilus influenzae,* and *Moraxella catarrhalis* are the organisms that should be considered when the antibiotic is selected. Several antibiotics are appropriate, including amoxicillin (e.g., Amoxil), trimethoprim-sulfamethoxazole (TMP-SMX) (Septra, Bactrim), erythromycin-sulfisoxazole (Pediazole), cefaclor (Ceclor), amoxicillin-clavulanate (Augmentin), cefixime (Suprax), loracarbef (Lorabid), cefpodoxime (Vantin), cefuroxime axetil (Ceftin), and cefprozil (Cefzil).

The most common organisms involved in skin infections (cellulitis, impetigo) are *Staphylococcus aureas* and *Streptococcus pyogenes*, which can be treated effectively with several antibiotics, including erythromycin (e.g., Ilosone), dicloxacillin (Pathocil), cloxacillin (Tegopen), cephalexin (Keflex), cefaclor (Ceclor), amoxicillin-clavulanate (Augmentin), loracarbef (Lorabid), cefpodoxime (Vantin), and cefprozil (Cefzil).

The final choice therefore rests on the individual circumstance and features of a particular antibiotic that are most likely to ensure compliance in the patient and effectiveness against the organism. The following factors influence compliance with antibiotic medications and should influence the physician's decision regarding the appropriate antibiotic.

**I. Taste.** In general, most antibiotics have a bitter taste (especially penicillins) poorly masked by flavorings. Possible exceptions are the cephalosporins, which taste better but are more costly. Children vary in their willingness to accept unpleasant-tasting medicine; therefore, it is prudent to ask the parent how well the child accepts medicines and then consider the taste factor if needed (i.e., prescribing a more costly antibiotic that tastes better). A recent taste comparison (by adults) ranked the overall taste of oral suspensions of a series of brand name antibiotics as follows (from best to worst tasting): Lorabid, Keflex, Suprax, Ceclor, Cefzil, Augmentin, V-cillin K, Veetids, Vantin, Sulfatrim, Pediazole, and Dynapen.

**II. Frequency of administration.** Medications with a short half-life that must be given often may cause a problem with compliance. In general, the less often a medication is given, the more likely the parent is able to comply with the regimen. Antibiotics that require less frequent administration are cefixime (qd) and TMP-SMX, cefprozil, loracarbef, cefpodixime, and cefuroxime axetil (bid). Another strategy for improving compliance in medications that must be given more frequently is to try to relate the medication administration to some other life event as a reminder (e.g., with meals, on waking, at bedtime).

III. **Cost.** Prescriptions are paid for in many ways. Some insurance companies and Medicaid pay for the complete medication (especially if the medication requires a prescription). Some insurance companies require a copayment of $2–5 per prescription. Some parents must pay for the entire prescription. Before prescribing an antibiotic, the physician should ask the parent how prescriptions are paid for because the method of payment may affect the choice of prescription—for example, the newer cephalosporins tend to be costly, whereas the old standbys available as a generic brand are less expensive (e.g., amoxicillin, penicillin, sulfonamides).

IV. **Absorption with food.** Some antibiotics are poorly absorbed with food in the stomach and therefore must be given between meals. Others are unaffected. Since young infants tend to be fed frequently, medication absorption may be an issue in selecting an antibiotic. In general, the absorption of macrolides, amoxicillin with or without clavulanate, sulfonamides, and cephalosporins is unaffected by food in the stomach. The tetracyclines, penicillin G, cloxacillin, dicloxacillin, ampicillin, and nafcillin should be given 1 hour before or 2 hours after meals.

V. **Refrigeration requirement.** Most antibiotics that must be reconstituted with water at the time they are dispensed require refrigeration, which is indicated on the bottle. While this does not commonly present a problem, it may be a consideration for families who do not have access to refrigeration. Refrigeration is not required for the sulfonamides, TMP-SMX, erythromycin, griseofulvin, clindamycin, loracarbef, and tetracycline. All of the penicillins and most cephalosporins require refrigeration.

VI. **Drug interactions.** Relatively few drug interactions occur with antibiotics, but some may require consideration when prescribed:

- **A.** Tetracycline and antacids, anticonvulsants, or oral contraceptives
- **B.** Erythromycin and theophylline preparations, anticoagulants, digoxin, or Seldane
- **C.** Amoxicillin and oral contraceptives
- **D.** Chloramphenicol and anticonvulsants (phenobarbital, phenytoin) or acetaminophen
- **E.** Clindamycin and diphenoxylate-atropine
- **F.** Furazolidone and alcohol
- **G.** Griseofulvin and phenobarbital or anticoagulants
- **H.** Rifampin and anticoagulants, chloramphenicol, isoniazid, or barbiturates
- **I.** Sulfonamides and anticoagulants or phenytoin
- **J.** TMP-SMX and cyclosporine or anticoagulants

VII. **Physiologic interactions.** In children with chronic illnesses, attention should be paid to the mode of excretion of antibiotics when they are prescribed. Specifically, if the antibiotic is excreted in the urine (penicillins, aminoglycosides, cephalosporins), it should be used with caution in children with

**Table 52-1. Pediatric doses of commonly prescribed antibiotics based on weight**

| 1.0 ml/kg/day | | 30–50 mg/kg/day | |
|---|---|---|---|
| Antibiotic | Frequency | Antibiotic | Frequency |
| Erythromycin-sulfisoxazole (Pediazole—fixed combination) | qid | Penicillin V | qid |
| Trimethoprim-sulfamethoxazole (Septra, Bactrim—fixed combination) | bid | Amoxicillin | tid |
| Cefpodoxime (50 mg/5 ml) | bid | Amoxicillin-clavulanate (Augmentin) | tid |
| Clindamycin (75 mg/5 ml) | tid–qid | Cefaclor | tid |
| Nitrofurantoin (25 mg/5 ml) | qid | Cefprozil* | bid |
| | | Cefuroxime axetil | bid |
| | | Cephalexin | qid |
| | | Erythromycin (estolate)* | qid |
| | | Erythromycin (ethylsuccinate) | qid |
| | | Loracarbef* | bid |
| | | Tetracycline | qid |

*Dosage should be at lower end of dosing spectrum (30 mg/kg/day).

renal clearance abnormalities. Likewise, in children with significant liver disease, drugs excreted in the bile should be used with caution (erythromycin, tetracyclines, chloramphenicol).

**VIII. Adverse reactions.** The likelihood of an allergic reaction or other significant side effect should be considered, and a careful allergic history should be obtained. The following are examples of drug effects that may affect antibiotic choice:

**A.** Serum sickness-like reactions (3–5%) with cefaclor
**B.** Erythema multiforme with sulfonamides
**C.** Nausea with erythromycin (should be given with food)
**D.** Diarrhea with amoxicillin-clavulanate (Augmentin)

**IX. Remembering the dose of antibiotics.** Since most antibiotics prescribed for the pediatric population are dosed based on weight, Table 52-1 may be helpful in remembering doses of commonly prescribed antibiotics.

## Selected Readings

Craig CR, Stitzel RE. *Modern Pharmacology*. Boston: Little, Brown, 1990.

Demers DM, Chan DS, Bass JW. Antimicrobial drug suspensions: A blinded comparison of taste of twelve common pediatric drugs including cefixime, cefpodoxime, cefprozil, and loracarbef. *Pediatr Infect Dis J* 13:87, 1994.

Kaplan JM, Goretski SA, Keith S et al. Cost of antibiotic therapy for infants and children. *Pediatr Infect Dis J* 9:722, 1990.

Le CT. Choosing an antibiotic: Efficacy, side effects—and cost. *Contemp Pediatr* 8:11, 1991.

McCracken GH. Choosing among the orally administered antibiotics. *Pediatr Infect Dis J* 6:593, 1987.

Medical Letter. The choice of antibacterial drugs. *Med Lett* May 29, 1992.

Neu HC. Antibacterial therapy: Problems and promises. *Hosp Pract* May/June 1990, Pp 63–78/181–194.

Prober CG. Choosing an antibiotic: Is new always better? *Contemp Pediatr* 6:16, 1989.

Ruff ME, Schotik DA, Bass JW et al. Antimicrobial drug suspensions: A blind comparison of taste of fourteen common pediatric drugs. *Pediatr Infect Dis J* 10:30, 1991.

53

# Symptomatic Therapy of Children


## Raymond C. Baker


I. **Symptomatic therapy** refers to medications or treatments suggested or prescribed by a physician to alleviate patients' symptoms but that do not affect the disease process. Symptomatic therapy is in contrast to medications or treatments prescribed by physicians that effectively reverse a disease process, such as antibiotics for bacterial infection or steroids for asthma. Since so many illnesses of childhood are self-limiting and without specific treatment, symptomatic therapy is often the only therapy a physician has to offer a parent. Symptomatic therapy, like any other intervention, has both therapeutic advantages and disadvantages, however. The decision to use medications to treat symptoms should therefore be mitigated by several factors.

A. **Advantages of symptomatic therapy**

1. Subjective improvement with improved function
2. Placebo value to the child (and parent)
3. Something for parents to do to lessen their feelings of helplessness
4. Positive course of action
5. Symptomatic therapy may represent a compromise with the parents' demand for medication that will prevent them from seeking lower quality medical care.

B. **Disadvantages of symptomatic therapy**

1. Symptomatic medications may be expensive. Over-the-counter (OTC) symptomatic medications are usually less expensive than prescription medications and should be recommended whenever possible. The physician should be aware of the parents' financial status and method of payment when deciding whether to treat and in choosing between OTC and prescription medications. The majority of medications for symptomatic therapy are available OTC.
2. They are often relatively ineffective.
3. They have little impact on the course of the illness.
4. Some children resist taking medications of any kind.
5. Symptoms of advancing disease might be masked.
6. The false sense of security from the medication might make a parent (or physician) less vigilant.
7. Undesirable side effects.
8. Symptomatic therapy may create a mind-set in the parent that every symptom requires a medication.

II. The **ideal symptomatic medication** should be inexpensive (especially OTC), palatable, nontoxic, readily available (especially OTC), easy to administer (e.g., infrequent dose schedule, oral), and effective for the symptom being treated. Few symptomatic medications fulfill all these criteria, making the decision to treat a child with symptomatic therapy one that requires knowledge of the medication, the illness, the patient, and the family. For the following symptoms, available symptomatic medications are described in terms of effectiveness (not effective or placebo, somewhat effective, or effective), availability, and potential side effects. Whenever possible, home remedies also are suggested that might be helpful.

**III. Key**

**A. Trade name** medications are indicated by capitalization of the first letter of the medication (e.g., Benadryl).

**B. Generic** medications are medications having all lower case letters (e.g., phenylpropanolamine).

**C. Prescription** medications are indicated by italic letters (e.g., *Viscous Xylocaine*).

**IV. Cough.** Cough suppressants are somewhat effective and may be appropriate for cough that results from respiratory tract irritation due to viral inflammation and minor secretions if the cough interferes with the child's normal activities, such as sleep and feeding. Cough suppressants should not be used in bronchospasm or conditions in which large amounts of secretions are produced (e.g., cystic fibrosis).

**A. Non-narcotic cough suppressants** available include dextromethorphan (e.g., Robitussin DM), which is somewhat effective, and antihistamines, which may have minor cough-suppressant activity (e.g., diphenhydramine, Benadryl).

**B. Narcotic cough suppressants** include *codeine* and *hydrocodone,* usually in combination with other cold medications, such as decongestants and antihistamines. While the narcotic and synthetic narcotic cough suppressants (dextromethorphan, codeine, and hydrocodone) are somewhat effective, they are contraindicated in the infant younger than 6 months of age because of possible apnea, which has been reported as a rare side effect of these drugs. The more expensive prescription narcotics, *codeine* and *hydrocodone,* are not usually indicated in children less than 6 years of age.

**C. Expectorants** (e.g., guaifenesin, Robitussin) theoretically should be helpful in cough by thinning secretions, making cough more effective; however, these medications are not effective and should be considered only for their placebo value.

**V. Congestion** refers to blockage of upper respiratory passages secondary to viral or allergic inflammation. Treatment may be indicated if the symptoms interfere with sleep and feeding.

**A. Topical decongestants** are effective and relatively inexpensive. Short-acting phenylephrine (e.g., Neo-Synephrine) and long-acting oxymetazoline (e.g., Afrin) are available in both adult and pediatric strengths. They can cause rebound symptoms (rhinitis medicamentosa) if used for too long at a time, so their use in toddlers and children should be limited to the first 3–5 days of the illness. They are contraindicated in infants less than 6 months of age due to pronounced rebound and marked nasal obstruction following discontinuance that may occur in young infants who may be obligate nose-breathers.

**B. Oral decongestants** (e.g., pseudoephedrine, Sudafed, phenylpropanolamine) are also somewhat effective but less so than topicals. They are generally safe for use in infants and children over the age of 3–6 months. Decongestants are often combined with antihistamines, cough suppressants, or both, and sold as cold medications. Because of the wide variety of these medications available OTC, the physician must select the appropriate product for the symptom(s) to be treated.

A humidifier or vaporizer may be helpful to the congested infant to thin mucus and hydrate mucous membranes. A cool mist humidifier is preferred over a steam vaporizer, which can scald the curious child. In addition, cool mist humidifiers usually hold more liquid than steam vaporizers and can run nonstop all night. Saline nose drops also may be instilled in the congested infant's nares to loosen secretions for easier removal by a nasal aspirator.

**VI. Sore throat and sore mouth (stomatitis)**

**A. Topical analgesics** (benzocaine, diphenhydramine, *lidocaine*, phenol) are effective, but for sore throat pain are difficult to apply to the posterior pharynx, where the pain of pharyngitis is usually greatest. Some are available as a spray (Chloraseptic spray), which may reach the posterior pharynx in the cooperative older child, but are not easily applied to the younger child. Topical benzocaine (e.g., Cepacol, Chloraseptic) is available as lozenges and adequately soothes pain of the tongue and anterior structures of the mouth but is less effective in the posterior pharynx.

For the pain of stomatitis, topical analgesics are effective but may be difficult to apply in the uncooperative younger child, who is at the age most likely to get stomatitis. Topical benzocaine (Oragel), lidocaine (*Viscous Xylocaine*), diphenhydramine (Benadryl), and a 1:1:1 mix of diphenhydramine, Kaopectate, and *2% Viscous Xylocaine* are all effective if they can be applied. Sometimes a cotton- or sponge-tipped applicator can be used to apply these liquids in younger children; older children can swish and spit. These medications should not be swallowed due to systemic effects. Oral analgesics, such as acetaminophen and ibuprofen, may be somewhat effective if topical therapy is not feasible.

**B. Home remedies for sore mouth and throat**. Cold applied topically is probably just as effective as the above, although shorter-acting. Foods such as ice cream, Popsicles, cold pudding, and cold liquids may be better tolerated by young children and have the advantage of providing some nourishment that may be needed in the child whose intake is decreased due to the illness. Older children and teenagers may find some relief by gargling with a warm saline solution to soothe a painful throat.

**VII. Earache**. The pain of otitis media can be severe enough to significantly interfere with sleep (both infant and parents'), feeding, and play activities in the infant. Both topical and systemic effective pain relief are available for the pain of otitis media. Topical benzocaine (e.g., *Auralgan*) may be effective in some children, but because of the viscous nature of the vehicle, it may be difficult for parents to instill the product into the ear canal sufficiently to contact the tympanic membrane, which is necessary for the medication to be effective. A single application by the physician or nurse at the time of diagnosis may be appropriate. The physician should then recommend oral analgesics for the parent to administer at home. Satisfactory oral analgesia usually can be obtained with acetaminophen for mild pain and ibuprofen or *codeine* for more severe pain (see below).

Some infants may find relief from warm mineral oil applied topically as a home remedy, but this should not be recommended if a perforation could be present (ear drainage) or tympanostomy tubes are in place. Warm mineral oil may be particularly helpful for middle-of-the-night calls from anxious parents who have no oral analgesics available and may provide relief until the infant sees the physician the following morning. The wise physician (who also appreciates a good night's sleep) recommends that parents keep an oral analgesic in the home and know when and how to use it.

**VIII. Nausea and vomiting (infectious origin)**

**A. Oral medications** of the phenothiazine and antihistamine categories (e.g., *prochlorperazine, Compazine, promethazine, Phenergan,* diphenhydramine, Benadryl) for nausea and vomiting exist and may be somewhat effective but are contraindicated in young children due to their neurologic side effects (drowsiness, dystonic reactions). Furthermore, they are usually unnecessary, since vomiting is well-tolerated by young children and usually self-limiting due to its infectious etiology. In older children (over 6 years), these medications may be considered in some situations. The physician should be aware of young children in the home, however, and caution parents about appropriate security of these medications.

**B. Home remedies.** A more common practice in infants and young children, however, is to discontinue solid intake and replace with easily absorbed liquids to replace and maintain body fluids and decrease gastrointestinal activity. For this purpose, home remedies can be suggested, including clear liquids such as soft drinks, Kool-Aid, or broth. Electrolyte contents of the replacement fluid are not of great importance for the first 24–48 hours, and most vomiting has ceased by this time.

**IX. Diarrhea (infectious origin)**

**A. Oral medications** for diarrhea are available, usually of the opiate or anticholinergic categories (e.g., *Lomotil*, Immodium AD, Donnagel, *Paregoric*) and are effective in decreasing the numbers and volume of stool output; however, they are contraindicated for young children for several reasons. Most diarrhea is self-limiting and well-tolerated; the course of diarrhea in certain infectious etiologies may be prolonged; and "third spacing" may occur. In older children and teen-agers, they may be used, especially to maintain normal activities. Bismuth subsalicylate (e.g., Pepto-Bismol) is effective in large doses in enterotoxigenic diarrhea and in certain bacterial diarrheas (see Chap. 27).

**B. Home remedies.** It may be appropriate in infants with diarrhea of infectious origin to institute a clear liquid diet as above for similar reasons. Again, the electrolyte content of the liquids is probably not important unless the diarrhea exceeds 2–3 days' duration. If diarrhea has been present longer than 2–3 days, glucose-electrolyte oral rehydration solutions (e.g., Pedialyte, Rehydralyte, Ricelyte) in small, frequent amounts (daily dose is calculated based on losses and body weight) for 24 hours is appropriate. These are usually available in plain and flavored varieties. Oral rehydration is followed by return to a regular diet, although some physicians recommend a non–lactose-containing formula (e.g., Isomil, Prosobee) for an additional few days.

**X. Constipation** is a common complaint in infants and children and may require intervention, although most constipation is self-limiting. Before considering intervention, it is important to differentiate constipation (hard consistency) from infrequent passage or apparent difficulty in stool passage. Considerable variability in frequency of bowel movements exists in infants and children. Furthermore, infants, prior to successful toilet training, lack the mechanical advantage offered by the sitting position to have bowel movements. This often results in a greater effort to pass a bowel movement that may be interpreted by parents as constipation.

**A. Medications.** Many effective laxatives, mostly OTC, are available. **Stimulants** usually are reserved for older children rather than infants, as they are usually unnecessary and may be cramping. Examples of stimulant laxatives are bisacodyl (Dulcolax), phenolphthalein (Ex-Lax, Feen-A-Mint), and senna (Senokot). **Osmotic** laxatives, which act by drawing water into the bowel, are less cramping and are effective in older children (e.g., magnesium hydroxide, Fleets sodium phosphate). **Stool softeners** (e.g., mineral oil, docusate, Maltsupex, lactulose) and fiber medications (e.g., Metamucil) may be indicated in some children depending on the etiology of their constipation.

**B. Home remedies** commonly are suggested for constipation, especially in infants, and are somewhat effective. The addition of Karo syrup or molasses, 2–3 teaspoons per 4 oz, to infant formula is a time-honored suggestion that may be helpful. Other dietary manipulations include prune juice (stimulant), which is helpful in infants, and increased dietary fiber, such as bran cereals, popcorn, graham crackers, raisins, prunes, figs, spinach, carrots, and beets, in older children.

**XI. Pain.** There is a tendency among physicians to underestimate pain in infants and young children. Crying may be misinterpreted as fear and anxiety, and physicians may fear masking symptoms of advancing disease with effective pain management. In fact, pain management is clearly indicated in infants and children for the same reasons as in adults—to feel better and allay anxieties that are commonly expressed as crying and irritability in young children. The quantitation of pain in children requires innovative techniques, such as using a scale of 1–10 or a spectrum of cartoon faces, to determine the degree of pain management necessary. The parent is usually helpful in determining the degree of pain in children by interpreting visual cues and other signs that may elude the physician.

**A. Medications.** Many effective pain medications are available for children and should be selected based on the degree of pain that is present. For mild pain, acetaminophen, 15 mg/kg/dose q4–6h, or aspirin in similar doses is effective in infants and children. Aspirin is contraindicated for patients with influenza, varicella, reactive airways disease, and bleeding diatheses. For moderate pain, ibuprofen, 10 mg/kg/dose q6h (or other nonsteroidal anti-inflammatory agents), or *codeine*, 0.5–1.0 mg/kg/dose q4–6h, can be used. For severe pain, narcotic analgesics, orally or parenterally, including *morphine*, *meperidine (Demerol)*, and *hydromorphone (Dilaudid)*, are used with appropriate precautions and attention to underlying conditions that might contraindicate their use.

**B. Home remedies** for mild pain include cold or heat applied topically (e.g., for musculoskeletal pain, cellulitis).

**XII. Fever (infectious origin).** The treatment of fever as a symptom is controversial. There is evidence that fever of infectious origin may be beneficial by providing an environment unfavorable for the infecting organism. Fever also may produce some subjective benefits, such as encouraging decreased activity during the illness, and serving as an indicator of the illness's course. Furthermore, antipyretics are not without toxicities. On the other hand, treatment of fever may significantly improve the child subjectively, encouraging better oral intake. Treating fever may prevent febrile seizures, and antipyresis decreases insensible water losses.

**A. Medications.** Fever of infectious origin virtually always responds to acetaminophen in a dose of 15 mg/kg/dose PO or PR q4–6h. Failure to respond usually is secondary to inadequate dosing, either because the dose was too small, the child did not retain the dose, or heat loss was prevented by inappropriate wrapping. Aspirin is no longer recommended as an antipyretic. Ibuprofen is not superior to acetaminophen for fever reduction and is usually more expensive (the suspension form of ibuprofen, Children's Advil Suspension, requires a prescription). Ibuprofen, however, may last longer, requiring less frequent administration.

**B. Sponging with tepid water** is probably not any more effective than simply undressing the infant after an appropriate antipyretic has been given. If sponging is performed, it must not be started until 20–30 minutes after an appropriate oral or rectal antipyretic has been given to avoid shivering and an increase in the body core temperature. The exception is in the treatment of fever that is not of infectious origin, such as heat stroke, in which rapid lowering of body temperature is achieved solely with external cooling without antipyretics.

## Selected Readings

Means LJ. Pain relief for children: New concepts, new methods. *Contemp Pediatr* 11:70, 1994.

Schmitt, BD. *Your Child's Health* (rev ed). New York: Bantam Books, 1991.

Shelov SP (ed). *Caring For Your Baby and Young Child*. New York: Bantam Books, 1991.

Smith MBH, Feldman W. Over-the-counter cold medications: A critical review of clinical trials between 1950 and 1991. *JAMA* 269:2258, 1993.

# 54

# Management of the Infant Born to an HIV-Positive Mother

Raymond C. Baker

As the second decade of the acquired immunodeficiency syndrome (AIDS) epidemic begins, the mode of transmission of the human immunodeficiency virus (HIV) is shifting toward heterosexual activity and intravenous drug use, resulting in an increasing number of infants exposed prenatally and perinatally to HIV. The medical care of these infants is complicated by the fact that, although mother-to-infant transmission occurs in only about 25% of births, current laboratory evaluations are limited in their ability to establish the presence of infection in the infant in the early months of life. The standard HIV serology, which confirms infection in children over 2 years of age through adulthood, is virtually always positive in infants born to HIV-infected women due to passively acquired antibody. Seroreversion cannot be relied on to establish the absence of HIV infection until at least 15 months of life. More sophisticated tests, such as HIV culture and HIV polymerase chain reaction (PCR), are necessary to confirm infection in the early months of life. Because of this inherent delay in making a definitive diagnosis, the primary care physician must treat infants born to HIV-positive mothers as infected until testing proves otherwise.

I. The evaluation and management of the infant born to an HIV-infected woman begin with the **prenatal and perinatal history**, which should include specific HIV-related information as follows:

A. **Maternal history**

1. **Mode of HIV transmission to mother** (sexual, drug use, blood products)
2. **Symptoms of HIV infection.** The rate of HIV transmission is higher in mothers with more advanced disease.
3. **Sexually transmitted disease (STD) history** and prenatal STD screening. Maternal STDs are associated with a higher rate of HIV transmission both to sexual partners and infant.
4. **HIV therapy during pregnancy.** The rate of transmission is lower in women treated with zidovudine during the last two trimesters of pregnancy.
5. **CD4 count.** The rate of HIV transmission is higher with lower maternal CD4 counts.
6. **HIV status of other children.** The rate of HIV transmission is higher if previous children were HIV infected.
7. **Length of gestation.** The rate of premature delivery is higher in HIV-infected infants.

B. **Perinatal history**

1. **Length of labor and interval between rupture of membranes and delivery.**

2. **Type of delivery.** Cesarean-section (C-section) *may* be associated with decreased intrapartum HIV transmission.
3. **Delivery complications.**
4. **Apgar scores.** Early symptoms in HIV-infected infants are associated with prepartum transmission and a poorer prognosis than intrapartum transmission.

**II. The newborn physical examination** should be thorough with special attention to the following:

**A. Birth weight.** HIV-infected infants tend to have lower birth weights.

**B. Evidence of congenital cytomegalovirus (CMV), herpes, syphilis, or toxoplasmosis,** which may be associated with HIV infection.

**C. Head circumference.** HIV-infected infants may have smaller head circumferences.

**III. Laboratory evaluation**. The initial laboratory evaluation of the perinatally-exposed infant depends on the availability of laboratories with HIV culture and HIV PCR capabilities. Since the goal is to determine the presence of infection as soon as possible, HIV culture and HIV PCR should be performed three times during the first 6 months of life: at birth–2 months (an HIV culture or PCR should not be performed on cord blood due to the possibility of maternal contamination), 3–4 months, and 6 months. A positive PCR or HIV culture should be repeated to confirm the diagnosis unless both are positive. Other specific HIV testing that may be available include immune-complex dissociated p24Ag (ICD p24Ag) and IgA-specific anti-HIV antibodies.

If these are not available, HIV serology with Western Blot confirmation should be performed at 3- to 4-month intervals until seroreversion occurs and is confirmed. In the infant with persistently positive HIV serology beyond 15 months of age, HIV infection is likely. Other laboratory tests that may suggest HIV infection and can be performed at the same time as the HIV serologies are quantitative immunoglobulins (elevated in HIV infection), T cell subsets (HIV infection results in a decreased absolute CD4 count, decreased T4 to T8 ratio, and decreased percentage of T4 lymphocytes), and CBC (anemia, neutropenia, and thrombocytopenia may be associated with HIV infection).

**IV. Medical management**. In the period before HIV status is established, the infant should be presumed HIV-positive from a management perspective and undergo regular evaluation combining routine well-child procedures with expectant laboratory testing.

**A. Routine well-child care examinations** should be performed at regular intervals with special attention to possible early signs of HIV infection, such as failure to thrive, chronic diarrhea, lymphadenopathy, and recurrent monilial disease of the mouth and diaper area.

**B. Intercurrent illnesses**. HIV-infected infants tend to have a higher incidence of common infections such as otitis media, skin infections, pneumonia, and opportunistic infections.

**C. Immunizations** (see sec. **V.B.1.a**). The routine immunization schedule is followed except that the inactivated polio vaccine (IPV-Salk) is used rather than live oral polio vaccine (OPV-Sabin). IPV should be continued even if the infant is determined to be uninfected due to the small risk of the live virus vaccine to the HIV-positive mother.

D. ***Pneumocystis carinii* pneumonia (PCP) prophylaxis.** Most experts in pediatric HIV infection recommend PCP prophylaxis in the infant born to an HIV-positive mother until the infant's HIV status is known. Current recommendations for PCP prophylaxis are oral trimethoprim-sulfamethoxazole (TMP-SMX) suspension (first choice), 0.5 ml/kg PO bid 3 days a week (Monday, Tuesday, and Wednesday), or dapsone (second choice), 2 mg/kg PO qd, in children unable to tolerate TMP-SMX.

E. **Screening tests**. During the period before HIV status is known, infants should have routine screening for the following:

1. **Urine culture for CMV** at 2 and 6 months
2. **Toxoplasmosis titers at birth** (may be done on cord blood) and at 2–4 months
3. **Serologic testing for syphilis** if not documented negative in the mother during her prenatal care and at birth

V. **Medical management of HIV-infected infants and children.** While the medical management of HIV-infected infants and children is beyond the scope of this handbook, there are several principles that should be followed in providing their medical care.

A. **The HIV team**. The primary care physician for HIV-infected infants and children may be a generalist or specialist, depending on the physician's individual ability, availability, interest, and support (from colleagues, medical institution). Because of the many needs of families affected by HIV—both medical and psychosocial—the primary care physician must serve as the primary provider of care as well as a coordinator of care. The core HIV team should include the primary care physician, nurse, and social worker working closely with nutrition, psychology, and pharmacy professionals. Other disciplines often needed for consultation include infectious disease, immunology, pulmonology, hematology-oncology, and dentistry. Essential ancillary services needed include pharmacy, laboratory, and radiology.

B. **Medical care**

1. **Routine well-child care**

a. **Immunizations.** In addition to the substitution of IPV for OPV as above, other changes in the immunization schedule for HIV-infected infants include yearly influenza immunizations beginning at 6 months of age, pneumococcal vaccine at age 2 years and about every 3 years thereafter, and tuberculin skin testing as often as every 6 months depending on the local prevalence of HIV disease and tuberculosis.

b. **Nutrition and growth**. Monitoring growth and providing nutritional information are critical to the successful management of the HIV-infected infant. Increasing the caloric density of routine infant formulas, special high-density formulas (e.g., Pediasure, Ensure), and caloric additives such as Polycose may promote growth that has been slowed by the disease process. Each visit should include measurements of height, weight, head circumference, triceps skinfold thickness, and upper arm circumference.

c. **Development.** Careful monitoring of development by routine developmental examination and periodic neuropsychiatric testing are the most sensitive indicators of disease progression, which dictates therapeutic choices.

2. **Intercurrent illnesses and opportunistic infections.** HIV-infected infants and children have increased susceptibility to all of the common illness of childhood, especially recurrent otitis media, pneumonia, urinary tract infections, skin infections, and viral infections. Careful attention should be paid to prophylactic dental care to avoid complications of dental infections. Additionally, opportunistic infections, most commonly PCP, CMV disease, toxoplasmosis, *Mycobacterium avium* complex, and pulmonary tuberculosis, should be considered at each intercurrent illness and aggressively pursued.
3. **PCP prophylaxis** with oral TMP-SMX suspension, 0.5 ml/kg PO bid 3 days a week (Monday, Tuesday, and Wednesday), is recommended in HIV-infected children in the following circumstances:
   a. **History of previous episode(s) of PCP**
   b. **CD4 percentage less than 20% of total peripheral lymphocyte count**
   c. **CD4 count** lower than 1,500/μl (1–11 months of age), 750/μl (12–23 months), 500/μl (2–5 years), or 200/μl (6 years and older).

   In children unable to tolerate TMP-SMX, alternatives are oral dapsone (2 mg/kg/day) or aerosolized pentamidine.
4. **Intravenous gamma globulin (IVIG),** given monthly at a dose of 400 mg/kg/dose, has been shown to be effective in prophylaxis of bacterial infections in some circumstances including the following:
   a. **Hypogammaglobulemia**
   b. **Recurrent, serious bacterial infections**
   c. **Children who fail to form antibodies against common antigens**
   d. **Children living in geographic areas of high measles prevalence in whom measles antibody has not developed** after two doses of the mumps, measles, rubella (MMR) vaccine at least a month apart
5. **Antiretroviral chemotherapy**. The decision regarding when to begin antiretroviral chemotherapy is a complex one that does not yet have universal consensus. Some or all of the following criteria are used to determine when to initiate therapy with currently available nucleoside reverse transcriptase inhibitors (zidovudine [AZT, ZDV], didanosine [ddI], zalcitabine [ddC], stavudine [D4T], and lamivudine [3TC]):
   a. **Presence of an AIDS-defining illness.**
   b. **Failure to thrive** (crossing two percentiles).

c. **Progressive encephalopathy.**
d. **Malignancy.**
e. **Recurrent sepsis or meningitis.**
f. **Thrombocytopenia.**
g. **Hypogammaglobulinemia.**
h. **CD4 percentage** less than 30% (<12 mos), less than 25% (1–2 years), less than 20% (over 2 years).
i. **Low CD4 count.** CD4 counts in children are higher than in adults; therefore, the guidelines used for adults (200–500)) to begin antiretroviral therapy are inappropriate. Suggested guidelines for initiating antiretroviral therapy in children are as follows: less than 1,750/μl at younger than 1 year, less than 1,000/μl at 1–2 years, less than 750/μl at 2–6 years, and less than 500/μl at older than 6 years.
j. **Other symptoms** that may influence the decision to begin therapy independent of the CD4 count are the presence of lymphoid interstitial pneumonitis, parotitis, splenomegaly, persistent oral candidiasis, recurrent and/or chronic diarrhea, cardiomyopathy, nephropathy, hepatitis, endocrinopathy, recurrent and/or chronic bacterial infections (e.g., sinusitis, pneumonia), recurrent herpes simplex and/or varicella-zoster infection, neutropenia, anemia, and developmental delay.
k. **Other antiretroviral chemotherapeutic agents** currently being tested in adults include the nonnucleoside reverse transcriptase inhibitors (nevirapine and delavirpine) and protease inhibitors.

C. **Psychosocial care.** Social service plays an integral role in the care in HIV-affected families. Counseling, interacting with community social agencies to obtain services for families, and monitoring the family's psychological and emotional needs are necessary for the success of the HIV team.

D. **Terminal/hospice care**

## Selected Readings

Indacochea FJ, Scott GB. HIV-1 infection and the acquired immunodeficiency syndrome in children. *Curr Probl Pediatr* 22:166, 1992.

Lindegren ML, Hanson C, Miller K et al. Epidemiology of human immunodeficiency virus infection in adolescents, United States. *Pediatr Infect Dis J* 13:525, 1994.

Luzuriaga K, Sullivan JL. Pathogenesis of vertical HIV-1 infection: Implications for intervention and management. *Pediatr Ann* 23:159, 1994.

Stiehm ER, Frenkel LM (eds). AIDS. *Pediatr Ann* 22:399, 1993.

Task Force on Pediatric AIDS. Perinatal HIV testing. *Pediatrics* 89:791, 1992.

Working Group on Antiretroviral Therapy. National Pediatric HIV Resource Center. Antiretroviral therapy and medical management of the HIV-infected child. *Pediatr Infect Dis J* 12:513, 1993.

# III

# The Problem Visit—Behavioral

# 55

# Behavior Management and Discipline

Janet R. Schultz

Five to fifteen percent of children exhibit significant behavior problems associated with significant psychopathology. This does not include the more common, often irritating or worrisome behaviors or habits, such as temper tantrums, picky eating habits, thumb-sucking, and reluctance to do homework, that are not usually associated with significant psychopathology. Nor does it include other common biobehavioral concerns not usually associated with psychopathology, such as learning disabilities, enuresis, and encopresis. Up to 50% of all families in the United States have consulted their primary care provider at some point for mental health services for their children. With the growing role of primary care physicians as "gatekeepers," it is quite likely that a higher percentage of pediatric office visits will have at least some component of behavioral concern.

I. **Barriers to uncovering behavior problems during well-child care**
   A. **Parents may try to tell physicians their concerns, but they are not acknowledged.**
   B. **Parents may not mention their concerns.** Some studies indicate that about one-third of the time, parents do not express their greatest concern about their child's health and development, behavioral or otherwise. Primary reasons parents may not express their concerns to the physician are the following:
      1. They perceive physicians as too busy, not interested, or not qualified to be of assistance with the problem.
      2. They are embarrassed or fear they will be blamed for their child's problem.

II. **Methods the physician can use to elicit behavioral concerns from parents**
   A. **Being supportive** of parents, not critical
   B. **Being empathic** to the parents and showing interest in their child as a person
   C. **Asking about behavioral and emotional concerns directly**
   D. **Paying particular attention to the parent** while he or she talks about behavioral concerns by maintaining eye contact and being verbally responsive (phrases and reflections that show the physician is listening) during the interaction. Good listening by physicians has been shown to elicit more detailed illness-related information, disclosure of a larger number of patient concerns, greater parent satisfaction with office visits, reduction in parental concern, and increased compliance with the physician's recommendations.

III. **Goals of behavior management**
   A. **Prevention of behavior problems** through parent education and intervention

B. **Detection of early signs of growing behavior problems** or the development of mild but bothersome behavior patterns in which the physician can competently intervene

C. **Detection and identification of psychopathology or behavioral problems warranting referral to a specialist.** Many pediatric behavioral problems are best addressed by the joint efforts of the primary care physician and the consulting specialist. General criteria for referral might include the following:

1. The behavior(s), relationship(s), or emotional state(s) interfere with everyday life in a recurrent, substantial way, or the quality of family interactions has become predominantly negative.
2. The type or severity of the concerns is outside the range of the primary care physician's expertise, which depends on individual training, experience, and confidence.
3. The type or severity of the problem(s) is within the range of the physician's expertise, but resources, such as time, ready availability, back-up, and, perhaps, desire to treat these problems, are not present.

IV. **Context of behavior**. Behavior occurs in a complex context that needs to be considered when attempting to change behaviors. The following are important factors that have an impact on management:

A. **Child's temperament**

B. **Child's developmental level**

C. **Personality and general functioning of parents**

D. **Developmental level of the family** (e.g., first child, last child, settled marriage)

E. **Composition of and relationships** within the family

F. **Subcultural and cultural values**

G. **Particular life events for the family,** including stressors and helpful occurrences

**There is no one right way to raise a child. Different ways work for different families, but there are reliable themes for successful behavior management.**

V. **General principles of behavior management**

A. **Child behavior usually is maintained by its consequences.**

1. The sooner the consequence (positive or negative) follows the action, the more impact it will have.
2. Praise works best when it is specific (e.g., *"Every piece of dirty clothes is in the hamper and all your books are back on the shelf! That's what I call a good job cleaning up!"* is more instructive than *"nice job" or "good girl"*).
3. Punishment should "fit the crime" in magnitude and logic (e.g., a child who rides his bike in the street after being forbidden to do so might lose use of his or her bicycle for 3 days rather than losing television for a day).
4. Whether a consequence is positive or negative should be defined by the outcome, not by an *a priori* judgment. Some behaviors can be maintained by a parent's scolding the child if the attention is positive, even if the content is not.
5. Consistency is very important and must be maintained from parent to parent (e.g., if the mother does not allow

a snack just before dinner, the father should not allow it, even if the period just before dinner is the first opportunity he has had to play with the child), from situation to situation (e.g., a temper tantrum at the grocery should be handled the same way a temper tantrum is handled at home), and from time to time (e.g., name calling should be handled the same way Monday afternoon when the family is alone as it is on Sunday afternoon when the clergyman is visiting). Sometimes it matters less what the punishment is (within broad limits) than if it is done consistently.

**B. Child behavior tends to be governed by parents' actions,** not their words (e.g., a parent spanks a child and says, *"This will teach you to hit someone smaller than yourself!"* or a father smiles while discussing his son's aggression problem on the playground). Threats are not effective in managing behaviors and tend to leave parents feeling frustrated.

**C. Children learn much of their behavior by the examples set around them.** The more important the model, the bigger the impact. Examples include the behaviors of parents, other adults, other children, and television characters.

**D. Behavior occurs in a relationship.** If the relationship is positive, the child will behave better to please the adult (if the adult shows it) than in a negative relationship. Often before any major behavior change can occur, some positive activities need to be implemented. Suggestions include 15–20 minutes a day of playtime with the child during which the child directs the play rather than the parent. The parent should avoid demands or questions and simply make descriptive comments on the child's play during that special time. (e.g., *"The car crashed into the blocks"*).

**E.** In general, **punishment, especially physical punishment, tends to suppress behavior briefly, not eliminate the undesirable behavior** (*"I spank him and 15 minutes later, he's back doing the same thing"*). Punishment alone rarely conveys what behavior is expected from the child. Explanation (not complex reasoning or persuasion) and positive reinforcement (praise, tangible reward, hug, attention) for the desired behaviors are far more instructive.

**VI. Discipline**

**A. Definition.** The word *discipline* comes from the Greek word "to lead." Discipline is a teaching process, not a synonym for punishment. It is the process by which a child learns values; limits on behaviors in specific settings; general rules of interaction; and other familial, cultural, and societal expectations and rules. It can be thought of as the process of "civilizing" or socializing children. The process is lifelong, and with the right parental direction, children develop *self-discipline*, internalized controls on their own behavior in the absence of an externally provided structure or reacting to long-delayed consequences.

**B. Age.** Even as a newborn, the child begins to learn that crying has an impact on events, that certain things bring discomfort, and that others bring comfort and satisfaction. The process of discipline changes with the developmental age of the child, parents, and family.

C. **Aspects of developmentally targeted discipline**
   1. **Environmental "engineering,"** or structuring the environment to be conducive to good behavior (e.g., removing breakable figurines from a child's reach)
   2. **Behavior management techniques** matched to development
   3. **Recognizing normal developmental trends** that effect behavior (e.g., growing need for autonomy and accommodating that need)
   4. **Consistency of rules across settings** or at least clear discrimination between settings (*"That may be okay at Grandma's, but at home, we don't eat candy before dinner."*)

D. **The more positive behavior management methods are, the more positive the parent-child relationship.**

E. **General approach to behavioral problem solving**
   1. **Identify the patterns**. To do so, parents need to keep a chart of whenever the designated problem behavior occurs by date, time, location, activity, persons present, and outcome of the behavior.
   2. **Analyze the pattern** to identify associated events and consequences.
   3. **Generate alternatives,** such as changing consequences, addressing associated events (e.g., changing nap times to avoid overfatigue) or teaching new, more desirable behaviors.
   4. **Implement alternatives** and evaluate their effectiveness by continuing to chart behaviors.

F. **Specific techniques that can be used across developmental ages**
   1. **Positive reinforcement** is a powerful force for shaping desired behaviors.
   2. **Differential attention** is a powerful technique for managing undesirable behaviors that do not hurt anyone else. Parents often feel that ignoring undesirable behavior is not enough or that other parents will judge them harshly. If the interest is in outcome, many small infractions of rules are best treated by ignoring, as long as desirable behavior is reliably receiving positive attention. Behavior to ignore includes temper tantrums, nonphysical struggles with siblings, and noise-making activities.

G. **Time-outs** can be introduced after 2 years of age, sooner or later depending on verbal development.
   1. **Time-outs should be used only for specific behaviors**. In the preschool range, there should only be a few, important behaviors that are followed by time-out, namely, when a child in this age range does something significantly out of bounds (e.g., hits a sibling or parent).
   2. The **purpose** of time-out is to remove the child from opportunities for positive consequences, break the behavior's flow, and teach the child limits to behavior.

3. **Method.** Parents should decide on a somewhat isolated place where the child cannot see television or play with toys but can be supervised by the parent. Sitting on a specified couch, chair, or stair-step is often successful. The child should be placed there *calmly* by the parent with the word "time-out" used in some way to label the event (e.g., "*When you hit you get a time-out*"). The parent should not threaten (e.g., "*Do you need a time-out?*" or "*If you do that again, you'll have to go to time-out*"). After introducing the rule, the time-out should be carried out without delay and without bargaining.
4. **Timing.** The child should sit in the designated place for about 1 minute per year of chronological age; most parents place children in time-out much too long. A mechanical digital or old-style baking timer is useful because it makes the timing more objective for both parties.
5. **Common pitfall—interacting with the child during time-out.** *Parents should not interact with the child during time-out.* During time-out, the child should be ignored. Parents should not allow themselves to be engaged (in conversation, body gesture, or glance) by the child during this period (e.g., "*But Mom, why do I have to sit here?*" "*Because you misbehaved, that's why*").
6. **Ending time-out.** The parent should restate the rule that was broken in a positive fashion (e.g., "*We are gentle with each other*" or "*We use words to show what we want*").
7. **Problem solving.** What about with the child who won't stay in time-out? Often, children who have been taught time-out at an early age learn to take "good" time-outs, but some children introduced to the concept later or more defiant children regardless of age of introduction may refuse to stay in the designated time-out spot. Sometimes, it is a direct result of parental inconsistency with or mishandling of time-outs (e.g., talking to the child). Three options are suggested for the child who refuses to sit in time-out:
   - **a.** The best option is to have a toy-free, hazard-controlled room prepared as back-up. If the child does not stay in a properly administered time-out spot, he or she should be told, "*Since you did not stay in the chair, you'll have to be by yourself.*" The parent should then lead the child to the room, leave the room's lights on, and close the door. All child behavior is ignored, and 60 seconds later, the child is led by the hand back to the chair for a full time-out. If the physician or parents feel uncomfortable about a child's being left alone with the door shut, a sheet of plywood slid across the open door and held in place by the parent is a good alternative. The rest of the procedure is carried out the same way. The parent must *not* interact with child. If the child makes a mess, the child is to return to the time-out chair, finish time-out, then be led back to the room to clean up the mess.
   - **b.** The second option for parents whose child refuses to stay in time-out is to hold the child in the time-out

chair. The parent should say, *"Since you didn't stay in time-out, I'll have to help you."* The child is returned to the chair in a businesslike fashion. The parent should be behind the chair reaching around to hold the child's wrists firmly crossed in front of the child. If the time-out chair has arms, the adult, from behind the chair, can lay one arm across the child's lap and grasp the chair arm firmly, essentially creating a seat belt. When the child's struggling decreases, the parent releases the hold with the statement, *"Now finish your time-out."* This is repeated as necessary.

**c.** The least desirable of the three options for a child who refuses to stay in time-out (but better than not having any effective behavior control) is spanking. The parent says, *"Since you did not stay in time-out, I'll have to spank you."* The parent then spanks the child twice with open hand on the child's clothed buttocks and then returns him or her to the time-out chair with the statement, *"Now finish your time-out."* This may need to be repeated. *This recommendation should be made only with careful consideration of the family and parental anger control.*

Usually several trials of any of the above teach the child to stay in the time-out chair. In turn, applied correctly, time-out is a portable, safe way of teaching children when they have violated a major rule.

**H. Spanking** is controversial and, as addressed above, tends to suppress behaviors, not teach desired behaviors. Nonetheless, it is estimated that more than 60% of parents spank their children. It is not uncommon for primary care physicians to recommend spanking for behavior control. Sometimes it is a good idea to address how to spank with parents, rather than to pretend it does not occur. The child should be spanked only on the clothed buttocks and never on the head or face. An open hand should be the only thing used—never paddles, extension cords, wooden spoons, or other objects. One stern spank is more effective than multiple light taps. Spanking works best (if at all) when saved for major infractions. The parent should wait until he or she calms down rather than spank the child in anger. In fact, the parent leaving the room to cool down can be thought of as a sort of time-out equivalent and may be just as effective without the spanking.

**VII. Discipline guidelines by age of child**

**A. Toddlers and preschoolers.** In the early years, much of discipline is environmental engineering, which includes baby-proofing for safety of the child and belongings, thereby reducing the frequency of frustration-producing *"no no's."* Behavior management also includes attending to the infant or toddler's physical needs to reduce the trouble times of fatigue and hunger. Physicians often can help parents examine their discipline methods, praise or complement them for their specific behaviors, and help them generalize the concept to problem-solve for their own specific family needs.

**1. Under 18 months.** *Teaching task*: To teach the child that the world is a safe, pleasant, reliable place in which his or her needs will be met. To teach that some behaviors have different consequences than others.

The physician should help parents recall that developmentally, the child cannot possibly do things purposefully to irritate the parents. The toddler is cognitively incapable of sophisticated analysis of a situation, including putting himself or herself in the place of the parent. Things a child does may irritate the parent or "push his or her buttons" but that is not *why* the child does them. When parents attribute this kind of intent, they almost inevitably feel the child must be punished to teach them not to defy parental authority. This is not helpful and may set the stage for long-term power struggles. The physician should help parents not to expect too much. Instead, environmental planning is key so that the child is safe to explore without unnecessary frustration on the part of adult or child.

Physical punishment should be avoided with children this age because the behaviors being punished are generally a result of normal development (e.g., urge to explore; tendency to put objects in the mouth; experimentation with the world, including throwing things). Redirection of the child's activity or physically moving the child away from the forbidden object or activity is more educational and effective.

Language is not yet controlling for toddlers, so parents should be given the anticipatory guidance that *"no, no"* is a temporary deterrent at best. There is a point in development around 18 months at which some children respond to any sort of linguistic command by speeding up the behavior rather than stopping it. This is related to neuropsychological development of language functioning in which language may facilitate rather than inhibit behavior.

2. **18–36 months.** *Teaching task*: The child begins to learn that there are rules and limits and that he or she can do and learn for himself or herself. The child begins to learn to use words and to modulate self-expression. The child can begin to learn to be independent.

   Language is developing, but frustration tolerance is very limited. Children this age can delay only for a minute or so. When dealing with the rigidity and inflexibility of this age (*"I want what I want when I want it"*), it is helpful for parents to avoid head-on confrontation and use environmental engineering. Parents should simplify routines, not offer too many (or too complex) choices, and allow the child to express the growing urge to be independent using self-help skills. Positive statements of rules are more effective than negative (e.g., *"We walk in the house"* rather than *"no running"*).

   Frequent disciplinary issues include temper tantrums and physical aggression, especially hitting and biting. Both are almost inevitably linked to the child's frustration by an adult, the child's limitations, a toy, or another child.

3. **3–5 years.** *Teaching task*: To help the child learn to use words to delay gratification, avoid physical aggression, and meet his or her own needs.

Prevention of behavior problems becomes more verbal at this level of development. Children can say "*yes,*" not just "*no*" and "*we*" instead of just "*me.*" Rituals are less necessary. Language is very powerful, and behavior can be influenced by words such as "*new,*" "*different,*" "*help,*" and "*guess.*" Many preschoolers love to please and conform as far as they are capable. They can listen to spoken directions but need them to be specific (e.g., "*We sit quietly in church*") rather than general (e.g., "*Be good*"). This is a "*me too*" age, and children are motivated by the behavior of others, especially if they see another child praised for desirable behaviors. Reasoning now enters into discipline but cannot be depended on. Fantasy is big at this age, and it can be used by parents to engage cooperation by their entering into the game (e.g., "*Can the engineer drive the train all the way back to the toy box?*"). Indirect approaches often work well—for example, a parent might get a child this age to take off his or her outer clothing by guessing what color his or her socks are (of course, by guessing all the wrong colors first). Whispering or exaggerating can be helpful too. The parent will be more effective if he or she avoids asking the child to do something if the intent is a command.

Especially when children are older than 4 years of age, firm limits that are consistently and fairly administered are important to help them limit their actions and keep them safe. Many children feel far more secure with clear limits at this age because their own feelings and actions may scare them in their intensity. Clear, specific expectations should be announced before entering new situations. Time-outs should be used through this age period but seasoned with a heavy allotment of praise, rewards, and affection. Star charts and public admiration are attractive at this age. Heroes are important too, so parents should consider their exposure carefully. Children this age will model their heroes' behaviors.

If a preschool child does something wrong, it is especially helpful to have the "punishment fit the crime" (e.g., if a child leaves the toys all over the playroom, he or she not only has to clean up the room but cannot use the toys for 1 day). Similarly, a child who damages the belongings of another should make up for it in some way. Besides making sense to the child, this kind of approach allows the child to regain some dignity through restitution.

Preschool children who do not readily comply with adults' requests and commands are at greater risk for developing behavior disorders during the school years. This does not mean preschoolers should be always obedient little automatons; however, parents should be able to get their preschoolers to do what they need them to do with a minimum of repetition and time-outs.

**B. School-age children.** *Teaching task*: To help children learn the behavioral expectations outside the home and channel their energy for learning, working, socializing, and having fun into constructive directions.

The same behavioral principles apply, but because of the child's developmental level, there is greater capacity to delay gratification. Praise and punishment also can be a little further removed in time from the behavior that earned it. Unfortunately, typical parents tend to use praise less often with school-age children than younger ones. There is also a tendency to praise outcomes more than the behaviors that led to the outcomes—for example, good quarter grades may be praised more than the daily studying and working that led to the grades.

Time-outs may lose their effectiveness after age 8 years. Removal of privileges becomes more powerful for older kids as they acquire more privileges and opportunities to venture outside the family. Although money becomes a more powerful positive reinforcer for school-age children, parental time is often equally or more effective—for example, the child makes his or her bed every day for a week and earns an extra amount of time with parents or a special activity with them, such as playing Monopoly or another game that a parent might not otherwise play.

Anticipatory guidance at this age should include the warning against assuming that since children always seem so busy and tied up with friends that they no longer need positive time with parents. The child needs to interact with the parent at play and work. Doing tasks together cooperatively rather than in a parallel fashion helps keep the relationship positive. This, in turn, encourages the child to want to please the parent. Communication without criticism or judgment threat is also imperative. Asking questions is generally the least effective way of learning about the child's life. Rather, having quiet, positive times together when the child can offer up small reports without criticism is more likely to help keep communication open.

School-age children still need supervision. There is clear evidence that children, especially ones who already have a history of acting out, will engage in far more frequent, unacceptable, and aggressive behaviors if left unsupervised at this age.

Preteens continue to need praise and generally respond to it more than punishment or threats of punishment. Praise has to be meaningful, not empty words. Genuine praise for an accomplishment that the young person believes required effort is a very positive act from the parent. Recognizing the child's particular struggles makes for powerful praise (e.g., a grade C in math that required hard study may be much more praiseworthy than the A in social studies that did not require as much effort). The values of friends become increasingly important; the presence of a constant set of parental values is an important balance. Values that are not lived but just spoken, however, will be seen by the child as hypocritical very rapidly. Parents and their own behaviors remain very important to their children throughout development.

## Selected Readings

American Academy of Pediatrics. *Report of the Task Force on Education.* Chicago: American Academy of Pediatrics, 1978.

Barkley R. *The Defiant Child: A Clinician's Manual for Parent Training.* New York: Guilford Press, 1987.

Campbell SB. *Behavior Problems in Preschool Children.* New York: Guilford Press, 1990.

Schmitt B. *Your Child's Health* (rev ed). New York: Bantam Books, 1991.

Wissow L, Roter D, Wilson M. Pediatrician style and mothers' disclosure of psychosocial issues. *Pediatrics* 93:289, 1994.

## Recommended Books for Parents

Clark L. *SOS: Help for Parents.* Bowling Green, KY: Parents Press, 1985.

Crary E. *Without Spanking or Spoiling: A Practical Approach to Toddler and Preschool Guidance.* Seattle: Parenting Press, 1979.

Leach P. *Your Baby and Child.* New York: Knopf, 1978.

Patterson GR. *Living With Children.* Champaign, IL: Research Press, 1976.

Sloane HN. *The Good Kid Book: How to Solve the 16 Most Common Behavior Problems.* Champaign, IL: Research Press, 1988.

# 56

# Sleep and Bedtime Behavior

**Janet R. Schultz**

Few parents realize there is an element of learning involved in sleep itself as well as in bedtime behavior. The behavioral factors and principles outlined in the previous chapter are relevant insofar as both the development and consequences of behavior need to be considered with regard to sleep.

**I. Newborns.** *Teaching tasks*: To help the child differentiate wakefulness from sleep and to sleep more at night than during the day.

Newborns typically sleep 16–22 hours a day; not much will make them sleep more or less. In the earliest days, babies tend to drift between states of alertness. To help them learn to be either completely awake or completely asleep, parents should have the child go to bed for sleep rather than be held or kept in a "pumpkin seat." The infant should be "gotten up" when he or she is awake, which also helps strengthen the association between bed and sleep.

Similarly, at night, it is helpful for the child to fall asleep in the place that will be the night's bed. Since rocking the baby to sleep is a pleasant ritual of parenthood, it may be difficult for parents to follow the recommendation that, whenever possible, the infant be placed in the crib while still somewhat awake but sleepy. Placing the drowsy child in the crib helps the child learn to fall asleep on his or her own.

Things that improve the quality of sleep at night include making sure the infant has been fed and burped, keeping the room warm, darkening the room so that even if bedtime is early in the evening, the room looks different than it does in the daytime, and swaddling the infant. There is some evidence that infants who have had more body contact during the day (e.g., in a front baby-carrier) sleep better at night and that, by contrast, infants who are not handled much have more difficulty sleeping. There is little evidence that in the first 6 months of life, an infant can make himself or herself stay awake.

Colic, of course, can complicate the bedtime ritual. In many instances, parents shift into a "making it through" mode during their infant's colic episodes, a totally understandable mind set. Parents need to know that colic is not a result of disease or poor parenting. It is also helpful for them to know that in general, colic lasts no more than 8 weeks and is directly related to the maturity of the child's nervous and digestive systems. Coping strategies include swaddling the child, using an infant swing (motion), and recognizing that sometimes nothing but time will stop the crying. Parents need adequate sleep at other times of the day so that they can remain relatively calm during the infant's colicky episodes. Getting support and hands-on assistance from other adults is useful (see Chap. 31).

**II. 6–18 months.** *Teaching task*: To help the infant learn to soothe himself or herself to sleep without adult help.

Babies in this age range need to have a short, simple, predictable bedtime routine; bedtime should be fairly consistent. As for younger infants, the baby should be put in the crib while still somewhat awake to learn to soothe himself or herself to sleep.

After 6 months of age, some children can keep themselves awake, and many more still need to learn to soothe themselves back to sleep when they wake up. Babies who are accustomed to an adult soothing them to sleep, (e.g., falling asleep while being rocked or cuddled by an adult) or have a history of illness that necessitated parental involvement during the night may need to learn to help themselves back to sleep. Otherwise, when the child's sleep lightens as a normal part of his or her sleep cycle and he or she reaches a relatively wakeful state, adult intervention may be required for the child to go back to sleep. The result is frequent wakenings without nutritive or other needs.

If a bedtime routine has not been established, one should be attempted, preferably for a week or more before intervening further in the baby's sleep. Most babies who still need help learning to put themselves back to sleep can learn to do this in less than a week if parents are willing and committed. At bedtime after feeding, the infant should be put in the crib while still somewhat awake. The parent should not "disappear," but instead putter around the room for a few minutes before leaving. The room should resemble the conditions that will be present when the infant wakens later in the night. It should be as dark or as light and as quiet or as filled with music as it is likely to be later. Favorite comfort items, such as a treasured toy or blanket, should be available. Whenever the child begins to cry, the parent should wait 5 minutes (by the clock) to respond. The parent then should check the child briefly to make sure there is no cause for discomfort and leave again. The child should be aware of the parent's presence, but the adult should not pick up, hug, or sing to the child. A few words to the infant should be the extent of the interaction. After the next 10 minutes (by the clock) of crying, the checking procedure should be repeated until the child falls asleep in the parent's absence. On succeeding nights, the waiting period is gradually lengthened. The usual time of waking in the morning and length of naps should be maintained during this learning period.

A commitment should be made to try this method for 4–5 days. Parents should be warned that the first night is almost always the worst because the child will continue to cry until he or she unlearns the old pattern of expecting a parent to put him or her to sleep and learns to do it himself or herself. If the family lives in an apartment, it may even be necessary to warn immediate neighbors that there may be some crying and why. A supportive call from the physician or the physician's staff can be very helpful to parents, especially the first morning after implementation. Rarely, an infant will cry until he or she vomits. If the infant does vomit, it should be treated with a matter-of-fact clean-up and the process resumed. For some parents, keeping track of when the baby awakens and for how long is a way to measure progress and reassure them that things are in fact getting better. Many parents prefer to start on a night (usually a Friday night) when there are no work obligations the following day and both parents can alternate participation.

About 20–30% of infants 12–36 months of age have trouble sleeping throughout the night. The same basic plan can be used throughout this age range if the problem is frequent awakenings.

**III. Toddlers and preschoolers.** *Teaching task*: To begin to recognize body clues of fatigue, become comfortable with the separation of bedtime, and go to bed and fall asleep without behavioral disruptions or unusual fears.

**A. Resisting bedtime**. As children move into toddler and preschool years, the emphasis shifts from getting the child to fall asleep to getting the child to go to bed and stay there. In this age period, having a set bedtime and a well-established bedtime routine (ritual) are important for teaching the children that it is safe and even pleasant to separate from the many interesting, exciting, and comforting elements of the waking environment. Physical needs (e.g., *"I want a glass of water!"* and *"I gotta go potty"*) should be addressed during the bedtime routine.

Parents also need to understand that they can legislate bedtime but cannot control sleep. The goal of behavior management is to get the child to go to bed peacefully and stay there so that the possibility of sleep is increased and encouraged. It is often useful with a fearful or reluctant child to promise to return to check on the child 5 minutes after tucking the him or her in. The first few times, the child will stay awake to make sure parents keep their word, so it is important that parents not be waylaid by other tasks or children. At the checking time, parents should praise the child for staying in bed and tell the child they will check again later. Generally after a few nights, the child falls asleep sooner and the frequency of checking can be reduced.

**B. Not staying in bed**. For "jack-in-the box" children who pop out of their beds (and usually their bedrooms) as soon as they are put to bed, it is imperative that parents be consistent with management, or else this behavior can be hard to eliminate. The child should not be allowed "just this once" to stay up later, watch a television show, have a snack, or read another book. Calmly and quietly, the parent should take the child by the hand and walk the child back to bed without reassurance or reprimanding. The parent should tuck in the child and leave. This procedure should be repeated each time the child gets out of bed. If a few evenings of this procedure (applied consistently) does not solve the problem, a behavioral program involving positive consequences for staying in bed should be implemented—for example, parents should tell the child they will return in 5 minutes to check on the child. At that point, if the child has stayed in bed, the child is praised and gets a star or sticker on a chart. The parent needs to continue this process, extending the time waited to check on the child, until the child is asleep. If the child remains in bed all night (except to get up to go to the bathroom), the child gets a bonus in the morning, perhaps eating a favorite food for breakfast or watching cartoons during breakfast.

C. **Trouble falling asleep**. If the child has trouble falling asleep but stays in bed, allowing tapes, books, or other quiet activities can be helpful. Use needs to be monitored because some children stay awake longer just to do those things. Children who are afraid of the dark often do well with a room light left on rather than just a night-light, which can create scary shadows. Children in the 4- to 5-year age range love flashlights, which may help them feel some personal control over checking out fears. Many times, children who have been roughhousing just before bedtime or had caffeinated drinks at bedtime are too "wired" to sleep; reconsidering the evening routine and intake can reduce or eliminate these problems. If a child consistently does not fall asleep while in bed but still gets up the following morning at the necessary hour without seeming tired, bedtime may need to be readjusted.

D. **Children who join their parents during the night.** Parents need to evaluate their own feelings about this behavior. Some like it, for a variety of reasons, although they may not freely admit it to themselves. If there is a desire to end this pattern, when the child comes to a parent's bed during the night, the parent should get out of bed and quietly but firmly take the child back to bed. The parent should check on the child's comfort needs, tuck the child in, say *"good-night,"* and return to his or her own bed, again with the promise of returning to check on the child in a few minutes. Generally, this will end the behavior if consistently applied. The star chart and bonus may be employed as well to reward positive consequences for the desired behaviors. If a parent says that he or she does not wake up when the child arrives and, for this reason, cannot take the child back to bed consistently, the parent should hang a string of jingle bells, a couple of empty cans on a string, or other noisemaker on the doorknob of the bedroom door. The door to the parents' bedroom should be kept closed or at least partially closed so that opening it makes enough noise to wake the parent. If a parent does not feel he or she can leave a very fearful child (this reluctance tends to give the child the idea there really is something to be frightened of), the child should be in the child's bed and the parent should stay in the child's room but not in the child's bed. The parent should sit on a chair near the bed for awhile. Then, gradually, each subsequent evening, the chair the parent sits on can be moved closer to the door and finally out the door.

IV. **School-age children**. Older children tend to have a more adult pattern of having their sleep affected by daily tensions. Avoiding disciplinary confrontations at bedtime, having a slow-down time prior to bedtime, keeping to a routine at bedtime, and positive quiet time with parents all can help children relax and sleep. Fears are still common for this age group;

however, while ghosts and monsters still play a role, more realistic fears regarding achievement, world events, burglars, kidnappers, and social rejection may emerge at bedtime.

Older children may resist going to bed. If the bedtime is appropriate for the child's school schedule or parents' needs, compliance can be improved by managing the consequences and rewarding desired behavior. Allowing activities in the bed, such as reading or listening to the radio for awhile, often makes the child's transition to bed easier. Dawdling as a way of delaying bedtime can be addressed by having the child "pay back" the time missed in bed by going to bed that much earlier the next night.

## Selected Readings

Guilleminault C (ed). *Sleep and Its Disorders in Children.* New York: Raven, 1987.

Kataria S, Swanson MS, Trevathan GE. Persistence of sleep disturbances in preschool children. *Behav Pediatr* 110:642, 1987.

## Recommended Books for Parents

Ferber R. *Solve Your Child's Sleep Problems.* New York: Simon and Schuster, 1985.

Leach P. *Your Baby and Child.* New York: Knopf, 1978.

Schaefer C, Petronko M. *Teach Your Baby to Sleep Through the Night.* New York: Putnam and Sons, 1987.

# 57

# Eating and Mealtime Behavior

Janet R. Schultz

Normal weight gain is the greatest in the first year of life (about 15 lbs). As children grow older, the growth curve becomes more gradual, and they tend to eat less while expressing their personal tastes, preferences, and behavioral inclinations more. Parents may be concerned about some of their child's eating changes and need reassurance from the physician that their child is growing at a normal rate. This reassurance reduces the pressure parents impose on their children to eat and makes mealtimes more pleasant and less likely to result in major power struggles. The more the food becomes part of a power struggle, the more frustrated the parents and child are and the less likely the child is to eat the desired quantity or selection of food.

I. **Toddler and preschoolers**. During the toddler years, it is not unusual for children to go on "food jags," during which they want to eat only a narrow range of foods over and over. Many parents may interpret this behavior as the child's being picky. It is an important time for parents to model good eating habits by offering a variety of nutritious (not "junk") foods. Over time, most healthy children will not only eat an adequate amount of food but also eat a relatively balanced diet. During the preschool years, snacks remain an important source of calories and nutrition. Appropriately chosen foods offered at times and in quantities that do not interfere with mealtimes are healthy additions.

If parents do not give in to their child's food fads or become anxious about their child's picky eating, the child generally will continue to grow well. Even though eating itself is usually a positive experience for the majority of healthy children, mealtime behaviors are still subject to the normal principles of behavior:

**A.** Insisting that preschoolers remain at the table more than 15–20 minutes may make mealtime unpleasant and increase the likelihood of avoidance behaviors. Once the child leaves the table, the child should not be allowed more mouthfuls or to return to the table under most circumstances. It should be made clear to the child that once he or she leaves the table after eating, the meal is over.

**B.** A child should not be forced to eat. If the child chooses not to eat, there should be no snack or other foods available until the next time food is normally offered, whether a planned snack time or meal. While a child's particular dislikes can be respected, it is often helpful for the child to be expected to take a "hello" bite of a new or infrequently offered dish.

**C.** Coaxing children to eat can backfire. Children may eat even less and learn that the way to guarantee their parents' intense involvement with them is to avoid eating. Coaxing a few, last bites can undo the whole attempt to encourage eating.

**D.** The behavioral equivalent of verbal coaxing should be discouraged as well. Sometimes parents become very invested in behavioral coaxing and spend excessive amounts of time trying to make delectable and visually tempting food. Then, when the child doesn't eat the food, the parent who spent so much time preparing it is more likely than ever to be angry, frustrated, or worse, hurt or rejected.

**E.** Mealtimes should be pleasant times, without undue emotional arousal (e.g., no exciting television programs or yelling about events that occurred earlier in the day). The focus should be on the behaviors desired from the child rather than on his or her negative behaviors. Mealtime is an especially good time for parents to use "differential attention," during which they pay attention to the child when he or she eats and behaves in the desired fashion and less or no attention during the periods when the child does not.

**F.** Young children often eat more when allowed to feed themselves. This independence can be facilitated by serving finger foods, providing child-sized utensils, and cutting difficult-to-manage foods (meat, spaghetti) ahead of time.

**G.** Allowing children to help choose and prepare foods may increase their intake. Even healthy but marginally attractive foods (e.g., bran muffins) tend to be eaten with more enthusiasm if the child has been the chef and added his or her own special touches.

**H.** When possible, parents should be discouraged from using food as a reward, punishment, or threat (e.g., "*If you don't eat this spinach, you won't get any dessert*"). Especially in families in which food has become an issue, this extra emotional baggage tends to make things worse. Food should not be linked to "good" or "bad" status.

**I.** For a resistant child, serving very small amounts (or allowing the child to serve himself or herself) on a small plate may make the task of eating less overwhelming. The child always can have seconds.

**J.** Most preschoolers are "purists"—that is, they generally do not care for foods that are mixed together as much as they like the foods they can identify and separate. Hence, foods such as casseroles and stews may be less appetizing than the components served separately.

**II. School-age children**. Older children often have a different issue with eating. There is strong evidence that some boys and many more girls develop concerns about being overweight while in the third to fifth grades. Many times, their parents share some of their children's fears, emphasize not becoming fat, and model strong concerns for their own weight. Pressure to meet model standards of appearance surround the child but are particularly meaningful when there is pressure in the home. If obesity is a problem from the physician's perspective, minimizing the availability of junk food, reducing television viewing (a sedentary occupation that tends to be associated with snacking), and increasing physical activity are better than dieting except in unusual cases. Emphasizing healthy eating and exercise habits as a general health promotion effort is better than overemphasizing appearance. If being underweight is the problem, careful behavioral and intake records need to be examined because school-age children can develop eating disorders. Similarly, family dynamics and general attitudes about appearance, body type, and the child's performance are relevant.

## Selected Readings

Birch LL, Mailin DW. I don't like it: I never tried it: Effects of exposure on two-year-old children's food preferences. *Appetite* 3:353, 1982.

Eppright ES. Eating behavior of preschool children. *J Nutr Ed* 1:16, 1969.

Frank D, Silva M, Needleman R. Failure to thrive: Mystery, myth, and methods. *Contemp Pediatr* 10:104, 1993.

Satter EM. The feeding relationship. *J Am Diet Assoc* 86:352 1986.

Satter EM. Childhood eating disorders. *J Am Diet Assoc* 86:357, 1986.

## Recommended Books for Parents

Satter EM. *How to Get Your Child to Eat . . . But Not Too Much.* Emeryville, CA: Publishers Group West, 1987.

# 58

# School-Related Problems

Janet R. Schultz

I. **School readiness.** Having a child begin school before he or she is ready can contribute cognitively, emotionally, socially, and behaviorally to problems, such as school refusal, lack of enjoyment of school, poor school achievement for both early and later grades, and behavioral problems.

Many schools now screen potential incoming kindergartners, and some have special programs for children who do not seem ready for school but are of chronological age. When parents ask physicians about the readiness of their children for school, the physician's opinion should be based on several sources of information, including the following:

A. **The physician's observation of the child and the child's relationship with the parent(s),** specifically, the ease of separation of child from parent, speech development, and frequency of physical complaints. Can the child copy a square, triangle, and circle? Can the child print his or her first name? Can the child state his or her first name, last name, address, and phone number?

B. **The parent's opinion and observations at home or with other caregivers.** Can the child play well with other children? Does the parent trust the child in the backyard alone, occasionally monitoring from inside the house? Is the child trusted to stop at a street corner or curb and wait for an adult? Can the child be trusted to cross a low-traffic, good visibility street on his or her own? Has the child shown interest in books or letters and numbers?

C. **The child's history of separation from parents and success in preschool settings.** Preferably, the history includes the opinion of the child's preschool teacher regarding readiness.

D. **The child's chronological age and sex.** While the relationship between school readiness and these demographics is not perfect, generally a child does better in kindergarten if his or her birthday is at least 4–6 months before the beginning of school. Also, girls are usually ready for school earlier than boys.

E. **The child's developmental history.** Has the child generally been in the average range of development, or has the child been in the slower range?

F. **Knowledge of the proposed program for the child.** Kindergartens that emphasize academics demand greater readiness than specially designed developmental programs or more traditional kindergarten programs. School readiness is in part a question of fit or match.

G. **Screening devices available.** An easy screening device for parents to perform is the Child Development Inventory (Ireton, revised 1993), a series of true-false questions requiring about 30 minutes or less to complete.

**II. Homework** is an area of recurrent tension in many homes but should be viewed as a teaching opportunity. If parents handle homework issues appropriately, completing homework serves two purposes: The child learns the academic material and about responsibility and organization at the same time.

**A.** Homework is the child's problem, not the parents'; hence, parents should not do the child's homework or take primary responsibility for seeing that it is completed.

**B.** After school, the parent and child should look over papers and materials sent home from school. It is a good time for praise, or at least encouragement, whenever possible. It is useful for parents to join younger children in looking over the homework for the evening, estimating how much time assignments will take, and setting an order in which they will be completed. Some families believe homework should be completed right after school so that the rest of the evening is clear. Others believe the child should have a break after a day of scholastic activity. When the child does homework is less important than ensuring consistency and an established routine for doing it.

**C.** With many younger children, homework goes better if parents ask to see each assignment as it is finished. Parents should give *positive* feedback on accuracy and praise whenever possible. Older children who generally do their homework without parental intervention should have a choice about showing each completed assignment to parents.

**D.** Emphasis should be on developing good study habits, which means taking pride in work; having a quiet place to study that is equipped with the child's needs; and learning to organize work, set priorities, and check for accuracy. For some children, developing good study habits includes learning how to break down assignments into manageable pieces. Reviewing notes even when no exam is imminent can be introduced at the junior high school level unless the school's academic demands indicate otherwise.

**E.** Children generally do more homework and perform better in school when their parents are in contact with teachers and know the school's expectations. Parent involvement with the school and its activities (e.g., PTA, open house, musical performances) is associated with better achievement by a child and enhanced self-esteem.

**F.** If an older child routinely has no homework, a telephone call to the teacher may be in order. If a child does not complete assigned homework, the teacher, parents, and often the child need to be in communication. Some teachers prefer that the problem of incomplete homework be handled between teacher and student only, which often serves to remove the aspect of rebelling against parents out of the struggle and emphasizes that homework is the child's responsibility, not the parents'.

Especially with younger students, parents may want to establish an assignment book between the teacher and parent in which the child records assignments, which are initialed by the teacher at the end of the day to confirm accuracy. Parents initial assignments as they are finished. A reward system also may be implemented. In general, rewards are more helpful if they focus on short-term work rather than quarterly report cards. Children perform better when the emphasis is placed on learning for the sake of knowledge and pleasure rather than for stars, stickers, and money. Some children, however, ultimately need extrinsic rewards if the intrinsic ones do not motivate adequately.

Most children who do not do homework operate in an avoidance paradigm: The reward for not doing homework is the avoidance of the task itself and having the freedom it brings to do other things. Sometimes, avoiding homework is based on anxiety about or dislike for the assignment, especially if the child does not understand it. Sometimes, the child's failure to complete work is an indication of academic problems rather than a cause of them. Parent (or sometimes physician) contact with teachers may help clarify the problem (see Chaps. 62 and 63).

III. **School refusal** is a newer term for what previously was called school phobia. The terminology has changed because school phobia implies a limited etiology (fear of school), whereas school refusal implies that children avoid school for reasons other than fear. The term does not include occasional, deliberate acts of truancy, which is distinguished from school refusal based on where the child stays when not at school but should be. School refusers tend to be home or in the care of family friends or relatives. Truant children are out on the street or in the home of friends, usually without adult supervision.

A. **Etiology.** School refusal is, in most respects, a problem of avoidance. The child avoids the unpleasant or anxiety-provoking situations of separating from home (and usually parent) and attending, performing, and socializing in school. Sometimes nurturance that accompanies any physical symptoms helps maintain the pattern; however, avoidance tends to be the most powerful force underlying school refusal.

B. **Presentation.** School refusers often present to primary care physicians offices with physical symptoms, such as stomachaches, headaches, or general malaise, rather than with the complaint of school refusal. Often the symptoms are vague, vary from day to day, and recur on Sunday evenings or Monday mornings, having disappeared over the weekend. If certain academic courses engender more anxiety than others, the onset of symptoms may vary and match the child's class schedule. This behavior tends to be more characteristic of older children.

C. **Prevalence and patterns**. The incidence of school refusal is difficult to establish because many school refusers are not diagnosed as such; it has been estimated at 1–2%. Unlike many childhood behavior problems, school refusal is not identified primarily in boys. Some studies indicate equal incidence by sex; others suggest it may be more frequent in girls. There are no clear socioeconomic correlations or differences in occurrence by birth order. School refusers are intelligent, and their achievement scores are no different than those of their schoolmates. The data are somewhat unclear, but there may be three peaks of school refusal: age 5–6 years (beginning elementary school), around 11 years (often during middle school or transition into junior high), and around 14 years (beginning high school). Generally, the older the child, the more difficult the problem is to treat.

**D. Onset**. Although separation anxiety is a well-known contributor, there are other sources of school refusal that should be routinely considered.

1. The onset of school refusal may be linked to a clear precipitant for the family or child, including a death, a separation or divorce, birth of a sibling, or a change of teacher. Given the apparent association of transition times with peaks of symptoms, new school routines with unclear expectations and social challenges also may be involved.
2. There are "reality-based" considerations for school refusal as well—for example, a child may be the target of an intimidating child (the class "bully") or adult and fear for his or her own safety. Similarly, children whose lunches or lunch money are stolen regularly or who must walk to school through neighborhoods with intimidating people (or animals) may develop aversions and fears. Some children may have motion sickness from riding the bus or dislike the lengthy or unruly school bus ride with older children on board.

**E. Detection of school refusals**

1. Sometimes, the diagnosis of school refusal is clear because the child says outright that he or she refuses to go to school and clings to the parent when it is time to go.
2. Sometimes, physical symptoms predominate, and the physician must rule out physical illness first and then consider school-related problems. The latter may be suggested by patterns of symptoms relative to school attendance and questions to the parent about school (e.g., *"Does your child's illness usually keep him home from school?" "How many days of school has the child missed in the last month?" "Is the child usually better on weekends until Sunday evening?"*). Other occurrences of mild illness that resulted in school absences, especially associated with Mondays or the day of return to school after holidays, should raise the index of suspicion. Many cases of recurrent abdominal pain include a component of school refusal.

**F. Managing school refusal**

1. *The most important part of treating school refusal is to get the child back to school as soon as possible*. Getting the child to return to school sometimes involves intervention during the events that provoke fear or avoidance in the child, especially if the events are clear. If the fear or avoidance is more generalized, returning the child to school may take one of several formats, including the following:
   a. Sometimes just hearing that the child should be in school motivates parents to get the child there. It should be made clear, however, that the child is not

faking symptoms so that there is no punitive edge to the parents' actions. Motivating parents by ruling out major illness is most successful when the child has not yet missed much school.

**b.** Often, parents and, at times, the physician should contact school personnel to inform them that the child is well enough to attend school and to enlist their assistance. Many schools, especially elementary schools, have dealt with such problems and have a protocol, which usually involves having the parent hand the resisting child over to the teacher and leaving promptly. School personnel then take over, with reassurance and firmness.

**c.** If the school does not have a protocol and the child has been out for several days already, a good proposal is for the child to come to school late and be there only part of the day. The child always should leave with the other children, which is much better than repeating the problem pattern that often has happened already, namely that the child goes to school with the children in the morning and leaves early. Over a week, the child's school day should be extended gradually until the child is there all day. Parents or the physician should notify the school that the child not be sent home. If the child is "too sick" to stay in class, the child should remain at school, preferably in the nurse's office (without TV or positive reinforcement from a well-meaning nurse or secretary). The physician should set an objective rule with the school (e.g., a temperature higher than 100.4°F or vomiting) for sending the child home.

If the parent is not sure whether the child is too sick to attend school, the same or a similar objective rule should be enforced to avoid ambivalence. Sometimes keeping breakfast light (but making sure the child eats something) helps the child's nausea or motion sickness.

**2.** For several weeks, the child will need follow-up appointments to monitor his or her progress. The appointments, however, should not be scheduled in such a way that they interrupt school attendance. It also should be made clear to parents that the purpose of the follow-up appointments is to monitor the child's progress, not to "make sure that nothing organic was missed."

**3.** Although the child may resume school attendance, the physician should explain to the parent that school refusal occurs for a reason that may still remain. To prevent recurrence and deal with what is behind the symptoms' development, the parent needs to be in contact with the school and consider the home situation to determine major stressors and contributions.

**4.** If the physician and parent together cannot identify the problem's source and determine how to address it, a referral to a psychiatrist, psychologist, or other therapist who addresses biobehavioral issues may be indicated. Similarly, if the child does not resume regular attendance promptly, a referral is indicated. The longer the child is out of school, the more difficult it is to get the child to return. Children who have a history of repeated episodes of school refusal are difficult to treat and should be referred as well.

## Selected Readings

Durlak JA. School Problems of Children. In CE Walker, MC Robert (eds), *Handbook of Clinical Child Psychology* (2nd ed). New York: Wiley, 1992.

Ireton H. *Child Behavior Inventory*. Minneapolis: Behavior Science Systems, 1992.

Last CG, Francis G. School Phobia. In B Lahey, AE Kasdin (eds), *Advances in Clinical Child Psychology*. New York: Plenum, 1988.

## Recommended Books for Parents

Rosemond, J. *Ending the Homework Hassle*. Kansas City: Andrews and McMeel, 1990.

Sloane HN. *The Good Kid Book: How to Solve the 16 Most Common Behavior Problems*. Champaign, IL: Research Press, 1988.

# 59

# Temper Tantrums

## Janet R. Schultz

Temper tantrums usually occur when children are 12 months to 5 years old, with a peak between 18 and 48 months. While not all children have the lay-down-and-kick-and-scream variety of tantrum, most children have some angry outbursts their parents see as tantrums. One study shows that 15% of parents report that their 1-year-olds have tantrums every day. Another study suggests that children who have daily tantrums at 2 years of age are likely to continue to have frequent tantrums at 3, and a third of them will continue to have tantrums at 4 and 5 years of age. An estimated 5% of children have "breath-holding spells" as part of their tantrums. The prime candidates for recurrent tantrums are those 10% of children whose temperament is sometimes described as "difficult" or, in a more positive light, "spirited." These children often had a history of head-banging and head-bumping at earlier ages and tended to express desires and needs in a physical fashion. Delays in verbal development may increase the likelihood of tantrums by limiting more acceptable means of getting needs met.

**I. Preventing tantrums.** In the toddler years, the goal should be preventing tantrums rather than figuring out the best response to them. Generally, tantrums occur when children are particularly frustrated by limits set on their behavior, limits placed on them by their own development, or the challenges of their environment.

Problem solving should begin with charting all temper tantrums for several days. Parents should keep track of tantrums by day, time, place, person present, activity at the time of the tantrum, and what happened as a result of the tantrum. Patterns usually emerge from these observations and commonly indicate that the tantrums occur most often at a specific time of day. This time of day should be considered in terms of hunger; fatigue; and changes in the environment, such as a decrease in the caregiver's availability (e.g., during dinner preparation) or an increase in activity and competition for attention (e.g., older children coming home from school). Sources of frustration operating at the time also should be considered.

Whatever the tantrums' pattern, it provides information as to their prevention. Snack or nap times may need to be altered; plans for entertaining small children while the parent is otherwise occupied may need to be made. Often, better environmental engineering ("baby-proofing") needs to be implemented to reduce the frequency of the child's frustration. Often, parents can pay attention to the pattern and, using their own observations of the child's behavior, learn to detect when tension is mounting. Parents then can prevent tantrums by distracting the child with a less frustrating or safer activity. Other times, children need more physical outlets for their energy. Verbal children need to be coached on how to put their desires and reactions into words to which the parents must be at least willing to listen. Generally, routines, warnings of approaching transitions (e.g., *"In a few minutes, we will have to stop playing and go pick up Jimmy from school"*), and use of **limited** choices (e.g., *"Do you want your bunny or your tiger to sleep with you?"* rather than *"Are you ready for nap, now?"*) help prevent tantrums.

**II. Responding to tantrums.** When tantrums cannot be prevented, parents should try to appear calm and businesslike. In general, unless children are endangering themselves or encroaching substantially on the rights of others (e.g., screaming and kicking in church), the best approach is to reduce the positive reinforcement children receive by having tantrums and ignore the negative behavior (e.g., by leaving the room in which the tantrum is occurring). This means not giving in to the child's demands or paying attention to the child during the tantrums. If necessary, the child can be moved out of the public path (e.g., church). In this circumstance, the parent should continue to remain calm and, as soon as the child is moved, resume ignoring the behavior. When the child is calm, there is opportunity to discuss with the child other ways to ask for things and to handle anger and frustration.

Children should not be allowed to hurt anyone, including parents, during the tantrum. The intensity of their own feelings often scares them. When children later realize they have done something genuinely hurtful, it may frighten them further. Not being prevented from hurting someone else may undermine a child's sense of security in the parents' ability to protect him or her.

Many children respond well to positive attention, including cuddling and soothing after the tantrum, but it should be restricted to when the tantrum is over rather than used as a means to get the tantrum to stop. Otherwise, the child may learn to get these special reactions by throwing tantrums.

## Selected Readings

Chess S, Thomas A. *Temperament in Clinical Practice*. New York: Guilford Press, 1986.

Needlman R, Howard B, Zuckerman B. Temper tantrums: When to worry. *Contemp Pediatr* 6:12–34, 1994.

## Recommended Books for Parents

Crary E. *Without Spanking or Spoiling: A Practical Approach to Toddler and Preschool Guidance*. Seattle: Parenting Press, 1979.

Leach P. *Your Baby and Child*. New York: Knopf, 1978.

Patterson GR. *Living With Children*. Champaign, IL: Research Press, 1976.

# Toilet Training

Janet R. Schultz

Toilet training involves teaching children to recognize their body's physical cues signaling the need to empty the bowel and bladder and encouraging them to maintain bowel and bladder continence until the potty chair or toilet can be used.

**I. Readiness**. Although having the first child on the block to be toilet-trained seems to be important to a parent's self-esteem, a child's ability to be toilet-trained depends largely on his or her overall development level. Even the most skillful trainer cannot teach a child to reliably initiate independent toileting if the child is not ready.

Generally, a child is ready for toilet training when he or she is in the 24- to 36-month age range. The child should be showing interest in the task before it is begun in earnest. Readiness depends on motor, cognitive, and emotional maturation. The following screening items are useful in determining if a child is ready for toilet training. The child should be able to accomplish at least eight of the following items before toilet training is begun.

- **A.** The child should be able to point to his or her (1) eyes, (2) nose, (3) mouth, and (4) hair.
- **B.** The child should be able to follow verbal instructions to (5) sit down in a chair; (6) stand up; (7) walk with the parent to a particular place, such as another room; (8) imitate the parent in a simple task (e.g., playing "pat-a-cake"); (9) bring the parent a familiar object (e.g., a toy); and (10) place one familiar object with another (e.g., "*Put your teddy bear by the book*").

**II. Training techniques.** The child should be trained for daytime dryness and cleanliness before nighttime. Many children who have regular bowel movements find it easier to master bowel control first because bowel movements are less frequent and give more warning to parent and child. Constipation complicates learning and may contribute to refusal to use the toilet or potty for defecation. Children can learn to control bowels and urination in either order or together.

It is often easier for the child to use a child-sized potty; parents may accustom the child to using it by having the child sit on it fully clothed. The potty then can be placed in the bathroom, where the child is encouraged to sit on it while older siblings and parents use the toilet (with or without clothes on the child). Once the child is comfortable with the potty, he or she should be told (not asked) at intervals convenient to the caregiver (45 minutes to an hour) that *"it is time to go to the potty"* and brought to sit on it. To facilitate bowel training by capitalizing on the gastrocolic reflex, the child should sit on the potty after meal(s). Parents also can add sitting times when behavioral signals of impending defecation are noted. Part of preparing for toilet training is noting behavior in children that predicts urination or defecation (e.g., becoming quiet; straining or turning red in the face; passing flatus; time of day; or timing near an event, such as bath time).

The child should be praised for sitting and praised again if he or she has a result in the potty. Stickers, star charts, and small candies can help the process. If the child does not produce, he or she should be encouraged ("*maybe next time*") and not made to sit more than a few minutes. If sitting slightly longer seems to help, the parent should come prepared with books or toys to keep the sitting pleasant. There should be no punishment for "accidents" because toilet training is a skill building time, not a struggle of wills.

Some children virtually train themselves when given access to proper equipment, whereas others take months to learn these skills. Reluctant or very verbal children often benefit from books such as *I'm a Big Kid Now* or Mr. Rogers's book, *Going to the Potty*, about toileting.

It is generally easier to teach a boy to urinate sitting down first and then move to standing. Potties usually have splashguards to accommodate the male anatomy.

**III. Diapers and training pants.** Diapers can be used during the training period, but training pants generally facilitate learning because they are easier for the child to lower independently and give quicker feedback about wetness. Some diaper services deliver training pants if parents do not want to wash them themselves. There are, of course, disposable training pants available, which have the advantage of being able to be ripped down the sides and removed like diapers if the child soils them. In warm weather, having the child naked from the waist down sometimes makes training easier, albeit messier. Diapers still can be used at night during training and, if they are not used during the day, the child can make the discrimination between expectations relatively readily.

If the parents and children go out during training, parents should be vigilant to keep sitting schedules and watch for nonverbal (or verbal, if they are lucky) clues that the child needs to visit a bathroom. They should come prepared with extra clothes and treat accidents calmly. Many novices are more comfortable if their parents bring a portable potty seat along.

By 36 months, around 80% of children are dry reliably through the day. Almost all children who do not have urologic problems or major developmental delays are dry during the day in time for school. Nighttime dryness may come later, however.

## Selected Readings

Azrin N, Fox R. *Toilet Training in Less Than a Day*. New York: Simon and Schuster, 1974.

Brazelton TB. A child-oriented approach to toilet training. *Pediatrics* 29:121, 1962.

Matson JL, Ollendick TH. Issues in toilet training normal children. *Behav Therapy* 8:549, 1977.

Schmitt B. *Your Child's Health* (rev ed). New York: Bantam Books, 1991.

## Recommended Books for Parents

Brooks JG. *I'm A Big Kid Now: A Book About Toilet Training (For Parents and Child).* Neenah, WI: Kimberly-Clark Corp., 1993.

Leach P. *Your Baby and Child.* New York: Knopf, 1978.

# 61

# Sibling Rivalry

**Janet R. Schultz**

Sibling rivalry is a universal issue dating back to Cain and Abel. There are few families in which children cooperate and are caring to each other all the time. Children who are cooperative and caring all of the time are the exception rather than the rule, and many times, mutually aggravating behavior between or among siblings is a major challenge for parents. These relationship problems may or may not represent dysfunction. More often than not, these behaviors become habits maintained by their consequences, regardless of their origin.

**I. Etiology.** While the most well-known formulation of sibling rivalry is the theory of displacement from the sole (or at least youngest) position, children can have rivalrous feelings about older *or* younger siblings. In fact, the sibling may be still in utero and evoke rivalrous feelings. Most research suggests, however, that the etiology may be the change in the parent-child relationship (especially the mother-child relationship) after a baby is born. Even parents who try very hard not to be different with their older child(ren) have been documented to have changes in expectations, time availability, and patience (often related to "new baby fatigue"). Practically speaking, behaviors that were once acceptable, even admired (e.g., making siren noises while playing with a toy fire engine) may now be disruptive or forbidden. Things *are* different when a new baby arrives!

**II. Preventing sibling rivalry**. Parents can do several things to prevent sibling rivalry from occurring (proactive management) or at least from becoming a significant problem (reactive management), including the following:

**A.** Prepare older children for the new sibling's arrival by talking, reading children's books together, and reminiscing about what they were like as infants, preferably with pictures of their early days. Parents should describe what a baby's behavior will be like.

**B.** Friends and family often bring gifts for the new baby and pay much attention to the new arrival to the exclusion of the older children. Encourage extended family members to pay attention to the older children and perhaps take them for a few hours to help out. Gifts brought home from the hospital "from the baby" also can help balance the attention being given. Paying attention to the older child's new status as a big brother or sister helps as well and should include some new status symbol (e.g., staying up 15 minutes later) and being included in the baby's care (e.g., getting diapers, pushing the stroller, helping burp the baby).

**C.** Avoid comparing children to each other, even for motivation.

**D.** Accept siblings' feelings about each other, even unpleasant ones, and help the children put them into words. There should be limits on behavioral expressions of their feelings, however.

**E.** Parents need to have some positive time with each child, even if not always alone.

**F.** As soon as the second sibling is verbal, try to coach verbal ways of requesting things (e.g., "*May I have the train?*") instead of grabbing for them, managing anger (e.g., "*I'm really mad at you for calling me a brat*") instead of hitting the other sibling, and negotiating (e.g., "*I'll trade you the ball for the Barbie*"). Siblings are perfect partners to practice social skills relevant to everyone outside the home.

**G.** With children less than 5 years of age, put their names on possessions in readily visible locations. In the preschool years, a printed name develops into greater proof of ownership than does use. It is easier for a child to share things that are indisputably marked as the child's own.

**H.** Not all possessions need to be shared. Special toys can be designated as for one child's use only, but then the child must play with them in a private place or when the other child is not present. This practice often frees the child to share other, less precious toys.

**I.** Parents should not "play favorites." Trying to avoid playing favorites does not mean buying each child a pair of socks because one child needs a pair; however, it does mean avoiding behavioral expressions of emotional favoritism, such as praising one child's behavior or accomplishment while ignoring the same or similar achievement in another.

**J.** Set limits on expressions of rivalry or other disagreements. Parents should model these behaviors in their interactions with the children. Possible rules include no hitting, breaking things, or calling names. Follow-through and consequences are necessary.

**K.** Parents should try to stay out of their children's arguments, especially the arguments of school-age children. When parents involve themselves in the children's arguments, children sometimes learn that arguing is a way to engage parents. There is rarely an easy solution for parents. If the arguing annoys parents, they should tell the children to resolve their differences quietly or in another place. If they do not comply, the children can be sent outdoors or geographically separated. There is one exception to not becoming involved in children's arguments: If an argument becomes physically aggressive, parents should stop the fight, geographically separate the children, and treat them as equally responsible. Physical fights left without intervention tend to escalate and are often unfairly matched.

**L.** Like most behaviors, bickering can be addressed by the suggested general problem-solving paradigm. Effective together are positive reinforcement for getting along and "response cost" for arguing (i.e., awarding points for playing cooperatively and getting along for specific periods of time and penalizing them a certain number of points for arguing; the remaining points are redeemable for a joint reward).

**M.** Sometimes it is helpful for parents to think about their own positions in their families of origin. Often, when two parents interpret situations consistently differently and have conflict over these views, it reflects their own experiences as children. Other times, one of the children reminds a parent of his or her own sibling, himself or herself, or a former spouse; thus, reactions lose objectivity.

**N.** *Tattling*, a form of sibling rivalry, is a very powerful tool siblings use to "get even" with each other. A rule that allows "telling" only when the sibling or someone with the sibling could get hurt may prevent or minimize tattling. A response, such as *"thank you for letting me know"* or *"it really bugs you when he does that, doesn't it,"* is an equally clear message to the tattling child that the parent is not allowing himself or herself to be engaged in the power play.

## Selected Readings

Faber A. Mazlish E. *Siblings Without Rivalry*. New York: W.W. Norton, 1987.

Schmitt B. When Siblings Quarrel. *Contemp Pediatr* 8:74–75, 1991.

## Recommended Books for Parents

Crary E. *Kids Can Co-operate*. Seattle: Parenting Press, 1988.

Kingsley EP. *A Baby Sister for Herry. A Sesame Street/Golden Press Book*. New York: Western Publishing, 1984.

Leach P. *Your Baby and Child*. New York: Knopf, 1978.

# Attention Deficit Hyperactivity Disorder

Rosemary E. Schmidt

Hyperactivity is a common complaint heard by primary care physicians and professionals who deal with the behavioral problems of school children. Usually, when an appointment is made for the child, the school has contacted the parent and suggested having the child evaluated for hyperactivity due to behavior difficulties at school. The most common age at which children are referred for evaluation is 6–8 years of age, when the structured setting of school tends to bring this kind of behavior into focus. The term *hyperactivity* has been used variously to describe a symptom, a symptom complex, and a specific disorder, which is now termed *attention deficit hyperactivity disorder* (ADHD).

I. **The definition for ADHD** in the *Diagnostic and Statistical Manual of Mental Disorders* (3rd edition, revised) (DSM-III-R) is a disturbance of behavior of at least 6 months duration that (1) began before 7 years of age, (2) does not meet the criteria for a pervasive developmental disorder, and (3) is associated with at least eight of the following behaviors:

**A.** Often fidgets with hands or feet or squirms in seat (in adolescents, may be limited to subjective feelings of restlessness)

**B.** Has difficulty remaining seated when required to do so

**C.** Is easily distracted by extraneous stimuli

**D.** Has difficulty awaiting turn in games or group situations

**E.** Often blurts out answers to questions before they have been completed

**F.** Has difficulty following through on others' instructions (e.g., fails to finish chores). This difficulty is not due to oppositional behavior or failure of comprehension.

**G.** Has difficulty sustaining attention in tasks or play activities

**H.** Often shifts from one uncompleted activity to another

**I.** Has difficulty playing quietly

**J.** Often talks excessively

**K.** Often interrupts or intrudes on others (e.g., "butts" in on other children's games)

**L.** Often does not seem to listen to what is being said to him or her

**M.** Often loses things necessary for tasks or activities at school or at home (e.g., toys, pencils, books, assignments)

**N.** Often engages in physically dangerous activities without considering the possible consequences (e.g., runs into the street without looking). The child does not engage in these activities for the purpose of thrill-seeking.

The above items are listed in descending order of discriminating power based on data from a national field trial of the DSM-III-R criteria for disruptive behavior disorders. The above criteria are considered to be met only if the behavior is considerably more frequent in the child than in most children of the same mental age.

**II. Criteria for severity of ADHD**

**A. Mild.** Few, if any, symptoms in excess of those required to make the diagnosis and only minimal or no impairment in school and social functioning.

**B. Moderate**. Symptoms or functional impairment intermediate between "mild" and "severe."

**C. Severe.** Many symptoms in excess of those required to make the diagnosis and significant, pervasive impairment in functioning at home and school with peers.

**III.** The **differential diagnosis** for hyperactive behavior is extensive and may include the following:

**A.** Specific learning disabilities
**B.** Adjustment disorders
**C.** Disorders of mood (dysthymia, depression)
**D.** Anxiety disorders
**E.** Pervasive developmental disorders such as autism
**F.** Absence seizures
**G.** Visual or hearing impairment

**IV. Conditions that often accompany ADHD**

**A.** Speech and language disorders
**B.** Enuresis
**C.** Sleep disturbances
**D.** Borderline intelligence
**E.** Coordination difficulties
**F.** Specific learning disabilities
**G.** Oppositional defiant disorder
**H.** Conduct disorder
**I.** Symptoms of depression or anxiety

**V. Evaluation.** The diagnosis of ADHD requires an extensive **history and physical examination**, with particular attention to the neuropsychiatric examination. Both parents and teachers should report on the child's behaviors at home and in the classroom. Several **behavior rating scales** are available for these purposes, including the Taylor Parent Behavior Rating Scale and the Connors Teacher Rating Scale (Table 62-1), commonly used because of its simplicity. Most children should undergo specific **IQ and achievement testing,** such as the Wechsler Intelligence Scale for Children and the Woodcock-Johnson Psychoeducational Battery, to ensure appropriate school placement. **Psychological evaluation** may be necessary to identify behavioral components that may affect treatment significantly.

**VI. Treatment** for children diagnosed with ADHD must be tailored to the child's individual needs and may include appropriate school grade (re)placing, tutoring, language therapy, and drug therapy. It almost always requires behavioral management for the child and frequently the family. Medication is never the only intervention. The most commonly used drugs prescribed by the primary care physician are methylphenidate (Ritalin) and dextroamphetamine (Dexedrine). The former is preferred because dextroamphetamines have a significant abuse potential. Medications are usually begun with a small dose (2.5–5.0 mg) given at breakfast and lunchtime and grad-

**Table 62-1. Connors Abbreviated Teacher Rating Scale**

| Behavior | None (0) | Pretty little (1) | Very much (2) | Much (3) |
|---|---|---|---|---|
| Restless (overactive) | ___ | ___ | ___ | ___ |
| Excitable, impulsive | ___ | ___ | ___ | ___ |
| Disturbs other children | ___ | ___ | ___ | ___ |
| Fails to finish things (short attention span) | ___ | ___ | ___ | ___ |
| Fidgeting | ___ | ___ | ___ | ___ |
| Inattentive, distractable | ___ | ___ | ___ | ___ |
| Demands must be met immediately, gets frustrated | ___ | ___ | ___ | ___ |
| Cries | ___ | ___ | ___ | ___ |
| Mood changes quickly | ___ | ___ | ___ | ___ |
| Temper outbursts (explosive, unpredictable) | ___ | ___ | ___ | ___ |
| Total score* | ___ | ___ | ___ | ___ |

*≥ 15 significant.
Source: Adapted from CK Connors. *Conners' Rating Scales Manual*. North Tonawanda, NY: Multi-Health Systems, 1990.

ually increased until either satisfactory results are obtained or side effects develop (maximum dose, 1.0 mg/kg/day). Once an effective dose is determined, the sustained-release Ritalin or a combination of sustained-release and short-acting Ritalin may be more suitable depending on the circumstances. Ritalin shows results very quickly, and therefore dosage can be adjusted weekly to monthly until the optimal dose is determined. Follow-up discussions and evaluations from teachers and parents are necessary to determine the drug's effectiveness. Although careful monitoring of growth is recommended, it is usually not a long-term problem in the usual recommended dose. If Ritalin is ineffective, the primary care physician in most instances should consider a referral to a specialist in childhood ADHD and behavior disorders.

## Selected Readings

Adesman AR, Wender EH. Improving the outcome for children with ADHD. *Contemp Pediatr* 8:122–139, 1991.

American Psychiatric Association. *Diagnostic and Statistical Manual of Mental Disorders-III-Revised*. Washington, DC: American Psychiatric Association, 1987.

Cantwell DP, Baker L. Differential diagnosis of hyperactivity. *JDCP* 8:159, 1987.

Levine MD, Jordan NC. Learning disorders: The neurological underpinnings. *Contemp Pediatr* 4:16, 1987.

Levine MD. *Developmental Variation and Learning Disorders*. Toronto: Educators Publishing Service, 1987.

Silver LB. Controversial proposals to treating learning disabilities and attention deficit disorder. *Am J Dis Child* 140:1045, 1986.

Taylor B. Syndrome of Overactivity and Attention Deficit. In M Rutter, BA Hersov (eds), *Child and Adolescent Psychiatry* (2nd ed). Oxford, England: Blackwell, 1985.

Wechsler D. *Wechsler Intelligence Scale for Children-Revised Manual (WICS-R)*. New York: Psychological Corporation, 1974.

Woodcock RW, Johnson MB. *Woodcock-Johnson Psychoeducational Battery*. Bingham, MA: Teaching Resources Corporation, 1977.

# School Failure

Rosemary E. Schmidt

Children who are underachieving in school often are referred to their primary care physician, often at the suggestion of the school, to determine the cause. Some parents may overlook obvious reasons due to their own subjectivity, and the physician may in fact be able to provide assistance. For example, identifying poor vision in a child too embarrassed or proud to admit he or she is having trouble to seeing the blackboard or uncovering a school bully who is intimidating a child may come to light fairly easily in the office setting. More commonly, however, the problem of underachievement is more complex, such as a learning disability or a significant emotional problem, that parents, in fact, do recognize, or at least suspect. These impediments to learning usually require the help of other professionals to provide a diagnostic and therapeutic regimen.

I. **Causes of school failure**
   - **A.** Mental subnormality
   - **B.** Disorders of communication (hearing, speech, or language)
   - **C.** Emotional disorders (e.g., child abuse, depression)
   - **D.** Truancy
   - **E.** School refusal (school phobia)
   - **F.** Unrealistic parental or teacher expectations
   - **G.** Attention deficit hyperactivity disorder (ADHD) and learning disabilities
   - **H.** Lack of motivation (often without parental involvement to encourage the child)
   - **I.** Environmental circumstances (e.g., unsupportive, chaotic home; child not permitted to do homework due to baby-sitting or work responsibilities; malnutrition)
   - **J.** Poor teaching
   - **K.** Acute or chronic health problems

II. **Evaluation** of a child's poor school performance begins with a careful history, including birth history, significant past medical history, early developmental history, family history of school achievement and mental abilities, psychosocial and environmental history, and a review of systems. A detailed physical examination should include a careful neurologic examination with a search for "soft" neurologic findings and difficulties in communication. Vision and hearing testing are imperative. Other medical tests are ordered as indicated from the history and physical examination (e.g., CBC to rule out anemia, EEG, urinalysis, blood chemistries, thyroid studies, urine chromatography, chromosomal analysis).

   Information must be obtained from the child's school to determine the school faculty's primary concerns, results of previous testing, available resources, and suggestions for improvement. An example of a form designed to obtain specific educational and behavioral information from the school is indicated in Fig. 63-1. A commonly used standardized questionnaire to obtain specific behavioral information from the

Date ____________

SCHOOL PERFORMANCE RECORD

Name ____________ Grade ____________
Date of Birth ____________ Homeroom Teacher ____________
School ____________ Visiting Teacher ____________
School Phone # ____________ Principal ____________

Achievement: Reading Level / Reading Method

| Subject | Very Good | Average | Barely Passing | Failing | Subject | Very Good | Average | Barely Passing | Failing |
|---|---|---|---|---|---|---|---|---|---|
| | | | | | | | | | |
| | | | | | | | | | |

Do you think this child is working up to his mental capacity? ____________
What special placement or help has he had? ____________
What special provisions would you recommend? ____________
Is this special help or placement available? ____________

PLEASE CHECK MAJOR AREAS OF CONCERN IN BLOCK TO RIGHT OF ITEM

LANGUAGE:
A. Difficulty following verbal directions
B. Difficulty following written directions
C. Difficulty following the child's conversation
D. Difficulty understanding the child's words

BEHAVIOR:
A. Disrupts classroom thru aggressive behavior
B. Difficulty coping with frustration
C. Difficulty establishing peer relationships
D. Poor self-image
E. Poor group participation
F. Other

ATTENTION CENTER FUNCTIONS:
A. Overactive
B. Underactive
C. Distractible
D. Overreacts to touch and/or noise
E. Poor Attention Span
F. Unable to organize independent work
G. Other

MOTOR SKILLS:
A. Gross Motor-Skipping/playground activities
B. Fine motor (writing)
C. Hesitant to participate in physical games and activities
D. Clumsy - poor body coordination
E. Other

REVERSALS
A. Difficulty determining right & left in games
B. Tends to reverse printing letters, numbers
C. Tends to reverse reading letters, numbers, words
D. Tends to draw or read from left to right
E. Other

FORM & SPACE PERCEPTION
A. Difficulty with puzzles, etc
B. Poorly spaced & messy papers
C. Difficulty recognizing shapes, letters, words
D. Poor sense of direction
E. Poor awareness of self in space
F. Poor math concepts (larger than, smaller than, etc)
G. Difficulty with spelling

Poorly established hand dominance (switching
Poor eye tracking (skips letters, words, lines in reading

Have psychological studies been done? ____________
If so, may we please have a copy? ____________

Impression of home situation ____________

**Fig. 63-1. Sample school performance record.**

child's teachers is the Connors Teacher Rating Scale (see Chap. 62). Behavioral information also should be sought from parents to understand the child's behavior in the home, and that appraisal should be compared with behavioral and educational information from the school. There are also standardized tools, such as the Connors Parent Symptom Questionnaire or the Taylor Parent Behavior Scale, for obtaining parental information.

Minimal psychometric testing should include a basic intelligence test, such as the Wechsler Intelligence Scale, and achievement testing, such as the Woodcock-Johnson Psychoeducational Battery. If serious learning disabilities are suspected, a learning skills test is mandatory. Public Law 1029–119 requires all schools in the United States to either provide appropriate testing for children experiencing school failure or pay for private testing if such testing is not available in the school district.

If the work-up and treatment plan are complex, the physician should arrange a conference with parents to review the results of testing and make recommendations to the family and school. The physician, family, and school must work as a team to develop an individual educational plan that allows the child to draw on his or her strengths to compensate for weaknesses. Strategies may include appropriate class placement, tutoring, speech-language therapy, or medication and counseling for the child with ADHD. The physician should coordinate the educational, therapeutic, consultative, and counseling services necessary as the evaluation and treatment progress. The physician should be an advocate for the child and the family in the community and the provider of specific medical treatment. Physicians must be aware of special referral sources in the community, such as psychologists, speech-language pathologists, and diagnostic centers, and select these as carefully as a cardiologist or other specialist might be selected.

## Selected Readings

Connors CK. Parent Symptom Questionnaire. *Psychopharmacol Bull* 21:835, 1985.

Connors CK. Teacher Questionnaire. *Psychopharmacol Bull* 21:823, 1985.

Jordan NC, Levine MD. Learning disorders: Assessment and management strategies. *Contemp Pediatr* 4:31, 1987.

Levine MD, Jordan NC. Learning disorders: The neurological underpinnings. *Contemp Pediatr* 4:16, 1987.

Levine MD. *Developmental Variation and Learning Disorders*. Cambridge, MA: Educators Publishing Service, 1987.

Silver LB. Controversial proposals to treating learning disabilities and attention deficit disorder. *Am J Dis Child* 140:1045, 1986.

Taylor E. Syndrome of Overactivity and Attention Deficit. In M Rutter, BA Hersov (eds), *Child and Adolescent Psychiatry* (2nd ed). Oxford, England: Blackwell, 1985.

Wechsler D. *Wechsler Intelligence Scale for Children-Revised Manual (WICS-R)*. New York: Psychological Corporation, 1974.

Woodcock RW, Johnson MB. *Woodcock-Johnson Psychoeducational Battery*. Bingham, MA: Teaching Resources Corporation, 1977.

# Appendixes

# Appendix A. Drug Dosages

**Table A-1. Medication dosage guidelines**

| Medication[a] | Available | Dosing[b] |
|---|---|---|
| Acetaminophen (multiple) | Drops 10 mg/ml<br>Elixir 160 mg/5 ml<br>Chewable tablets (80-mg)<br>Tablets (325-, 500-mg) | 15 mg/kg PO q4h |
| Acyclovir (Zovirax) | Capsules (200-mg)<br>Suspension 200 mg/5 ml<br>Ointment 5%<br>Parenteral solution (500 mg/10 ml) | *Genital HSV*<br>5 mg/kg IV q8h for 5–7 days<br>400 mg PO tid for 7–10 days (not to exceed 80 mg/kg/day)<br>*HSV (immunocompromised)*<br>5–10 mg/kg IV q8h for 7–14 days<br>*HSV encephalitis*<br>10 mg/kg IV q8h for 14 days<br>*Varicella-zoster (immunocompetent)*<br>20 mg/kg PO qid for 5–7 days (maximum dose 3,200 mg)<br>10 mg/kg IV q8h for 7–10 days<br>*Varicella-zoster (immunocompromised)*<br>10 mg/kg IV q8h for 7–10 days |
| Albuterol (Proventil, Ventolin) | Elixir 2 mg/5 ml<br>Tablets (2-, 4-mg)<br>Inhaler<br>Nebulized solution 5 mg/ml<br>Ampules 2.5 mg in normal saline | 0.1 mg/kg PO q6–8h<br><br>1–2 puffs q4–6h<br>0.5 ml in normal saline q6–8h |

**Table A-1.** (continued)

| Medication[a] | Available | Dosing[b] |
|---|---|---|
| Amantidine (Symmetrel) | Suspension 50 mg/5 ml<br>Capsules (100-mg) | 3–4 mg/kg PO q12h for 2–7 days (maximum of 150 mg/day) |
| Aminophylline (Somophylline) | Elixir 105 mg/5 ml<br>Tablets (100-, 200-mg) | 3–5 mg/kg q6h |
| Amoxicillin-clavulanate (Augmentin) | Suspension 125, 250 mg/5 ml<br>Tablets (125-, 250-mg)<br>Chewable tablets (250-, 500-mg) | 10–12 mg/kg PO tid |
| Amoxicillin (multiple brand names) | Suspension 125, 250 mg/5 ml<br>Chewable tablets (125-, 250-mg)<br>Capsules (250-, 500-mg) | 12–20 mg/kg PO tid |
| Aspirin | Chewable tablets (80-mg)<br>Tablets (325-, 500-mg)<br>Suppository 60, 120, 325, 650 mg | 15 mg/kg PO q4h |
| Beclomethasone (Vanceril, Beclovent) | Inhaler | 2 puffs q6–8h |
| Bisacodyl (Dulcolax) | Tablets (5-mg)<br>Suppository 10 mg | 0.3 mg/kg PO<br>5 mg (≤ 2 yrs) PR<br>10 mg (>2 yrs) PR |
| Carbamazepine (Tegretol) | Suspension 100 mg/5 ml<br>Chewable tablets (100-mg)<br>Tablets (200-mg) | 2–3 mg/kg PO tid<br>(maximum 20 mg/kg/day <6 yrs)<br>(maximum 200 mg/day ≥ 6 yrs) |
| Cefaclor (Ceclor) | Suspension 125, 187, 250, 375 mg/5 ml<br>Capsules (250-, 500-mg) | 15–20 mg/kg PO bid |
| Cefadroxil (Duracef) | Suspension 125, 250, 500 mg/5 ml<br>Capsules (500-mg)<br>Tablets (1-g) | 15 mg/kg PO q12h |

| | | |
|---|---|---|
| Cefixime (Suprax) | Suspension 100 mg/5 ml<br>Tablets (200-, 400-mg) | 8 mg/kg PO qd |
| Cefprozil (Cefzil) | Suspension 125, 250 mg/5 ml<br>Tablets (250-, 500-mg) | 15 mg/kg PO bid |
| Cefuroxime axetil (Ceftin) | Tablets (125-, 250-, 500-mg) | 125–250 mg PO bid (≤ 12 yrs)<br>250–500 mg PO bid (>12 yrs) |
| Cephalexin (Keflex) | Suspension 125, 250 mg/5 ml<br>Capsules (250-, 500-mg) | 6–12 mg/kg PO qid |
| Chloral hydrate | Elixir 250, 500 mg/5 ml<br>Capsules (250-, 500-mg)<br>Suppository 325, 500, 650 mg | *Sedative dose*<br>5–15 mg/kg PO q8h<br>*Hypnotic dose*<br>50–70 mg/kg PO or PR (maximum 1 g/dose, 2 g/day) |
| Clindamycin (Cleocin) | Elixir 75 mg/5 ml<br>Capsules (75-, 150-, 300-mg) | 4–8 mg/kg PO tid |
| Clotrimazole (Lotrimin, Mycelex) | Cream 1% | Topical qd (vaginal), bid (other) |
| Codeine | Elixir 12 mg/5 ml (with acetaminophen 120 mg/5 ml)<br>Tablets (15-, 30-, 60-mg; (also with acetaminophen, 300-mg) | 0.5–1.0 mg/kg PO q4–6h |
| Dextroamphetamine (Dexedrine) | Sustained-release capsules (5-, 10-, 15-mg) | Begin with 5 mg PO qAM, advance 5 mg per dose weekly to a maximum dose of 40 mg (>6 yrs) |
| Diphenhydramine hydrochloride (Benadryl) | Elixir 12.5 mg/5 ml<br>Capsules (25-, 50-mg) | 1 mg/kg PO q6h |
| Docusate (Colace) | Elixir 20 mg/5 ml<br>Tablets (50-, 100-mg) | 40–200 mg/day PO divided qd–qid |

**Table A-1.** (continued)

| Medication[a] | Available | Dosing[b] |
|---|---|---|
| Doxycycline (Vibramycin) | Capsules or tablets (50-, 100-mg)<br>Elixir 50 mg/5 ml<br>Suspension 25 mg/5 ml | 1–2 mg/kg PO bid |
| Erythromycin ethylsuccinate (E.E.S.) | Suspension 200, 400 mg/5 ml<br>Tablets (200-, 400-mg) | 12–15 mg/kg PO with food tid |
| Erythromycin estolate (Ilosone) | Suspension 125, 250 mg/5 ml<br>Chewable tablets (125-, 250-mg)<br>Capsules 125, 250 mg | 10 mg/kg PO with food tid |
| Ethosuximide (Zarontin) | Suspension 250 mg/5 ml<br>Capsules (250-mg) | 8–20 mg/kg PO bid (maximum 1,500 mg/day) |
| Fluconazole (Diflucan) | Tablets (50-, 100-, 200-mg) | 3–6 mg/kg PO qd |
| Fluoride (Luride) | PO drops 0.125 F/drop (18 drops/ml)<br>Tablets (1.0-, 0.5-, 0.25-mg F) | [c] |
| Gamma benzene hexachloride (Lindane, Kwell) | Shampoo 1% | Apply to dry hair enough to wet, leave on 5–10 min, lather, rinse. Repeat 1 wk later. |
| | Lotion 1% | Apply after bath, leave on 6 hours, wash off. Repeat 1 wk later. |
| Griseofulvin (Grifulvin V) | 125 mg/5 ml | 12–15 mg/kg PO qd with fatty food |
| Hydroxyzine (Atarax, Vistaril) | Elixir 10 mg/5 ml<br>Tablets (10-, 25-, 50-mg) | 0.5 mg/kg PO q6h |
| Ibuprofen (Advil) | Suspension 100 mg/5 ml<br>Tablets (200-, 400-, 600-, 800-mg) | 10 mg/kg PO q6h |
| Imipramine (Tofranil) | Tablets (10-, 25-, 50-mg) | 10–25 mg PO qhs to start (for enuresis); not recommended for children <8 yrs of age |

| | | |
|---|---|---|
| Iron | $FeSO_4$ drops (Fer-in-Sol) 15 mg Fe/0.6 ml | 1–2 mg Fe/kg PO tid (for treatment of iron-deficiency anemia) |
| | $FeSO_4$ elixir (Feosol) 44 mg Fe/5 ml | |
| Isoniazid (INH) | Suspension 50 mg/5 ml | 10–20 mg/kg PO qd (maximum 300 mg) |
| | Tablets (50-, 100-, 300-mg) | |
| Ketoconazole (Nizoral) | Tablets 200 mg | 5–10 mg/kg PO qd |
| Lactulose (Cephulac) | Elixir 10 g/15 ml | 1–3 ml PO tid (infants) |
| | | 15–30 ml PO tid (older children) |
| Loracarbef (Lorabid) | Suspension 100, 200 mg/5 ml | 15 mg/kg PO bid |
| | Capsules (200-mg) | |
| Magnesium hydroxide (Milk of Magnesia) | Suspension 400 mg/5 ml | 0.5 ml/kg PO (children) |
| | | 30 ml/dose PO (adults) |
| Metaproterenol (Alupent, Metaprel) | Elixir 10 mg/5 ml | 0.5 mg/kg PO q6h |
| | Tablets (10-, 20-mg) | 0.5 mg/kg PO q6h |
| | Inhaler | 2 puffs q4–6h |
| | Nebulized solution 5% | 0.3 ml in 2.5 ml normal saline q4–6h |
| | Vials 0.6% (2.5 ml) | |
| Methylphenidate (Ritalin) | Tablets (5-, 10-, 20-mg) | 0.25 mg/kg PO bid to start |
| | Slow-release tablets (20-mg) | One PO qAM to start |
| Metronidazole (Flagyl) | Tablets (250-, 500-mg) | See Tables A-2 and A-3 |
| Mupirocin (Bactroban) | Ointment 2% | Apply tid |
| | 15-g and 30-g tubes | |
| Naproxen (Naprosyn) | Suspension 125 mg/5 ml | 5 mg/kg PO bid (for juvenile rheumatoid arthritis) |
| | Tablets (250-, 375-, 500-mg) | 250 mg PO tid (for dysmenorrhea) |
| Nitrofurantoin (Furadantin, Macrodantin) | Tablets (50-, 100-mg) | 1–2 mg/kg PO qid (treatment) |
| | Suspension 25 mg/5 ml | 1–2 mg/kg PO qd (prophylaxis) |

**Table A-1.** (continued)

| Medication[a] | Available | Dosing[b] |
|---|---|---|
| Nystatin (Mycostatin) | Suspension 100,000 U/ml | One dropper (2 ml) PO qid |
| | Cream, ointment, powder 100,000 U/g | Topical bid–tid |
| | Vaginal tablets 100,000 U | 1 tablet qhs for 10 days |
| Pediazole (erythromycin plus sulfisoxazole) | Suspension 200, 600 mg/5 ml | 0.25–0.30 ml/kg PO q6h |
| Pemoline (Cylert) | Chewable tablets (37.5-mg)<br>Tablets (18.75-, 37.5-, 75-mg) | Start at 37.5 mg PO qd in the morning, increase as needed at 18.75 mg/wk to maintenance of 1–3 mg/kg (maximum 112.5 mg/day) |
| Penicillin V (Pen•Vee K) | Suspension 125, 250 mg/5 ml<br>Tablets 125, 250, 500 mg | 8–12 mg/kg PO qid (maximum 3 g/day) |
| Procaine penicillin G | 300,000 and 600,000 U/ml | 25,000–50,000 U/kg IM (maximum 4.8 MU) |
| Benzathine penicillin G | 300,000 and 600,000 U/ml | 40,000–50,000 U/kg IM (maximum 2.4 MU) |
| Phenobarbital | Elixir 20 mg/ml<br>Tablets (15-, 30-, 60-, 100-mg) | 5–8 mg/kg PO qd (infants and children) |
| Phenytoin (Dilantin) | Suspension 30, 125 mg/5 ml<br>Chewable tablets (50-mg)<br>Capsules (30-, 100-mg) | 2–4 mg/kg PO bid |
| Prednisone | Elixir 5 mg/5 ml<br>Tablets (1-, 2.5-, 5-, 10-, 20-, 50-mg) | 0.5–2.0 mg/kg PO qd (for reactive airways disease, anti-inflammatory) |
| Prochlorperazine (Compazine) | Elixir 5 mg/5 ml<br>Suppository 2.5, 5, 25 mg<br>Tablets (5-, 10-, 25-mg)<br>Parenteral solution 5 mg/ml | 0.1 mg/kg PO q6h PO, PR, or IM |

| | | |
|---|---|---|
| Promethazine (Phenergan) | Elixir 6.26, 25 mg/5 ml<br>Tablets (12.5-, 25-, 50-mg)<br>Suppository 12.5, 25, 50 mg<br>Parenteral solution 25, 50 mg/ml | 0.25–0.50 mg/kg PR, IM (for nausea and vomiting) q4–6h |
| Propranolol (Inderal) | Tablets (10-, 20-, 40-, 60-, 80-mg)<br>Sustained-release capsules (60- ,80- ,120-, 160-mg) | 10–20 mg PO bid (<35 kg)<br>20–40 mg PO bid (>35 kg)<br>(migraine prophylaxis) |
| Rifampin (Rimactane, Rifadin) | Capsules (150-, 300-mg) | *Tuberculosis (all ages)*<br>10–20 mg/kg PO qd<br>*Neisseria meningitis* prophylaxis<br>10 mg/kg PO bid for 2 days<br>5 mg/kg PO bid for 2 days (<1 mo old)<br>*Haemophilus influenzae* prophylaxis<br>20 mg/kg PO qd for 4 days (maximum 600 mg qd)<br>10 mg/kg PO qd for 4 days (<1 mo old) |
| Sulfisoxazole (Gantrisin) | Suspension 500 mg/5 ml<br>Tablets (500-mg) | Start at 75 mg/kg PO for 1 dose, then 35 mg/kg PO q6h<br>25–35 mg/kg PO bid (otitis prophylaxis) |
| Terfenadine | Tablets (60-mg) | 60 mg PO bid (>12 yrs old) |
| Tetracycline | Elixir 125 mg/5 ml<br>Capsules (250-, 500-mg) | 10 mg/kg PO q6h (maximum 500 mg q6h) |
| Trimethoprim-sulfamethoxazole (Septra, Bactrim) | Suspension 40 mg TMP/200 mg SMX/5 ml<br>Tablets 80/400 (single strength), 160/800 (double strength) | 0.5 ml/kg PO bid |

**Table A-1.** (continued)

| Medication[a] | Available | Dosing[b] |
|---|---|---|
| Valproic acid | Elixir 250 mg/5 ml<br>Capsules (250-, 500-mg) | Start 10–15 mg/kg/day qd–tid, increase by 5–6 mg/kg/day weekly to maintenance of 30–60 mg/kg/day qd–tid |
| Vancomycin | Capsules (125-, 250-mg) | 10 mg/kg PO q6h (maximum 500 mg) (for colitis) |

MU = million units.
[a]Generic (trade name).
[b]All medication amounts are per dose unless otherwise indicated.

[c]

| Fluoride content of drinking water | 6 mos–3 yrs | 3–6 yrs | 6–16 yrs |
|---|---|---|---|
| <0.3 ppm | 2 gtts | 4 gtts | 8 gtts |
| 0.3–0.6 ppm | 0 | 2 gtts | 4 gtts |

(If >0.6 ppm, supplementation is not indicated.)

Sources: Adapted from G Peter (ed). *1994 Red Book: Report of the Committee on Infectious Diseases* (23rd ed). Elk Grove Village, IL: American Academy of Pediatrics, 1994; KB Johnson (ed). *The Harriet Lane Handbook* (13th ed). St Louis: Mosby-Year Book, 1993; JD Nelson (ed). *Pocket Book of Pediatric Antimicrobial Therapy* (11th ed). Baltimore: Williams & Wilkins, 1995; *Physicians' Desk Reference*. Montvale, NJ: Medical Economics, 1995; United States Pharmacopeial Convention. *United States Pharmacopeia Dispensing Information*. Taunton, MA, 1993.

**Table A-2. Antimicrobial drugs for the treatment of sexually transmitted diseases**

| Disease | Drug | Dose | |
|---|---|---|---|
| | | **<45 kg (100 lbs)** | **>45 kg and ≥ 9 yrs** |
| **Gonorrhea (uncomplicated vulvovaginitis, urethritis)** | Ceftriaxone (reconstitute with lidocaine per package insert) | 125 mg IM one time | 125 mg IM one time |
| | Cefixime (Suprax) | 8 mg/kg PO one time | 400 mg PO one time |
| | Spectinomycin | 40 mg/kg IM one time (2 g maximum) | 2 g IM one time |
| ***Chlamydia trachomatis*** | Erythromycin estolate | 30–40 mg/kg/day PO qid for 7 days | — |
| | Doxycycline | — | 100 mg PO bid for 7 days |
| | Azithromycin | — | 1 g PO one time |
| **Syphilis** | | | |
| Congenital | Aqueous penicillin G | 100,000–150,000 U/kg/day IV q8–12h for 10–14 days; 200,000–300,000 U/kg/day (older infants) IV q6h for 10–14 days | |
| Acquired (early): | Benzathine penicillin G | 50,000 U/kg (maximum 2.4 million units) IM one time | |
| >1 year's duration | Benzathine penicillin G | 50,000 U/kg (maximum 2.4 million units) IM weekly × 3 weeks | |
| Neurosyphilis | Aqueous penicillin G | 2–4 million units IV q4h for 10–14 days | |
| **Pelvic inflammatory disease** | | | |
| Outpatient management: | | | |
| *Option 1* | | *Option 2* | |
| Cefoxitin 2 g IM or ceftriaxone 250 mg IM plus probenecid 1 g PO one time plus doxycycline 100 mg PO bid for 14 days | | Ofloxacin 400 mg PO bid for 14 days plus clindamycin 450 mg PO qid for 14 days or metronidazole 500 mg PO bid for 14 days | |
| Inpatient management: | | | |
| Cefoxitin, 2 g IV q6h, plus doxycycline, 100 mg PO or IV q12h for 14 days. Cefoxitin may be discontinued and patient discharged on doxycycline alone after at least 48 hrs of clinical improvement. | | | |

Source: Adapted from G Peter (ed). *1994 Red Book: Report of the Committee on Infectious Diseases* (23rd ed). Elk Grove Village, IL: American Academy of Pediatrics, 1994.

**Table A-3. Antiparasitic medication guidelines**

| Organism (disease) | Drug[a] | Available | Dosing[b] |
|---|---|---|---|
| *Ascaris lumbricoides* (roundworm) | Mebendazole (Vermox) | Chewable tablets (100-mg) | 100 mg PO bid for 3 days |
| *Necator americanus* or *Ancylostoma duodenale* (hookworm) | Mebendazole (Vermox) | Chewable tablets (100-mg) | 100 mg PO bid for 3 days |
| *Ancylostoma braziliense* (cutaneous larva migrans) | Thiabendazole (Mintezol) | Oral suspension 500 mg/5 ml<br>Chewable tablets (500-mg) | 25 mg/kg (maximum 3 g/day)<br>PO bid for 2–5 days |
| *Entamoeba histolytica* (amebiasis) | | | |
| Asymptomatic | Iodoquinol (Yodoxin) | Tablets (210-, 650-mg) | 10–12 mg/kg PO tid for 20 days |
| Symptomatic with intestinal symptoms, dysentery, extraintestinal | Metronidazole (Flagyl) | Tablets (250-, 500-mg) | 12–15 mg/kg PO tid for 10 days |
| *Enterobius vermicularis* (pinworms) | Mebendazole (Vermox) | Chewable tablets (100-mg) | 100 mg once; repeat in 2 wks |
| *Giardia lamblia* | Metronidazole (Flagyl) | Tablets (250-, 500-mg) | 5 mg/kg PO tid for 5 days |
| | Furazolidone (Furoxone) | Oral suspension 50 mg/15 ml | 1.5 mg/kg PO qid for 7–10 days |
| *Pediculus humanus capitis* (head lice) | Permethrin (Nix) | Cream rinse | Use after regular shampoo one time, then remove nits. |
| | Lindane (Kwell) | Shampoo | Shampoo one time, then remove nits.<br>Repeat in 1 wk. |
| | Pyrethrins (A-200, RID) | Shampoo | Shampoo one time, then remove nits.<br>Repeat in 1 wk. |
| *Phthirus pubis* (pubic lice) | Lindane (Kwell) | Shampoo | Shampoo one time, then remove nits. |
| | | Lotion | Apply, leave overnight then wash off (one time). |
| | Pyrethrins (A-200, RID) | Shampoo | Shampoo twice, 1 week apart, then remove nits. |

| | | | |
|---|---|---|---|
| *Pneumocystis carinii* (pneumocystic pneumonia) | Prophylaxis: trimethoprim-sulfamethoxazole (Septra, Bactrim) | Oral suspension 40/200/5 ml | 0.5 ml/kg PO bid 3 days per week |
| | | Tablets, SS, DS (80/400 and 160/800) | 1 DS PO qd or bid 3 days per week |
| | Treatment: trimethoprim-sulfamethoxazole | IV solution 80/400/5 ml | 4–5 mg TMP-SMX/kg IV or PO qid for 14–21 days |
| | | Oral suspension or tablets as above | |
| | Pentamidine | IV solution | 3–4 mg/kg IV qd for 14–21 days |
| *Sarcoptes scabiei* (scabies) | Elimite (Permethrin) | 5% cream | Apply to entire body, leave overnight, wash off (safe for use in infants). |
| | Lindane (Kwell) | Lotion | Apply to entire body, leave on overnight (only 6 hours for infants and children), wash off. |
| *Strongyloides stercoralis* (strongyloidiasis) | Thiabendazole (Mintezol) | Oral suspension 500 mg/5 ml | 25 mg/kg (maximum 3 g/day) |
| | | Chewable tablets (500-mg) | PO bid for 2 days |
| *Toxocara canis/cati* (visceral larva migrans) | Diethylcarbamazine (Hetrazan) | Tablets (200-, 400 mg) | 2 mg/kg PO tid for 7–10 days |
| *Toxoplasma gondii* (toxoplasmosis) | Pyrimethamine (Daraprim) *plus* | Tablets (25-mg) | 2 mg/kg PO qd for 3 days, then 1 mg/kg PO qd (maximum 25 mg/day) for 4 weeks |
| | Sulfadiazine | Tablets (500-mg) | 25–50 mg/kg PO qid for 3–4 weeks |
| *Trichinella spiralis* (trichinosis) | Mebendazole (Vermox) plus steroids for central nervous system symptoms or severe symptoms | Chewable tablets (100-mg) | 200–400 mg PO tid for 3 days, then 400–500 mg tid for 10 days (adults and children ≥ 2 yrs of age); dosage for infants <2 yrs of age has not been established |

**Table A-3.** (continued)

| Organism (disease) | Drug[a] | Available | Dosing[b] |
|---|---|---|---|
| *Trichomonas vaginalis* (trichomoniasis) | Metronidazole (Flagyl) | Tablets (250-, 500-mg) | 2 g PO one time *or* 250 mg PO tid for 7 days |
| *Trichuris trichiura* (whipworm) | Mebendazole (Vermox) | Chewable tablets (100-mg) | 100 mg PO bid for 3 days |

SS = single strength; DS = double strength.
[a]Treatment of choice listed.
[b]All drugs listed as mg/dose unless otherwise indicated.
Source: Adapted from G Peter (ed). *1994 Red Book: Report of the Committee on Infectious Diseases* (23rd ed). Elk Grove Village, IL: American Academy of Pediatrics, 1994.

# Appendix B. Infant Formula Composition

**Table B-1. Infant formula composition**

| Formula | Calories (per oz) | Protein | Carbohydrate | Fat | Solute load (mOsm/kg) |
|---|---|---|---|---|---|
| Cow's milk | 20 | Casein 80% and whey 20% | Lactose | Butter fat | 260 |
| Human milk | 20 | Casein 20% and whey 80% | Lactose | Human milk fat | 290 |
| Enfamil+Fe | 20 | Nonfat cow's milk and whey | Lactose | Coconut, soy, and sunflower oil, palm olein | 300 |
| Similac+Fe | 20 | Nonfat cow's milk | Lactose | Coconut and soy oil | 300 |
| SMA+Fe | 20 | Nonfat cow's milk and whey | Lactose | Coconut, soy, oleo, oleic, and safflower oil | 300 |
| Isomil+Fe | 20 | Soy protein isolate | Corn syrup, sucrose | Coconut and soy oil | 240 |
| Nursoy+Fe | 20 | Soy protein | Sucrose | Coconut, soy, and safflower oil | 266 |
| Prosobee+Fe | 20 | Soy protein isolate | Corn syrup solids | Coconut, soy, and safflower oil, palm olein | 200 |

Source: Adapted from KB Johnson (ed). *The Harriet Lane Handbook* (13th ed). St. Louis: Mosby-Year Book, 1993.

**Table B-2. Special infant formula composition**

| Formula | Calories (per oz) | Protein | Carbohydrate | Fat | Solute load (mOsm/kg) |
|---|---|---|---|---|---|
| Alimentum | 20 | Hydrolyzed casein | Sucrose, modified tapioca starch | MCT, safflower oil, and soy oil | 370 |
| Ensure | 31 | Casein, soy protein | Corn syrup, sucrose | Corn oil | 470 |
| Isocal | 32 | Casein, soy protein | Maltodextrins | Soy and MCT oil | 300 |
| Nutramigen | 20 | Hydrolyzed casein, AA | Corn syrup solids, corn starch | Corn oil | 320 |
| Pediasure | 30 | Casein, whey | Hydrolyzed corn starch and sucrose | Safflower, soy, and MCT oil | 325 |
| Portagen | 20 | Casein | Corn syrup solids, sucrose, lactose | Corn oil, MCT oil | 230 |
| Pregestimil | 20 | Hydrolyzed casein, cystine, tyrosine, tryptophan | Corn syrup solids, glucose, corn starch | MCT oil, corn oil, safflower oil | 320 |
| Sustacal | 30 | Casein, soy protein | Sucrose, corn syrup solids | Partially hydrolyzed soy oil | 620 |

MCT = medium-chain triglycerides.
Source: Adapted from KB Johnson (ed). *The Harriet Lane Handbook* (13th ed). St. Louis: Mosby-Year Book, 1993.

# Appendix C. Oral Rehydration Solution Composition

**Table C-1. Composition of commercially available oral rehydration solutions and selected clear liquids**

| Name | Carbohydrate | Kcal (per oz) | Na (mEq/liter) | K (mEq/liter) | Cl (mEq/liter) | Base (mEq/liter) | Osmolality (mOsm/liter)[a] |
|---|---|---|---|---|---|---|---|
| Pedialyte | Glucose | 3 | 45 | 20 | 35 | 30 | 270 |
| Rehydralyte | Glucose | 3 | 75 | 20 | 65 | 30 | 300 |
| Infalyte | Rice syrup/ glucose polymer | 3 | 50 | 25 | 45 | 34 | 200 |
| WHO solution | Glucose | 3 | 90 | 20 | 80 | 30 | 310 |
| Gatorade[b] | Fructose/glucose | 5 | 20 | 3 | 17 | 3 | 330 |
| Cola[b] | Sucrose corn syrup | 12 | 2 | N | N | 13 | 550 |
| Kool Aid (sweetened)[b] | Sucrose | 13 | N | N | N | N | 334 |

N = negligible (<2.0 mEq/liter).
[a]Osmolality <300–320 recommended to prevent osmolar diarrhea.
[b]Not recommended for rehydration.

# Appendix D. Recommended Dietary Allowances

**Table D-1. Recommended dietary allowances, revised 1989**

| Category | Age (yr) or condition | Weight | | Height | | Protein (g) | Fat-soluble vitamins | | | Water-soluble vitamins | | | | | | | |
|---|---|---|---|---|---|---|---|---|---|---|---|---|---|---|---|---|---|
| | | kg | lb | cm | in | | Vitamin A (μg RE) | Vitamin D (μg) | Vitamin E (mg α-TE) | Vitamin K (μg) | Vitamin C (mg) | Thiamin (mg) | Riboflavin (mg) | Niacin (mg NE) | Vitamin $B_6$ (mg) | Folate (μg) | Vitamin $B_{12}$ (μg) |
| Infants | 0.0–0.5 | 6 | 13 | 60 | 24 | 13 | 375 | 7.5 | 3 | 5 | 30 | 0.3 | 0.4 | 5 | 0.3 | 25 | 0.3 |
| | 0.5–1.0 | 9 | 20 | 71 | 28 | 14 | 375 | 10 | 4 | 10 | 35 | 0.4 | 0.5 | 6 | 0.6 | 35 | 0.5 |
| Children | 1–3 | 13 | 29 | 90 | 35 | 16 | 400 | 10 | 6 | 15 | 40 | 0.7 | 0.8 | 9 | 1.0 | 50 | 0.7 |
| | 4–6 | 20 | 44 | 112 | 44 | 24 | 500 | 10 | 7 | 20 | 45 | 0.9 | 1.1 | 12 | 1.1 | 75 | 1.0 |
| | 7–10 | 28 | 62 | 132 | 52 | 28 | 700 | 10 | 7 | 30 | 45 | 1.0 | 1.2 | 13 | 1.4 | 100 | 1.4 |
| Males | 11–14 | 45 | 99 | 157 | 62 | 45 | 1,000 | 10 | 10 | 45 | 50 | 1.3 | 1.5 | 17 | 1.7 | 150 | 2.0 |
| | 15–18 | 66 | 145 | 176 | 69 | 59 | 1,000 | 10 | 10 | 65 | 60 | 1.5 | 1.8 | 20 | 2.0 | 200 | 2.0 |
| | 19–24 | 72 | 160 | 177 | 70 | 58 | 1,000 | 10 | 10 | 70 | 60 | 1.5 | 1.7 | 19 | 2.0 | 200 | 2.0 |
| | 25–50 | 79 | 174 | 176 | 70 | 63 | 1,000 | 5 | 10 | 80 | 60 | 1.5 | 1.7 | 19 | 2.0 | 200 | 2.0 |
| | 51+ | 77 | 170 | 173 | 68 | 63 | 1,000 | 5 | 10 | 80 | 60 | 1.2 | 1.4 | 15 | 2.0 | 200 | 2.0 |
| Females | 11–14 | 46 | 101 | 157 | 62 | 46 | 800 | 10 | 8 | 45 | 50 | 1.1 | 1.3 | 15 | 1.4 | 150 | 2.0 |
| | 15–18 | 55 | 120 | 163 | 64 | 44 | 800 | 10 | 8 | 55 | 60 | 1.1 | 1.3 | 15 | 1.5 | 180 | 2.0 |
| | 19–24 | 58 | 128 | 164 | 65 | 46 | 800 | 10 | 8 | 60 | 60 | 1.1 | 1.3 | 15 | 1.6 | 180 | 2.0 |
| | 25–50 | 63 | 138 | 163 | 64 | 50 | 800 | 5 | 8 | 65 | 60 | 1.1 | 1.3 | 15 | 1.6 | 180 | 2.0 |
| | 51+ | 65 | 143 | 160 | 63 | 50 | 800 | 5 | 8 | 65 | 60 | 1.0 | 1.2 | 13 | 1.6 | 180 | 2.0 |
| Pregnant | | | | | | 60 | 800 | 10 | 10 | 65 | 70 | 1.5 | 1.6 | 17 | 2.2 | 400 | 2.2 |
| Lactating | First 6 mos | | | | | 65 | 1,300 | 10 | 12 | 65 | 95 | 1.6 | 1.8 | 20 | 2.1 | 280 | 2.6 |
| | Second 6 mos | | | | | 62 | 1,200 | 10 | 11 | 65 | 90 | 1.6 | 1.7 | 20 | 2.1 | 260 | 2.6 |

| Category | Age (yr) or condition | Weight | | Height | | Minerals | | | | | | |
|---|---|---|---|---|---|---|---|---|---|---|---|---|
| | | kg | lb | cm | in | Calcium (mg) | Phosphorus (mg) | Magnesium (mg) | Iron (mg) | Zinc (mg) | Iodine ($\mu g$) | Selenium ($\mu g$) |
| Infants | 0.0–0.5 | 6 | 13 | 60 | 24 | 400 | 300 | 40 | 6 | 5 | 40 | 10 |
| | 0.5–1.0 | 9 | 20 | 71 | 28 | 600 | 500 | 60 | 10 | 5 | 50 | 15 |
| Children | 1–3 | 13 | 29 | 90 | 35 | 800 | 800 | 80 | 10 | 10 | 70 | 20 |
| | 4–6 | 20 | 44 | 112 | 44 | 800 | 800 | 120 | 10 | 10 | 90 | 20 |
| | 7–10 | 28 | 62 | 132 | 52 | 800 | 800 | 170 | 10 | 10 | 120 | 30 |
| Males | 11–14 | 45 | 99 | 157 | 62 | 1,200 | 1,200 | 270 | 12 | 15 | 150 | 40 |
| | 15–18 | 66 | 145 | 176 | 69 | 1,200 | 1,200 | 400 | 12 | 15 | 150 | 50 |
| | 19–24 | 72 | 160 | 177 | 70 | 1,200 | 1,200 | 350 | 10 | 15 | 150 | 70 |
| | 25–50 | 79 | 174 | 176 | 70 | 800 | 800 | 350 | 10 | 15 | 150 | 70 |
| | 51+ | 77 | 170 | 173 | 68 | 800 | 800 | 350 | 10 | 15 | 150 | 70 |
| Females | 11–14 | 46 | 101 | 157 | 62 | 1,200 | 1,200 | 280 | 15 | 12 | 150 | 45 |
| | 15–18 | 55 | 120 | 163 | 64 | 1,200 | 1,200 | 300 | 15 | 12 | 150 | 50 |
| | 19–24 | 58 | 128 | 164 | 65 | 1,200 | 1,200 | 280 | 15 | 12 | 150 | 55 |
| | 25–50 | 63 | 138 | 163 | 64 | 800 | 800 | 280 | 15 | 12 | 150 | 55 |
| | 51+ | 65 | 143 | 160 | 63 | 800 | 800 | 280 | 10 | 12 | 150 | 55 |
| Pregnant | | | | | | 1,200 | 1,200 | 320 | 30 | 15 | 175 | 65 |
| Lactating | First 6 mos | | | | | 1,200 | 1,200 | 355 | 15 | 19 | 200 | 75 |
| | Second 6 mos | | | | | 1,200 | 1,200 | 340 | 15 | 16 | 200 | 75 |

Source: Reprinted with permission from the National Academy of Sciences. Recommended Dietary Allowances (10th ed). Washington, DC: National Academy Press, 1989.

# Appendix E. Growth Charts

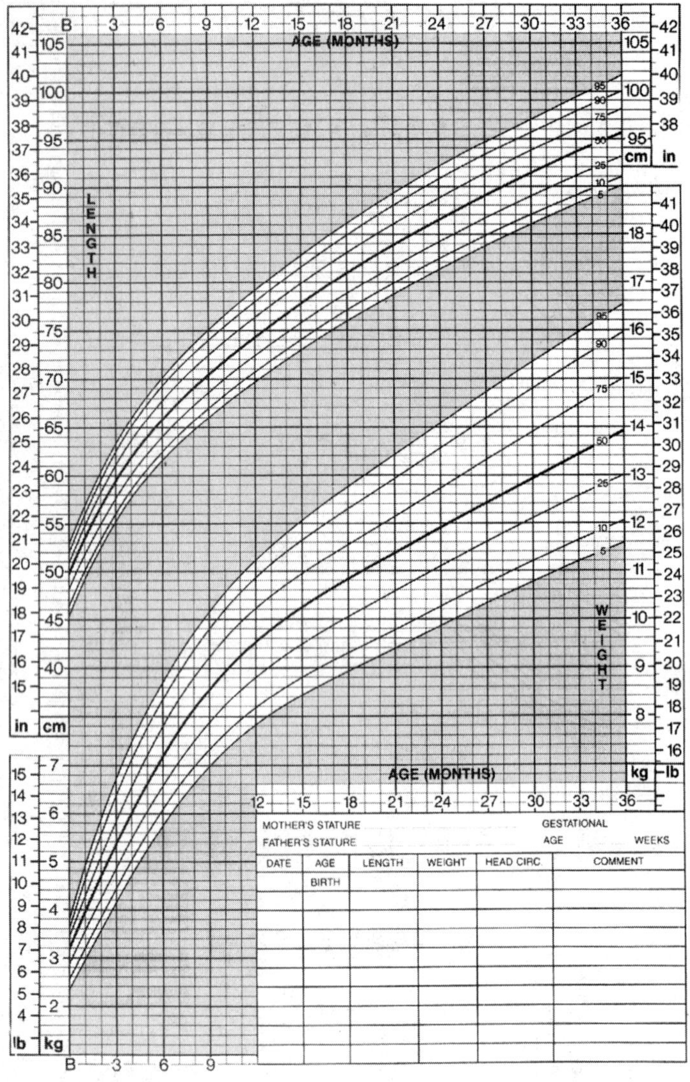


**Fig. E-1. Girls: birth to 36 months, length and weight. (Adapted from PVV Hamill, TA Drizd, CL Johnson et al. Physical growth: National Center for Health Statistics percentiles. *Am J Clin Nutr* 32:607, 1979.)**

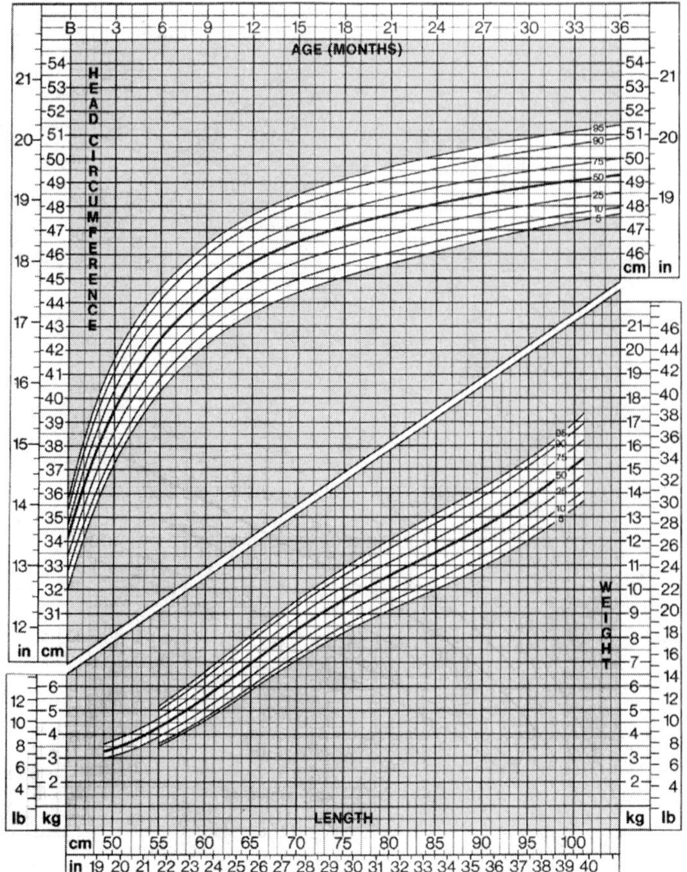


**Fig. E-2. Girls: birth to 36 months, head circumference. (Adapted from PVV Hamill, TA Drizd, CL Johnson et al. Physical growth: National Center for Health Statistics percentiles.** ***Am J Clin Nutr*** **32:607, 1979.)**

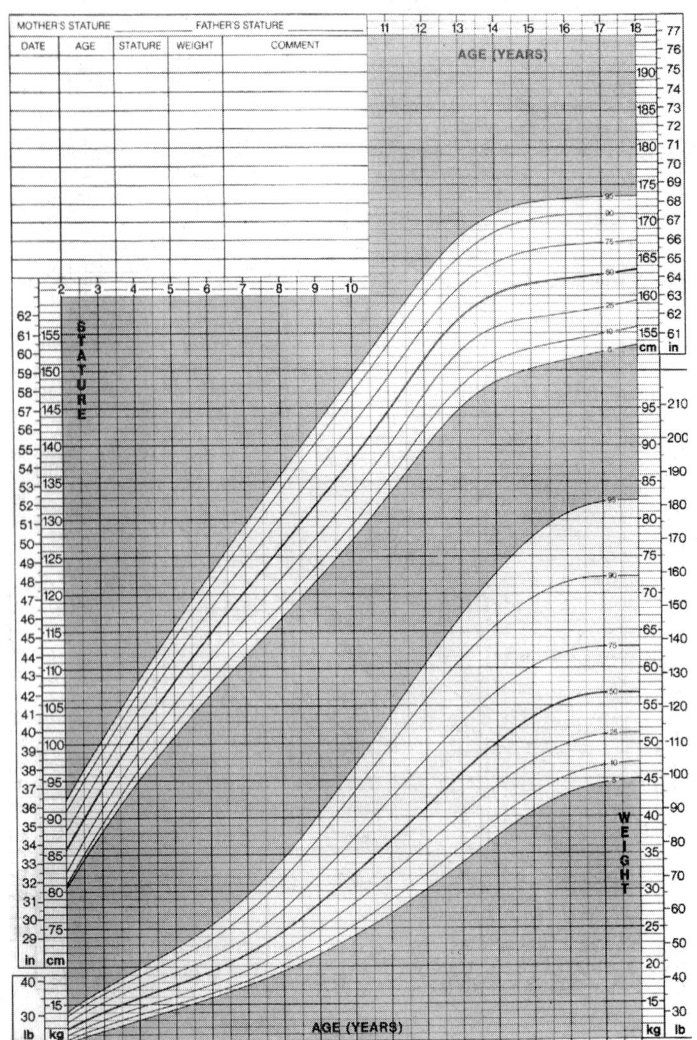


**Fig. E-3. Girls: 2–18 years, height and weight. (Adapted from PVV Hamill, TA Drizd, CL Johnson et al. Physical growth: National Center for Health Statistics percentiles. *Am J Clin Nutr* 32:607, 1979.)**

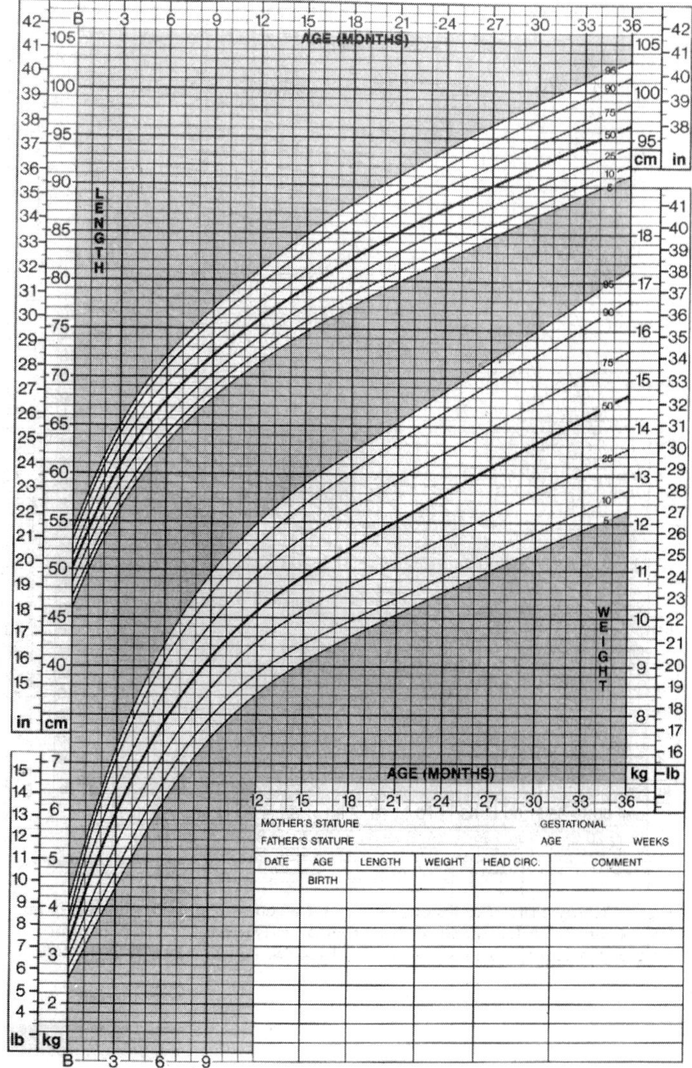


**Fig. E-4. Boys: birth to 36 months, length and weight. (Adapted from PVV Hamill, TA Drizd, CL Johnson et al. Physical growth: National Center for Health Statistics percentiles.** ***Am J Clin Nutr*** **32:607, 1979.)**

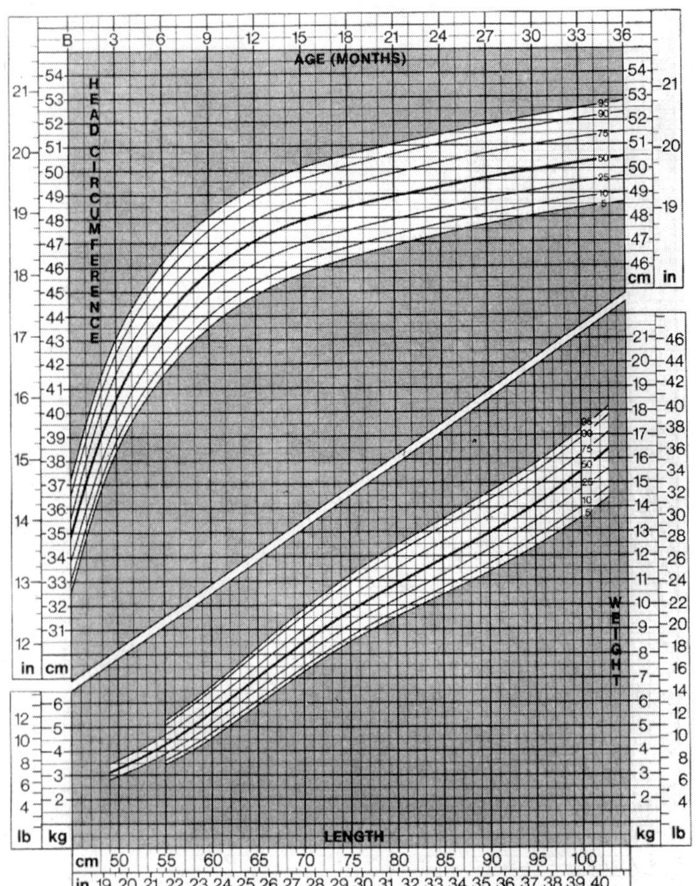


**Fig. E-5. Boys: birth to 36 months, head circumference. (Adapted from PVV Hamill, TA Drizd, CL Johnson et al. Physical growth: National Center for Health Statistics percentiles. *Am J Clin Nutr* 32:607, 1979.)**

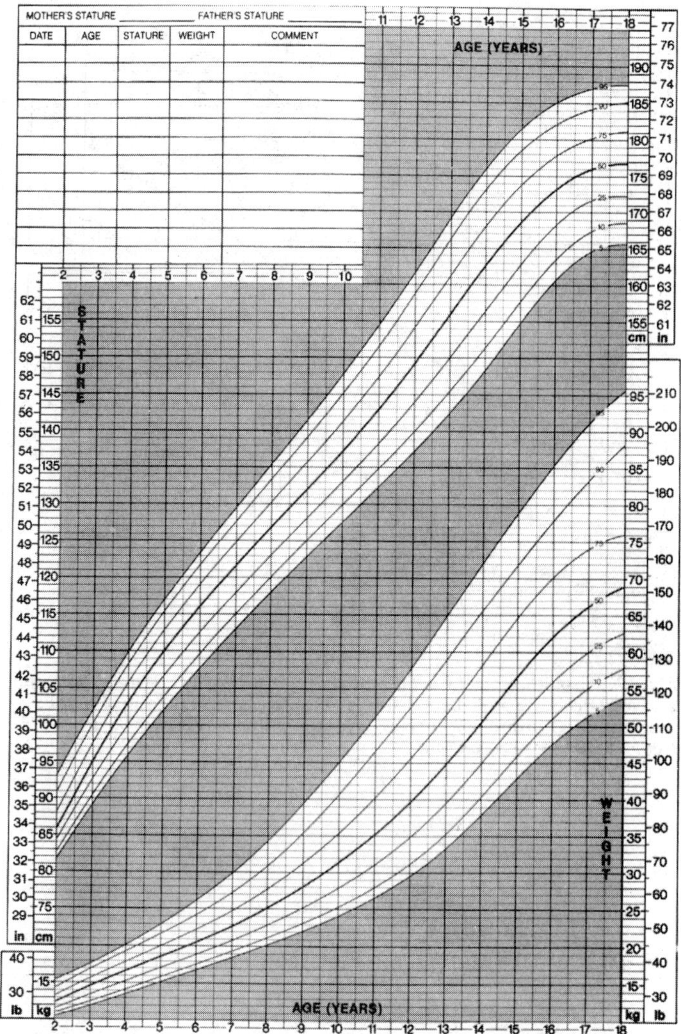


**Fig. E-6. Boys: 2–18 years, height and weight. (Adapted from PVV Hamill, TA Drizd, CL Johnson et al. Physical growth: National Center for Health Statistics percentiles. *Am J Clin Nutr* 32:607, 1979.)**

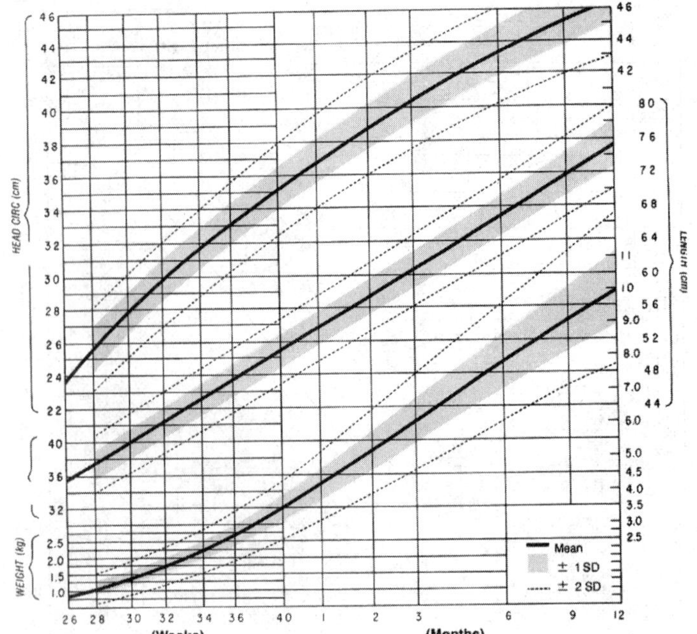


**Fig. E-7. Growth record for premature infants, birth to 1 year, male and female. (From SG Babson, GI Benda. Growth graphs for the clinical assessment of infants of varying gestational age. *J Pediatr* 89:814, 1976. Reproduced by permission.)**

# Appendix F. Blood Pressure Norms

**Table F-1. Blood pressure levels for the 90th and 95th percentiles of blood pressure for girls 1–17 years of age by percentiles of height**

| Age (yr) | Percentile | Systolic blood pressure (mm Hg) by percentile height | | | | | | | Diastolic blood pressure (DBP5) (mm Hg) by percentile height | | | | | | |
|---|---|---|---|---|---|---|---|---|---|---|---|---|---|---|---|
| | | 5% | 10% | 25% | 50% | 75% | 90% | 95% | 5% | 10% | 25% | 50% | 75% | 90% | 95% |
| 1 | 90th | 98 | 98 | 99 | 101 | 102 | 103 | 104 | 52 | 52 | 53 | 53 | 54 | 55 | 55 |
| | 95th | 101 | 102 | 103 | 104 | 106 | 107 | 108 | 56 | 56 | 57 | 58 | 58 | 59 | 60 |
| 2 | 90th | 99 | 99 | 101 | 102 | 103 | 104 | 105 | 57 | 57 | 58 | 58 | 59 | 60 | 60 |
| | 95th | 103 | 103 | 104 | 106 | 107 | 108 | 109 | 61 | 61 | 62 | 62 | 63 | 64 | 64 |
| 3 | 90th | 100 | 101 | 102 | 103 | 104 | 105 | 106 | 61 | 61 | 61 | 62 | 63 | 64 | 64 |
| | 95th | 104 | 104 | 106 | 107 | 108 | 109 | 110 | 65 | 65 | 66 | 66 | 67 | 68 | 68 |
| 4 | 90th | 101 | 102 | 103 | 104 | 106 | 107 | 108 | 64 | 64 | 65 | 65 | 66 | 67 | 67 |
| | 95th | 105 | 106 | 107 | 108 | 109 | 111 | 111 | 68 | 68 | 69 | 69 | 70 | 71 | 71 |
| 5 | 90th | 103 | 103 | 105 | 106 | 107 | 108 | 109 | 66 | 67 | 67 | 68 | 69 | 69 | 70 |
| | 95th | 107 | 107 | 108 | 110 | 111 | 112 | 113 | 71 | 71 | 71 | 72 | 73 | 74 | 74 |
| 6 | 90th | 104 | 105 | 106 | 107 | 109 | 110 | 111 | 69 | 69 | 69 | 70 | 71 | 72 | 72 |
| | 95th | 108 | 109 | 110 | 111 | 113 | 114 | 114 | 73 | 73 | 74 | 74 | 75 | 76 | 76 |
| 7 | 90th | 106 | 107 | 108 | 109 | 110 | 112 | 112 | 71 | 71 | 71 | 72 | 73 | 74 | 74 |
| | 95th | 110 | 111 | 112 | 113 | 114 | 115 | 116 | 75 | 75 | 75 | 76 | 77 | 78 | 78 |
| 8 | 90th | 108 | 109 | 110 | 111 | 112 | 114 | 114 | 72 | 72 | 73 | 74 | 74 | 75 | 76 |
| | 95th | 112 | 113 | 114 | 115 | 116 | 117 | 118 | 76 | 77 | 77 | 78 | 79 | 79 | 80 |
| 9 | 90th | 110 | 111 | 112 | 113 | 114 | 116 | 116 | 74 | 74 | 74 | 75 | 76 | 77 | 77 |
| | 95th | 114 | 115 | 116 | 117 | 118 | 119 | 120 | 78 | 78 | 79 | 79 | 80 | 81 | 81 |

**Table F-1** (continued)

| Age (yr) | Percentile | Systolic blood pressure (mm Hg) by percentile height | | | | | | | Diastolic blood pressure (DBP5) (mm Hg) by percentile height | | | | | | |
|---|---|---|---|---|---|---|---|---|---|---|---|---|---|---|---|
| | | 5% | 10% | 25% | 50% | 75% | 90% | 95% | 5% | 10% | 25% | 50% | 75% | 90% | 95% |
| 10 | 90th | 112 | 113 | 114 | 115 | 116 | 118 | 118 | 75 | 75 | 76 | 77 | 77 | 78 | 78 |
| | 95th | 116 | 117 | 118 | 119 | 120 | 122 | 122 | 79 | 79 | 80 | 81 | 81 | 82 | 83 |
| 11 | 90th | 114 | 115 | 116 | 117 | 119 | 120 | 120 | 76 | 77 | 77 | 78 | 79 | 79 | 80 |
| | 95th | 118 | 119 | 120 | 121 | 122 | 124 | 124 | 81 | 81 | 81 | 82 | 83 | 83 | 84 |
| 12 | 90th | 116 | 117 | 118 | 119 | 121 | 122 | 123 | 78 | 78 | 78 | 79 | 80 | 81 | 81 |
| | 95th | 120 | 121 | 122 | 123 | 125 | 126 | 126 | 82 | 82 | 82 | 83 | 84 | 85 | 85 |
| 13 | 90th | 118 | 119 | 120 | 121 | 123 | 124 | 124 | 79 | 79 | 79 | 80 | 81 | 82 | 82 |
| | 95th | 122 | 123 | 124 | 125 | 126 | 128 | 128 | 83 | 83 | 84 | 84 | 85 | 86 | 86 |
| 14 | 90th | 120 | 121 | 122 | 123 | 124 | 125 | 126 | 80 | 80 | 80 | 81 | 82 | 83 | 83 |
| | 95th | 124 | 125 | 126 | 127 | 128 | 129 | 130 | 84 | 84 | 85 | 85 | 86 | 87 | 87 |
| 15 | 90th | 121 | 122 | 123 | 124 | 126 | 127 | 128 | 80 | 81 | 81 | 82 | 83 | 83 | 84 |
| | 95th | 125 | 126 | 127 | 128 | 130 | 131 | 131 | 85 | 85 | 85 | 86 | 87 | 88 | 88 |
| 16 | 90th | 122 | 123 | 124 | 125 | 127 | 128 | 129 | 81 | 81 | 82 | 82 | 83 | 84 | 84 |
| | 95th | 126 | 127 | 128 | 129 | 130 | 132 | 132 | 85 | 85 | 86 | 87 | 87 | 88 | 88 |
| 17 | 90th | 123 | 123 | 124 | 126 | 127 | 128 | 129 | 81 | 81 | 82 | 83 | 83 | 84 | 85 |
| | 95th | 127 | 127 | 128 | 130 | 131 | 132 | 133 | 85 | 86 | 86 | 87 | 88 | 88 | 89 |

Source: B Rosner, RJ Prineas, JMH Loggie et al. Blood pressure nomograms for children and adolescents, by height, sex, and age, in the United States. *J Pediatr* 123:871, 1993. Reproduced with permission.

**Table F-2. Blood pressure levels for the 90th and 95th percentiles of blood pressure for boys 1–17 years of age by percentiles of height**

| Age (yr) | Percentile | Systolic blood pressure (mm Hg) by percentile height | | | | | | | Diastolic blood pressure (DBP5) (mm Hg) by percentile height | | | | | | |
|---|---|---|---|---|---|---|---|---|---|---|---|---|---|---|---|
| | | 5% | 10% | 25% | 50% | 75% | 90% | 95% | 5% | 10% | 25% | 50% | 75% | 90% | 95% |
| 1 | 90th | 94 | 95 | 97 | 99 | 101 | 102 | 103 | 49 | 49 | 50 | 51 | 52 | 53 | 54 |
| | 95th | 98 | 99 | 101 | 103 | 105 | 106 | 107 | 54 | 54 | 55 | 56 | 57 | 58 | 58 |
| 2 | 90th | 98 | 99 | 101 | 103 | 104 | 106 | 107 | 54 | 54 | 55 | 56 | 57 | 58 | 58 |
| | 95th | 102 | 103 | 105 | 107 | 108 | 110 | 110 | 58 | 59 | 60 | 61 | 62 | 63 | 63 |
| 3 | 90th | 101 | 102 | 103 | 105 | 107 | 109 | 109 | 59 | 59 | 60 | 61 | 62 | 63 | 63 |
| | 95th | 105 | 106 | 107 | 109 | 111 | 112 | 113 | 63 | 63 | 64 | 65 | 66 | 67 | 68 |
| 4 | 90th | 103 | 104 | 105 | 107 | 109 | 110 | 111 | 63 | 63 | 64 | 65 | 66 | 67 | 67 |
| | 95th | 107 | 108 | 109 | 111 | 113 | 114 | 115 | 67 | 68 | 68 | 69 | 70 | 71 | 72 |
| 5 | 90th | 104 | 105 | 107 | 109 | 111 | 112 | 113 | 66 | 67 | 68 | 69 | 69 | 70 | 71 |
| | 95th | 108 | 109 | 111 | 113 | 114 | 116 | 117 | 71 | 71 | 72 | 73 | 74 | 75 | 76 |
| 6 | 90th | 105 | 106 | 108 | 110 | 112 | 113 | 114 | 70 | 70 | 71 | 72 | 73 | 74 | 74 |
| | 95th | 109 | 110 | 112 | 114 | 116 | 117 | 118 | 74 | 75 | 75 | 76 | 77 | 78 | 79 |
| 7 | 90th | 106 | 107 | 109 | 111 | 113 | 114 | 115 | 72 | 73 | 73 | 74 | 75 | 76 | 77 |
| | 95th | 110 | 111 | 113 | 115 | 117 | 118 | 119 | 77 | 77 | 78 | 79 | 80 | 81 | 81 |
| 8 | 90th | 108 | 109 | 110 | 112 | 114 | 116 | 116 | 74 | 75 | 75 | 76 | 77 | 78 | 79 |
| | 95th | 112 | 113 | 114 | 116 | 118 | 119 | 120 | 79 | 79 | 80 | 81 | 82 | 83 | 83 |
| 9 | 90th | 109 | 110 | 112 | 114 | 116 | 117 | 118 | 76 | 76 | 77 | 78 | 79 | 80 | 80 |
| | 95th | 113 | 114 | 116 | 118 | 119 | 121 | 122 | 80 | 81 | 81 | 82 | 83 | 84 | 85 |
| 10 | 90th | 111 | 112 | 113 | 115 | 117 | 119 | 119 | 77 | 77 | 78 | 79 | 80 | 81 | 81 |
| | 95th | 115 | 116 | 117 | 119 | 121 | 123 | 123 | 81 | 82 | 83 | 83 | 84 | 85 | 86 |

**Table F-2** (continued)

| Age (yr) | Percentile | Systolic blood pressure (mm Hg) by percentile height | | | | | | | Diastolic blood pressure (DBP5) (mm Hg) by percentile height | | | | | | |
|---|---|---|---|---|---|---|---|---|---|---|---|---|---|---|---|
| | | 5% | 10% | 25% | 50% | 75% | 90% | 95% | 5% | 10% | 25% | 50% | 75% | 90% | 95% |
| 11 | 90th | 113 | 114 | 115 | 117 | 119 | 121 | 121 | 77 | 78 | 79 | 80 | 81 | 81 | 82 |
| | 95th | 117 | 118 | 119 | 121 | 123 | 125 | 125 | 82 | 82 | 83 | 84 | 85 | 86 | 87 |
| 12 | 90th | 115 | 116 | 118 | 120 | 121 | 123 | 124 | 78 | 78 | 79 | 80 | 81 | 82 | 83 |
| | 95th | 119 | 120 | 122 | 124 | 125 | 127 | 128 | 83 | 83 | 84 | 85 | 86 | 87 | 87 |
| 13 | 90th | 118 | 119 | 120 | 122 | 124 | 125 | 126 | 78 | 79 | 80 | 81 | 81 | 82 | 83 |
| | 95th | 121 | 122 | 124 | 126 | 128 | 129 | 130 | 83 | 83 | 84 | 85 | 86 | 87 | 88 |
| 14 | 90th | 120 | 121 | 123 | 125 | 127 | 128 | 129 | 79 | 79 | 80 | 81 | 82 | 83 | 83 |
| | 95th | 124 | 125 | 127 | 129 | 131 | 132 | 133 | 83 | 84 | 85 | 86 | 87 | 87 | 88 |
| 15 | 90th | 123 | 124 | 126 | 128 | 130 | 131 | 132 | 80 | 80 | 81 | 82 | 83 | 84 | 84 |
| | 95th | 127 | 128 | 130 | 132 | 133 | 135 | 136 | 84 | 85 | 86 | 86 | 87 | 88 | 89 |
| 16 | 90th | 126 | 127 | 129 | 131 | 132 | 134 | 134 | 81 | 82 | 82 | 83 | 84 | 85 | 86 |
| | 95th | 130 | 131 | 133 | 134 | 136 | 138 | 138 | 86 | 86 | 87 | 88 | 89 | 90 | 90 |
| 17 | 90th | 128 | 129 | 131 | 133 | 135 | 136 | 137 | 83 | 84 | 85 | 86 | 87 | 87 | 88 |
| | 95th | 132 | 133 | 135 | 137 | 139 | 140 | 141 | 88 | 88 | 89 | 90 | 91 | 92 | 93 |

Source: B Rosner, RJ Prineas, JMH Loggie et al. Blood pressure nomograms for children and adolescents, by height, sex, and age, in the United States. *J Pediatr* 123:871, 1993. Reproduced with permission.

# Appendix G. Clinical Stages of Pubertal Development (Tanner Stages)

**Table G-1. Clinical stages of pubertal development: Tanner stages**

| Tanner stage | Girls (breast) | Boys (genitalia) | Both sexes (pubic hair) |
|---|---|---|---|
| I | None | Prepubertal penis (<7 cm)<br>Testes <2.5 cm long | None |
| II | Budding less than diameter of areola | Prepubertal penis (<7 cm)<br>Scrotal thinning<br>Testes >2.5 cm long (4–6) ml in volume | Few dark, thick hairs over labia, mons, or both, or scotum, base of penis, or both |
| III | Breast greater than diameter of areola | Enlarging penis >7 cm<br>Testes 3–4 cm long (6–10 ml in volume) | Visible dark hairs over mons and labia or base of penis and scrotum |
| IV | Puffy areola | Larger penis with developed glans<br>Testes 4–5 cm long<br>(10–15 ml in volume) | Thick hair distribution over wider area |
| V | Adult | Adult | Adult |

Source: Adapted from WA Marshall, JM Tanner. Variations in the patterns of pubertal changes in boys. *Arch Dis Child* 45:13, 1970; and PC Sizonenko. Normal sexual maturation. *Pediatrician* 14:191, 1987.

# Appendix H. Sequence of Sexual Maturity

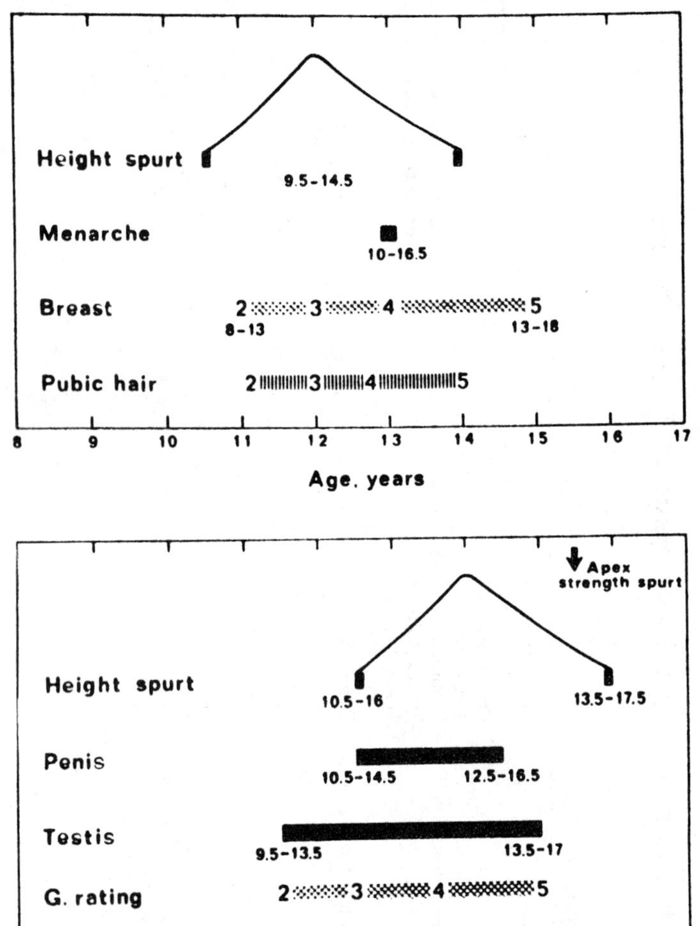


**Fig. H-1. Sequence of events at puberty in girls (top) and boys (bottom). (From WA Marshall, JM Tanner. Variations in the patterns of pubertal changes in boys. *Arch Dis Child* 45:22, 1970. Reproduced by permission.)**

# Appendix I. Denver Developmental Screening Test-II

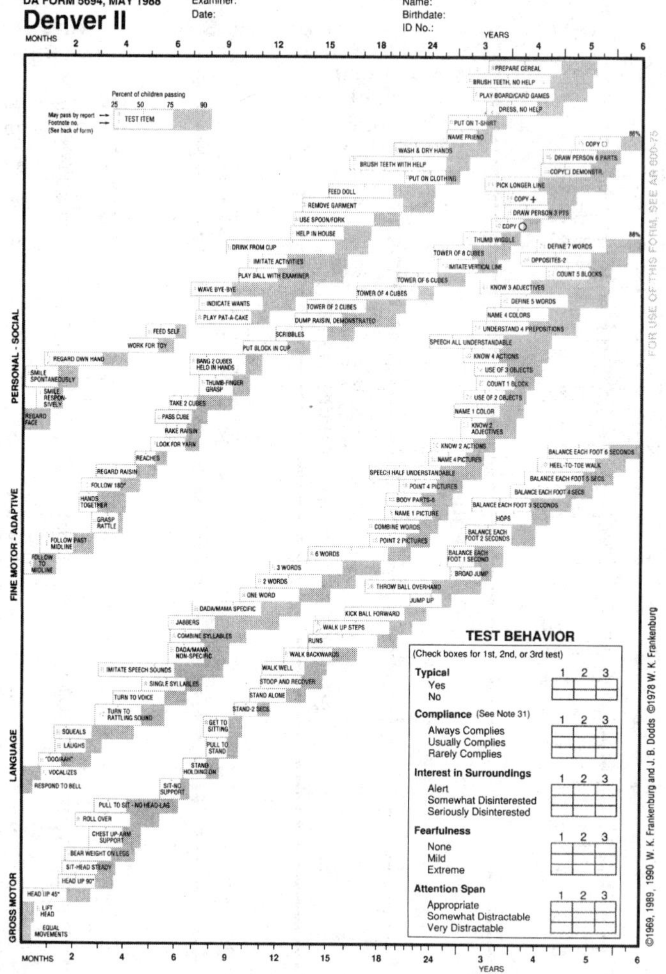


**Fig. I-1. Denver Developmental Screening Test-II. (From WK Frankenberg, J Dodds, P Archer et al. The Denver II: A major revision and restandardization of the Denver Developmental Screening Test. *Pediatrics* 89:91, 1992. Reproduced by permission.)**

# Appendix J. Surface Area Nomogram

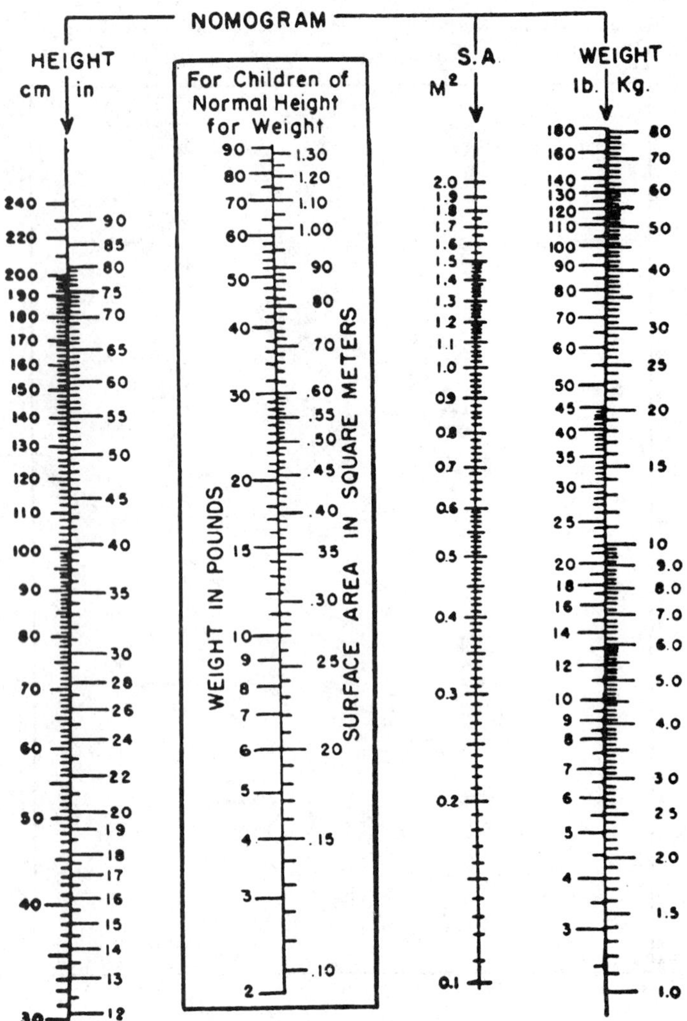


**Fig. J-1. Nomogram for estimation of body surface area. (From RE Behrman, RM Kliegman, WE Nelson et al. *Nelson Textbook of Pediatrics* [14th ed]. Philadelphia: Saunders, 1992. Reproduced by permission.)**

# Index

# Index


Abdomen
chronic pain of, 136
etiology of, 136, 137
history of, 136
physical examination for, 136–137
red flags suggesting organic etiology in, 136, 137t
treatment of, 137–138
of newborn, 18
trauma to from physical abuse, 228
in well-child examination, 16
Abstinence, 187
Abuse, 227. *See also* Physical abuse; Sexual abuse
Acetaminophen
dosage guidelines for, 305
for earache, 252
for fever, 254
for headache, 207–210
for pain, 253–254
for sore throat and mouth, 251
for vaso-occlusive sickle episode, 221
Acetazolamide (Diamox), 210
Achievement testing, 296
Acquired immunodeficiency syndrome (AIDS), 255
Acute chest syndrome, 222
Acyclovir (Zovirax)
dosage guidelines for, 305
for genital herpes simplex virus, 159
Adenovirus
in bronchiolitis, 120
in pertussis, 125
in pneumonia, 127
Adolescent
anticipatory guidance for, 42
in early adolescence, 56–58
in late adolescence, 59–60
in middle adolescence, 58–59
chlamydial infection in, 157
extracurricular activities of, 12
gonococcal infection in, 156–157
interview of, 11–12
nutritional requirements for, 36
physical examination of, 19–20
school behavior of, 12
sexual behavior of, 11–12, 185–190
social and emotional aspects of, 56
STDs in, 185–186
syphilis in, 158
Adrenarche
precocious, 167
premature, with increased ACTH, 182
Adrenocorticotropic hormone excess, 182
*Aeromonas* infections, 133, 135
Affect, 17
Affricate phonemes, 66
Age, caloric intake requirements and, 37t
Albuterol (Proventil, Ventolin), 305
Allen cards, 22
Allergy
in conjunctivitis, 109
food, 38–39
history
in comprehensive pediatric interview, 10
in ill-visit interview, 12
Alopecia, with tinea capitis, 92
Alstrom's syndrome, 181
Amantidine (Symmetrel), 306
Amblyopia, 22
Aminoglycoside interactions, 246, 248
Aminophylline (Somophylline), 306
Amitriptyline, 209t, 210
Amoxicillin (Amoxil)
for chlamydial infection, 157
cost of, 246
dosage guidelines for, 306
interactions of, 246
for otitis media, 98, 245
pediatric doses of, 247t
for pneumonia, 128
resistance to, 98
for sinusitis, 101, 102
Amoxicillin-clavulanate (Augmentin)
adverse reactions of, 248
dosage guidelines for, 306
for impetigo, 85
for otitis media, 99, 245
pediatric doses of, 247t
for sinusitis, 101
for skin infections, 245
Ampicillin
absorption of with food, 246
for gastroenteritis, 134
for pneumonia, 129
Anal examination, well-child, 17
Analgesia, patient-controlled, 221
Analgesics. *See also specific drugs*
for headache, 207–210
topical, for sore throat and mouth, 251
Anemia
iron deficiency, 217
screening for, 22
sickle cell, 221–224
Antibiotics. *See also specific drugs*
absorption of with food, 246
adverse reactions of, 248
antistaphylococcal, 87
broad spectrum, 245
for bullous impetigo of diaper area, 86
choice of, 245
cost of, 246
dose of, 248

Antibiotics—*continued*
drug interactions of, 246
frequency of administration of, 245–246
for gastroenteritis, 134–135
pediatric doses of, 247t
physiologic interactions of, 246, 248
for pneumonia
inpatient, 129
outpatient, 128
prophylactic, for urinary tract infections, 155
refrigeration requirement for, 246
for sinusitis, 102
taste of, 245
for urinary tract infections, 154
Anticholinergics, 252
Anticipatory guidance, 41
at 2 months, 46–47
at 4 months, 47
at 6 months, 47–48
at 9 months, 48–49
at 12 months, 49–50
at 15 months, 50–51
at 18 months, 51–52
at 2 weeks, 45–46
at 2 years, 52–53
at 3 years, 53–54
at 4 years, 54–55
at 5 years, 55
at 6–7 years, 55–56
for adolescent
early, 56–58
late, 59–60
middle, 58–59
components of, 42–43
for infant oral health, 62–63
for newborn, 44–45
in prenatal visit, 43–44
principles of, 41–42
for school-age children, 271
timing of, 42
for well child, 6–7
Antifungal agents, 85–86
Antihistamines
for allergic conjunctivitis, 109
for common cold, 105
for nausea and vomiting, 252
Antimicrobial drugs, 313
Antiparasitic drugs, 314–316
Antipyretics, 254
Antiretroviral chemotherapy, 258–259
Apgar scores, 256
Arrhythmia, headache with, 203
Arterial pulses, 16
Articulation
definition of, 64
development of
from 6–12 months, 65–66
from 12 months–3 years, 66
from 3–6 years, 66
from birth to 6 months, 64–65
referral guidelines for, 66
errors in, 66
Aspirin
contraindication for, 253–254
dosage guidelines for, 306
for pain, 253–254
Assessment, well-child, 6
Asthma, 117
crisis management for, 118
history of, 117
outpatient management of, 118
chronic mild, 118–119
chronic moderate, 119
chronic severe, 119
exercise-induced, 119
physical examination for, 117–118
precipitating factors in, 117
Asymmetric tonic neck reflex, 73–74
Atherosclerosis, prevention of, 37–38
Atopic dermatitis. *See* Dermatitis; Eczema
Attention deficit hyperactivity disorder, 295
conditions accompanying, 296
criteria for, 296
definition of, 295–296
differential diagnosis of, 296
evaluation of, 296
treatment of, 296–298
Auditory acuity testing, 22–23
Auditory brain stem response (ABR), 22
Autonomy, adolescent, 11
Azithromycin
for chlamydial infection, 157
for STD prophylaxis, 234

Babbling, 65–66, 68
Babinski reflex, 19
Baby, preparing older child for, 292
Backward parachute reflex, 77, 78f
Bacteremia, occult, 243
Bacteria
in conjunctivitis, 107–108
in gastroenteritis, 133, 134–135
in pneumonia, 127
Bacterial infections
serious (SBIs), 241
high-risk group for, 243
low-risk criteria for, 242–243
in young infants, 242
tracheitis differentiated from croup, 123
Bardet-Biedl syndrome, 181
Barlow test, 196, 197f
Bayley Scales of Infant Development, 72
Beclomethasone (Vanceril, Beclovent), 306
Bed, not staying in, 275–276
Bedtime
behavior at
at 6–18 months, 273–275
in newborns, 273

in school-age children, 276–277
in toddlers and preschoolers, 275–276
consistent routine at, 274
fears at, 276–277
resisting, 275, 277
Behavior
at 4 months, 47
at 6 months, 48
at 9 months, 49
at 12 months, 50
at 15 months, 51
at 18 months, 52
at 2 weeks, 46
at 2 years, 53
at 3 years, 53–54
at 4 years, 54
at 5 years, 55
at 6–10 years, 56
anticipatory guidance for, 43
bedtime, 273–277
consequence of, 264–265
examples for, 265
issues of in comprehensive pediatric interview, 11
management of
goals of, 263–264
positive, 266
principles of, 264–265
mealtime, 278–280
in mental status examination, 17
modification of, for obesity, 183
in newborn, 45
parents' actions and, 265
rating scales for, 296
in relationships, 265
Behavior problems
barriers to uncovering, 263
context of, 264
early detection of, 264
eliciting concerns about, 263
management of, 264–271
goals for, 263–264
prevention of, 263
school-related, 281–286
solving, 266
time-outs and, 267–268
Behavioral examination, newborn, 18
Benzathine penicillin G
dosage guidelines for, 310
for pharyngitis, 103
for syphilis, 158
Benzocaine
for earache, 251
for sore throat and mouth, 251
Beta$_2$-agonist, 119, 121
Beta-blockers, 210
Bilirubin, total serum level, 143
Birth control. *See* Contraception; *specific methods*
Birth cries, 64
Birth history
in failure to thrive, 176
past, 9
Bisacodyl (Dulcolax), 253
dosage guidelines for, 306
Bismuth subsalicylate, 252
Bites
animal, 228
human, 228–229
Bladder exercises, 151–152
Blood
analysis in well-child screening, 6
lead concentrations in, 23
Blood pressure
norms for, 329–332
routine, 21
at 3-year visit, 19
Blount's disease, 193
Body fat measures, 180
Body mass index (BMI), 180
Body surface, nomogram for estimating area of, 336
Body weight, caloric intake requirements and, 37t
Bone age
in delayed puberty, 168
in precocious puberty, 165
Bone pain, 221–222
*Bordetella parapertussis,* 125
*Bordetella pertussis,* 125
Bottle propping, 97
Bottle-fed infant
dental care of, 62
nutritional history of, 10
Bottle-feeding, 34
Bow legs. *See* Genu varum
Bowel
control of, 289–290
emptying for encopresis, 139–140
Brain growth velocity, 33
Breast milk
iron supplements in, 37
nutritional requirements in, 33–34
protective value of, 33
water in, 36
Breast-fed infant, nutritional history of, 10
Breast-feeding
dental care and, 62
jaundice associated with, 144
nutritional requirements with, 33–34
Breast(s)
development of
in childhood, 166
in infancy, 166
misconceptions about, 164
examination of, 20
of newborn, 18
in well-child examination, 16
Breath-holding spells, 287
Breech position, congenital hip dislocation with, 196

Bronchiolitis, 120
clinical course of, 120
diagnosis of, 121
etiology and pathophysiology of, 120
evaluation of, 120
prevention of, 121–122
treatment of, 121
Bronchodilator
for bronchiolitis, 121
for pneumonia, 128, 129
Bruises
accidental, 227–228
color of healing, 229t
from physical abuse, 227–228
Bullous impetigo, 87
of diaper area, 85, 86
Burn
from physical abuse, 228
third-degree, length of time to cause, 229t

Caloric intake
excess, 38
increased growth rate with, 172–173
inadequate, failure to thrive with, 175
Caloric loss, excessive, 175
Caloric requirements
by age, body weight, sex, 37t
in failure to thrive, 178
increased, 175
*Campylobacter* gastroenteritis, 133, 134–135
*Candida albicans* diaper dermatitis, 85
Carbamazepine (Tegretol), 306
Cardiovascular system
abnormalities with obesity, 181
in well-child examination, 16
CBC, 217
CD4 count
in HIV-positive mother, 255
in infant of HIV-positive mother, 259
Cefaclor (Ceclor)
adverse reactions of, 248
dosage guidelines for, 306
for nonbullous impetigo, 85
for otitis media, 99, 245
pediatric doses of, 247t
for skin infections, 245
Cefadroxil (Duracef), 306
Cefixime (Suprax)
dosage guidelines for, 307
frequency of administration of, 246
for gonorrhea, 156, 157
for otitis media, 99, 245
Cefotaxime
for gonococcal conjunctivitis, 107
for gonorrhea, 156
Cefoxitin, 159
Cefpodoxime (Vantin)
for nonbullous impetigo, 85
for otitis media, 99, 245
pediatric doses of, 247t
for skin infections, 245
Cefprozil (Cefzil)
dosage guidelines for, 307
for nonbullous impetigo, 85
for otitis media, 99, 245
pediatric doses of, 247t
for skin infections, 245
Ceftriaxone (Rocephin)
for gonococcal conjunctivitis, 107
for gonorrhea, 156, 157
for otitis media, 99
for PID, 159
for STD prophylaxis, 234
Cefuroxime, 129
Cefuroxime axetil (Ceftin)
dosage guidelines for, 307
for otitis media, 245
pediatric doses of, 247t
for sinusitis, 101–102
Cellulitis, facial, 112
Central nervous system event, 222
Cephalexin (Keflex)
dosage guidelines for, 307
for nonbullous impetigo, 85
pediatric doses of, 247t
for skin infections, 245
Cephalosporins
absorption of with food, 246
for bullous impetigo of diaper area, 86
interactions of, 248
taste of, 245
Cereal, in first year, 34
Cerebrospinal fluid pressure, 210
Cervical cap, 189
Chelation therapy, 220
Chemoprophylaxis, 155
Chemotherapy, antiretroviral, 258–259
Chest x-ray, 120
Chief complaint, 12
Child abuse. *See* Physical abuse; Sexual abuse
Child Development Inventory, 281
Child protective services (CPS)
reporting physical abuse to, 230
reporting sexual abuse to, 231
*Chlamydia* pneumonia, 127, 128
*Chlamydia trachomatis*
antimicrobial drugs for, 313
in neonatal conjunctivitis, 107
in pertussis, 125
Chlamydial infection
in adolescents, 157
in children, 157
Chloramphenicol interactions, 246, 248
Chlorpromazine (Thorazine), 208t, 210
Cholesterol
dietary intake of, 38
screening for, 37–38

serum level in well-child care, 22
Choral hydrate, 307
Chronic illness, 172
Cigarette burn, 228
Ciprofloxacin, 156, 157
Cleft palate, 97
Clindamycin (Cleocin)
dosage guidelines for, 307
interactions of, 246
pediatric doses of, 247t
for PID, 159
storage of, 246
Clotrimazole (Lotrimin, Mycelex), 307
Cloxacillin (Tegopen)
absorption of with food, 246
for nonbullous impetigo, 85
for skin infections, 245
Codeine
in cough suppressants, 250
dosage guidelines for, 307
for earache, 252
Cognitive development tests, 71–72
Cognitive function, 17
Cohen's syndrome, 181
Coitus interruptus, 190
Cold, common, 105
diagnosis of, 105
treatment of, 105
Colic
bedtime behavior and, 273
infantile, 145
definition of, 145
evaluation and treatment of, 146–147
natural history of, 146
Colonic evacuation, 139–140
Comprehensive pediatric interview, 9
allergy history in, 10
developmental history in, 10
family history in, 10–11
history of present illness in, 9
immunization history in, 10
medication history in, 10
nutritional history in, 10
past medical history in, 9–10
review of systems in, 11
social and environmental history in, 11
Computed tomographic scanning
for febrile seizures, 212
for headache, 205–206
Condom, 188–189
Confidentiality, 236
of adolescent interview, 11
heightened, 237
justified infringements to, 236
Congenital syndromes, 21, 174
Congestion, 250–251
Conjunctiva infections, 107–109
Conjunctivitis
allergic, 109
chemical, 107
*Chlamydia trachomatis,* 107
gonococcal, 107
herpes simplex, 108
infectious, 108
Connor Parent Symptom Questionnaire, 300
Connors Teacher Rating Scale, 296, 297t
for school failure evaluation, 300
Constipation
with chronic abdominal pain, 138
symptomatic therapy for, 253
Constitutional growth delay, 172
Contraception
chemical, 189
evaluation for, 185–187
laboratory tests for, 187
mechanical barrier, 188–190
medical and gynecologic history for, 186
methods of, 187–190
oral, 187–188
contraindications for, 186t
physical examination for, 187
primary care physician's role in, 185
Conversation, social rules of, 69
Cooing, 65
Cool mist humidifier, 251
for croup, 123
*Corynebacterium xerosis,* 107
Cough
suppressants of, 250
symptomatic therapy for, 250
Cranial nerves
examination in well-child visit, 17
neuropathies of in pseudotumor cerebri, 210
Cromolyn sodium, 109, 119
Croup, 123
membranous, 123
score, 124t
treatment of, 123–124
Crying
avoidable causes of, 146
at bedtime, 274
primary excessive, 145
Current medications, 12
Cushingoid features, 167
Cushing's syndrome, 181
Cyproheptadine (Periactin), 209t, 210
Cytomegalovirus infection
congenital, 174
in infant of HIV-positive mother, 258
*David Decides about Thumbsucking* (Heitler), 63
Decongestants
for allergic conjunctivitis, 109
for common cold, 105
oral, 250–251
topical, 250
Defecation retraining, 140

Dehydration, physical signs of, 134t
Demerol, 222
Dental care, infant, 61–63
Dental caries, 111–112
  in infant, 61–62
Dental history, infant, 61
Dental oral trauma, 112
Dental plaque, infant, 61
Dentist, first visit to, 61, 63
Denver Developmental Screening Test (DDST), 23, 71, 335
Dermatitis
  atopic, 83–84
  diaper, 85
    treatment of, 85–86
  moderate irritant, 85
  severe irritant, 85–86
Dermatologic disorders, 83–93. *See also specific conditions*
Desitin, 85–86
Desmopressin, 152
Development
  at 2 months, 46
  at 4 months, 47
  at 6 months, 48
  at 9 months, 48
  at 12 months, 49
  at 15 months, 50
  at 18 months, 51
  at 2 weeks, 45
  at 2 years, 52
  at 3 years, 53
  at 4 years, 54
  at 5 years, 55
  at 6–10 years, 55
  delays in
    global, 72
    identification of, 71
    screening for, 23
  in early adolescence, 56–57
  monitoring for infant of HIV-positive mother, 258
  motor and cognitive, 71–78
  of newborn, 44
  normal, anticipatory guidance for, 41
  screening tests in well-child care, 23
  stages of, anticipatory guidance for, 42
Developmental history, 10
Developmental milestones
  in failure to thrive, 176
  normal, 71
Dexamethasone, 123
Dextroamphetamine (Dexedrine)
  for attention deficit disorder, 296–298
  dosage guidelines for, 307
DHEAS level, 167
Diabetes
  chemical, obesity and, 182
  insulin-dependent mellitus
    inadequate caloric use in, 175
Diaper dermatitis, 85
  chafing, 85
  treatment of, 85–86
Diaphragm, 189
Diarrhea, 252–253
Diazepam, 214
Dicloxacillin (Pathocil)
  absorption of with food, 246
  for nonbullous impetigo, 85
  for skin infections, 245
Didanosine, 258–259
Diet
  for constipation, 253
  in failure to thrive, 177
  for obesity, 181, 182, 183
  special concerns in, 37–39
  vegetarian, 39
Dietary counsel, for failure to thrive, 178
Diethylcarbamazine (Hetrazan), 315
Differential attention, 265
Dimercaptosuccinic acid (DMSA) scanning, 155
Diphenhydramine (Benadryl)
  dosage guidelines for, 307
  for sore throat and mouth, 251
Diphenoxylate-atropine interactions, 246
Diphtheria immunization, 6
Diplopia, 203
Discipline
  at 4 months, 47
  at 6 months, 48
  at 9 months, 49
  at 12 months, 50
  at 15 months, 51
  at 18 months, 52
  at 2 weeks, 46
  at 2 years, 53
  at 3 years, 53–54
  at 4 years, 54
  at 5 years, 55
  at 6–10 years, 56
  age and, 265–266
  anticipatory guidance for, 43
  for behavior problems, 265–271
  definition of, 265
  developmentally targeted, 266
  of newborn, 45
  techniques of, 266
  time-outs in, 266–268
Disciplining guidelines, by age of child, 268–270
Dislocation, congenital hip, 196–198
Docusate (Colace)
  for constipation, 253
  dosage guidelines for, 307
Down's syndrome
  differentiation from failure to thrive, 174
  otitis media and, 97
Doxycycline (Vibramycin)
  for chlamydial infection, 157

dosage guidelines for, 308
for PID, 159
for STD prophylaxis, 234
for syphilis, 158
Drugs, dosage guidelines for, 305–316
DTaP vaccine, 29
DTP vaccination
common side effects of, 26–29
false contraindications to, 28t
with Hib conjugate vaccine, 30
recommended schedule for healthy infants and children, 26t, 27t, 28t

Earache, 251–252
Ears
disease of. *See specific disorders*
of newborn, 18
in well-child examination, 15
Eating
behavior, 278
in school-age children, 279–280
in toddler and preschooler, 278–279
patterns of
establishment of, 36
psychosocial-developmental issues relating to, 42
Eczema
description of, 83
treatment for, 83–84
Electroencephalography
for febrile seizures, 212
for headache, 206
Electrolytes
replacement in gastroenteritis, 133–134
with sports activities, 39
Elimite (Permethrin), 314
Emancipated minors, 237
Emergency treatment, informed consent and, 235
Emotional development, 56
Encopresis, 139
history of, 139
physical examination for, 139
treatment of, 139–140
Endocrine disorders, 163–190. *See also specific conditions*
increased growth rate with, 173
obesity and, 182
in poor growth, 172
Energy homeostasis, 181
*Enterobacter* infection, urinary tract, 153
Enuresis
alarm, 152
nocturnal, primary, 151
history of, 151
physical examination and laboratory evaluation of, 151
treatment of, 151–152
Environment
awareness of, 67
hazards of, 42–43
in obesity, 181
Epiglottitis, 123
Epilepsy
with febrile seizures, 213
triggered by fever, 212
Epstein's pearls, 110
Erythromycin estolate (Ilosone), 245
adverse reactions of, 248
for impetigo of diaper area, 86
for chlamydial infection, 157
for conjunctivitis, 107, 108
dosage guidelines for, 308
for eczema, 83
for gastroenteritis, 134–135
interactions of, 246, 248
for nonbullous impetigo, 87
pediatric doses of, 247t
for pertussis, 126
for pharyngitis, 104
for pneumonia, 128, 129
for STD prophylaxis, 234
Erythromycin ethylsuccinate
for chlamydial infection, 157
dosage guidelines for, 308
pediatric doses of, 247t
Erythromycin-sulfisoxazole (Pediazole)
dosage guidelines for, 310
for otitis media, 98, 245
for sinusitis, 101
*Escherichia coli*
fever with, 241
in urinary tract infections, 153
Ethical issues, outpatient, 235–237
Ethics, definition of, 235
Ethnic background, 97
Ethosuximide (Zarontin), 308
Exchange transfusion
for hyperbilirubinemia in term infant, 143
iron deficiency and, 217
Exercise
asthma with, 119
nutritional requirements and, 39
obesity and, 181, 183
poor growth with, 172
Expectorants, 250
Exposures, 12
Extracurricular activities, 12
Extremities, 16
Eyes
disease of. *See specific disorders*
infections of, 107–109
of newborn, 18

Face, examination of, 15
Facial cellulitis, 112
Facial expression, 67
Failure to thrive, 174
biologic conditions causing, 175
clinical assessment of, 176–178

Failure to thrive—*continued*
differential diagnosis of, 174
environmental factors in, 175–176
growth deficiency in, 174
laboratory evaluation for, 177–178
management of, 178–179
pathogenesis of, 174–175
physical examination for, 177
prevention of, 179
risk factors for, 175–176
Family
finances of, 11
support of
for failure to thrive, 178
for obesity, 183–184
Family history
in comprehensive pediatric interview, 10–11
in failure to thrive, 177
Fasting lipid profile, 22
Fat requirements, 38
Fatty acid requirements, 38
Fear
about school, 284
at bedtime, 276–277
Febrile seizures, 212
classification of, 212
evaluation of, 212
management of, 213–214
natural history of, 212–213
outcome in, 214
Fecal impaction, 139
Fecal soiling. *See* Encopresis
Feeding behavior
abnormal, in failure to thrive, 175–176
assessment of, 176
warning signs for problems with, 179
Feeding guidelines, first year of life, 35t
Feeding practices
anticipatory guidance for infants, 62
in infant dental health, 61
Femoral anteversion, 201–202
positions exacerbating, 202f
Ferritin levels, 22
in iron deficiency, 217, 218t
Fetal alcohol syndrome, 174
Fever
clinical assessment and management of
in infants 3–36 months, 243–244
in infants less than 3 months, 242–243
epidemiology of, 241
etiology of, 241–242
management strategies for, 241
in sickle cell anemia, 223–224
symptomatic therapy for, 254
Fiber
for constipation, 253
dietary, 38
Fifteen- and 18-month and 2-year visits, 19
First Amendment, 236
Fluconazole (Diflucan), 308
Fluid
replacement in gastroenteritis, 133–134
requirements with sports activities, 39
Fluoride (Luride)
anticipatory guidance for infants, 62–63
dosage guidelines for, 308
in infant dental health, 61
recommended daily intake in infants, 62t
supplement of, 37
Fluorosis, 111
Follicle-stimulating hormone
in delayed puberty, 168
in precocious puberty, 165
Follow-up, well-child, 7
Fontanelle
anterior, at 4 months, 19
examination at 4-month visit, 19
Food
allergies to, 38–39
antibiotic absorption with, 246
choice of, 279
jags, 278
junk, 279
solid, 34–36
Forensics, 232
Four-, 5-, and 6-year-old visits, 19
Fracture
mandibular, 113
from physical abuse, 228
Fricatives, 66
Fruits, 34
Frustration, 287
Fungal infection
in conjunctivitis, 107
in pneumonia, 127, 128
of scalp, 92–93
Furazolidone (Furoxone)
dosage guidelines for, 314
interactions of, 246
Furosemide (Lasix), 210
Fussiness, 145–147

Galactosemia screening, 21
Gamma benzene hexachloride (Lindane, Kwell), 308
Gamma globulin product, 24
*Gardnerella vaginalis,* 159
Gastroenteritis
acute
etiology of, 133
evaluation of, 133
treatment of, 133–134
bacterial, 134–135
Gastrointestinal tract disorders, 133–147

Gender, caloric intake requirements and, 37t
Generic medication, 250
Genetic disorders screening, 21
Genetics, in obesity, 181
Genital examination, well-child, 16
Genitalia
  abnormalities in urinary tract infections, 153
  determining sexual development stage from, 20
  examination for sexual abuse, 232–234
  of newborn, 18
Genitourinary tract disorders, 151–159. *See also specific disorders*
Gentamicin
  for conjunctivitis, 108
  for PID, 159
  for pneumonia, 129
Genu valgum, 193, 194f, 195f
Genu varum, 193
Gesell Developmental Schedule, 72
Gestures, 67
Gingivostomatitis, acute herpetic, 113
*Going to the Potty,* 290
Gonadal failure, delayed puberty, 167, 168
Gonadotropin
  in delayed puberty, 168
  in precocious puberty, 165
Gonococcal infections
  disseminated, 156–157
  uncomplicated, 156
Gonorrhea
  antimicrobial drugs for, 313
  in children, 157
  disseminated, 156–157
  uncomplicated, 156
Grease burn, 228
Griseofulvin (Grifulvin V), 92
  dosage guidelines for, 308
  interactions of, 246
  storage of, 246
  for tinea capitis, 92–93
Growth
  abnormal linear, 170–173
  abnormal rate of, 171
  assessment of, 33, 170–173
  catch-up, 170
  charting and interpreting data on, 170
  disorders of, 163–190. *See also specific conditions*
  monitoring in infant of HIV-positive mother, 257–258
  rate of
    decreased, 171–172
    in delayed puberty, 168–169
    increased, 171, 172–173
    normal, 170–171
  slow down in, 170
  spurt, 170
Growth charts
  for boys, 325–327
  for girls, 322–324
  for premature infants, 328
Growth factors, 172
Growth failure
  classification of, 175t
  differential diagnosis of, 174
  with failure to thrive, 174–179
Gums, 62
Gynecomastia
  definition of, 163
  physiologic pubertal, 164

*Haemophilus* conjunctivitis, neonatal, 107
*Haemophilus influenzae*
  in conjunctivitis, 107–108
  in otitis media, 98
  in sinusitis, 101, 102
  type B
    in croup, 123
    fever with, 241–242
    immunization for, 6, 30
  vaccine for, 243
Handwashing
  to prevent bronchiolitis, 121–122
  to prevent conjunctivitis, 109
Hazards, environmental, 42–43
Hb S-B thalassemia, 224
Hb SS, 224
$H_2$-blockers, 138
Head
  circumference of, 33
  injury from physical abuse, 229
  lice of, 89
  of newborn, 18
  in space reflex, 75
  in well-child examination, 15
Headache
  characteristics of, 204t
  diary, 207
  history of, 203–204
  incidence of, 203
  laboratory studies for, 205–206
  migraine, 204, 206–207
  neurologic examination for, 205
  past medical history with, 204–205
  pharmacotherapy for
    abortive, 207–210
    prophylactic, 210
  physical examination for, 205
  in pseudotumor cerebri, 210
  referral for, 210–211
  tension-type, 207
Health care coverage, family, 11
Health care providers, ethical issues for, 235–237

Health habits
in early adolescence, 57
in late adolescence, 59
in middle adolescence, 58
Health maintenance examination schedule, 8
Health maintenance supervision
anticipatory guidance in, 41–60
screening tests in, 21–23
Hearing testing in well-child care, 22–23
Heart
of newborn, 18
in well-child examination, 16
Heat stroke, 254
HEENT disorders, 97–113
Height, 171
*Helicobacter pylori* disease
chronic abdominal pain with, 137
treatment of, 138
Hematologic disorders, 217–224. *See also specific disorders*
Hematoma, eruption, 110–111
Hemoglobin, in iron deficiency, 217, 218t
Hemoglobin S
heterozygous, 223
homozygous, 223
Hemoglobin SC, 223
Hemoglobinopathy screening, 21
Hemorrhage, perinatal, 217
Hepatitis B vaccination, 6
common side effects of, 30–31
recommended doses of, 31t
recommended schedule for healthy infants and children, 26t, 27t, 28t
Herpangina, 103
Herpes simplex virus
genital, 159
in gingivostomatitis, 113
Hib conjugate vaccines, 30, 31t
Hib vaccination, recommended schedule, 26t, 27t, 28t
Hip
dislocation of, congenital, 196
confirmation and treatment of, 196–198
diagnosis of, 196
examination at 2-month visit, 19
instability of, 196–198
splinting or bracing of, 198
Hirschsprung's disease, 139
History
adolescent interview in, 11–12
comprehensive pediatric interview in, 9–11
goals of, 8
ill-visit, 12
nutritional assessment in, 33
prenatal interview in, 8–9
at routine well-child visit, 5
HIV culture, 255
HIV infection. *See* Human immunodeficiency virus
HIV serology, 255, 256
for infant of HIV-positive mother, 256
HIV team, 257
HIV-positive mother, managing infant born to, 255–259
Holophrastic words, 68
Home remedies
for constipation, 253
for diarrhea, 252–253
for nausea and vomiting, 252
for pain, 254
for sore throat and mouth, 251
Home visit, postdischarge, 5–6
Homework, problems with, 282–283
Homocystinuria screening, 21
Hormonal levels, 168. *See also* Sex steroid levels; *specific agents*
Hospital procedure, 8
Hospitalization
for croup, 123–124
for failure to thrive, 178–179
for pertussis, 126
for pneumonia, 128
Human bites, 228–229
Human immunodeficiency virus
symptoms of, 255
testing for, 159
transmission mode of, 255
Human parvovirus infection, 223
Hydration
for eczema, 83–84
for pneumonia, 129
Hydrocodone, 250
Hydrocortisone, 83
Hydromorphone (Dilaudid)
for pain, 254
for vaso-occlusive sickle episode, 221, 222
Hydroxyzine (Atarax, Vistaril), 308
Hyperactivity, 295–298
Hyperbilirubinemia
classification of, 142
criteria for investigation of, 142–143
direct, 144
history of, 142
indirect, 143–144
physical examination for, 142
in term infant, 142–144
treatment of, 143, 144
Hypercortisolism, 181
Hyperinsulinemia, 182
Hyperinsulinism, 181
Hypertension
obesity and, 181
screening tests for, 21
Hypogonadotropic hypogonadism, 167, 168
Hypothyroidism
congenital, screening for in newborn, 21
obesity with, 181

Ibuprofen (Advil)
dosage guidelines for, 308
for earache, 252
for fever, 254
for headache, 207–210
for pain, 254
for sore throat and mouth, 251
IGF-binding proteins, 172
Ill-child visit
for behavioral problem, 263–301
history in, 12
for medical problem, 83–259
*I'm a Big Kid Now* (Rogers), 290
Imipramine (Tofranil)
dosage guidelines for, 308
for nocturnal enuresis, 152
Immunization. *See also* Vaccines; *specific types*
active, 24
common side effects and special considerations in, 26–32
contraindications to, 25
government regulation of, 6
for infant of HIV-positive mother, 256–257
lapsed, 24
misconceptions about, 26
patient education on, 25
for pertussis, 126
for premature infants, 24
principles of, 24–25
religious exemption for, 236
requirements for, 3
routine childhood, 24
in those not up-to-date, 25–26
uncertain status of, 24
for well-child, 6
Immunization history
in comprehensive pediatric interview, 10
in ill-visit interview, 12
Immunoglobulin, 32
Impetigo
bullous, 87
of diaper area, 85, 86
nonbullous, 87
Incontinence, urinary, 151–152. *See also* Enuresis
Independence, 56
Infant
approach to physical examination of, 14–15
bedtime behavior in, 273–275
colic in, 145–147
conjunctivitis in, 108–109
dental care for, 61–63
anticipatory guidance for, 62–63
dental history of, 61
evaluating fever in, 241–244
hyperbilirubinemia in, 142–144
language development in, 67–69
oral examination for, 61–62
primitive reflexes in, 72–78
shifting growth in, 170
temper tantrums in, 287
Infant formula
changing for colicky baby, 147
composition of, 317–318
cow's milk, 97
for infant of HIV-positive mother, 257–258
iron supplements in, 37
nutritional requirements in, 33–34
water in, 36
Infections
in conjunctivitis, 108
of eczema, 83
headache with, 203–204
with sickle cell anemia, 223–224
Inflammation, eczema, 83
Influenza virus
immunization for infant of HIV-positive mother, 257
in pneumonia, 127
in sinusitis, 101
Informed consent
exemptions to, 235
process of, 235
Injury, from physical abuse, 227–229
Insulin growth factor I, 172
Intake visit, 4
Intelligence development, 71–72
Interim history, 9
Internal tibial torsion, 199–201
positions exacerbating, 202f
Intoeing, 199
femoral anteversion in, 201–202
internal tibial torsion in, 199–201
metatarsus adductus with, 199
physical examination for, 199
position for physical examination for, 200f
Intravenous gamma globulin, 258
Iodoquinol (Yodoxin), 314
IQ testing, 296
Iron
deficiency of, 217
diagnosis of, 217
pathogenesis of, 217
prevention and treatment of, 217
screening for, 22
signs and symptoms of, 217
stages of, 217
dosage guidelines for, 309
stores of, 217
supplement of, 37
in first year, 36
Iron sulfate, 217–218
Isoniazid (INH), 309
Itch, 83

Jargon, 66, 68
Jaundice
with breast-feeding, 144
in hyperbilirubinemia in term infant, 142–144

Jaundice—*continued*
physiologic of newborn, 143
Jenner, Edward, 24
Jugular veins, 16

Ketoconazole (Nizoral), 309
Ketorolac, 221
*Klebsiella* urinary tract infections, 153
Knock knees. *See* Genu valgum
Korotkoff's sound, fourth, 21
Kwell lotion. *See also* Lindane (Kwell)
for pubic lice, 90
for scabies, 91
Kwell Shampoo, 89

Laboratory tests
for delayed puberty, 168
for headache, 205–206
for infant of HIV-positive mother, 256
for urinary tract infections, 153–154
Lactation, dietary needs during, 34
*Lactobacillus* infection, 159
Lacto-ovo-vegetarianism, 39
Lacto-vegetarian, 39
Lactulose (Cephulac)
for constipation, 253
dosage guidelines for, 309
for encopresis, 140
Lamivudine, 258–259
Language. *See also* Speech
definition of, 64
delays in, audiology referrals for, 22–23
development of, 269
2–6 months, 66
6–12 months, 66–68
12–18 months, 68
18–24 months, 68–69
2–3 years, 69
3–6 years, 69
in newborns, 66
referral guidelines for, 69
early intervention for problems with, 70
expressive, 64, 67
milestones in development of, 65t
normal development of, 64–70
in preventing behavior problems, 270
receptive, 64
Laryngotracheobronchitis, acute viral, 123–124
Law, obligation to obey, 236
Laxatives
for constipation, 253
for encopresis, 139–140
stimulant, 253
Lead poisoning
classification and recommended action for, 219, 220t
definition of, 219
management of, 219–220
prevention of, 220
screening for, 219
in well-child care, 23
Leg length discrepancy, 196
Legal issues, 227–237
Length measurement, 170
Lice
head, 89
pubic, 89
Lidocaine, 251
Lifestyle, 181
Limits
consistent, 270
setting of, 43
Lindane (Kwell). *See also* Kwell lotion
dosage guidelines for, 314–315
for *Pediculosis capitis,* 89
for scabies, 91
Lingual frenum, 110
Liquid diet, 252–253
*Listeria monocytogenes,* 241–242
Loracarbef (Lorabid)
dosage guidelines for, 309
frequency of administration of, 246
for impetigo, 85
for otitis media, 99, 245
pediatric doses of, 247t
for skin infections, 245
storage of, 246
Lumbar puncture, 206
Lungs
of newborn, 18
in well-child examination, 16
Luteinizing hormone
in delayed puberty, 168
in precocious puberty, 165
Luteinizing hormone-releasing hormone
in delayed puberty, 168
in precocious puberty, 165
Lymphatic system, 15

Macrolide, 246
Magnesium hydroxide, 309
Magnetic resonance imaging
for febrile seizures, 212
for headache, 205–206
Malabsorption, 172
Maltsupex, 253
Mandible, fracture of, 113
Mantoux skin test, 22
Maternal history, for HIV-positive mother, 255
McCarthy Infant Observation Scale, 244
Mealtime atmosphere, 279
Mean corpuscular volume (MCV), 22
Meat, in first year, 34–36
Mebendazole (Vermox), 314–316
Medical management, for infant of HIV-positive mother, 257–259
Medication. *See also specific agents*
dosage guidelines for, 305–312

headache from, 205
history of in comprehensive pediatric interview, 10
symptomatic, 249–250. *See also* Symptomatic therapy
trade name, generic, and prescription, 250
Medicolegal issues, 227–237
Menarche, 163
Meningismus, 203
Meningitis
bacterial pathogens associated with, 241–242
*Haemophilus influenzae,* 123
in sickle cell anemia, 223
Mental retardation, 72
Mental status examination, 17
Meperidine (Demerol), 254
Metabolic disorders screening, 21
Metaproterenol (Alupent, Metaprel), 309
Metatarsus adductus, 200f
examination at 2-month visit, 19
treatment of, 199
Methylphenidate (Ritalin)
for attention deficit disorder, 296–298
dosage guidelines for, 309
Metronidazole (Flagyl)
dosage guidelines for, 309, 314
for PID, 159
for trichomoniasis, 158
*Microsporum* infection, 92–93
Migraine headache, 206–207
classification of, 207
management of, 207
pharmacotherapy for, 207–211
Migraine precipitants, 207
Mineral oil
for constipation, 253
for encopresis, 140
warm, for earache, 252
Mineral supplements, 37
Minors
emancipated, 237
mature, 237
MMR vaccination
common side effects of, 29–30
contraindications to, 30t
recommended schedule for healthy infants and children, 26t, 27t, 28t
Mood, 17
*Moraxella catarrhalis*
in otitis media, 98
in sinusitis, 101, 102
Moro's reflex, 73
Morphine
for pain, 254
for vaso-occlusive sickle episode, 221, 222
Morphine sulfate, 222
Motor development, 72
milestones for, 72
primary delays in, 72
primitive reflex in, 72–78
Motor system examination, 17
Mouth
of newborn, 18
in well-child examination, 15–16
Mumps immunization, 6
Mupirocin (Bactroban)
dosage guidelines for, 309
for nonbullous impetigo, 85
*Mycobacterium avium* complex, 258
*Mycoplasma hominis* vaginosis, 159
*Mycoplasma pneumoniae,* 120, 127, 128

Nafcillin
absorption of with food, 246
for pneumonia, 129
Naproxen (Naprosyn)
dosage guidelines for, 309
for headache, 207–210
Narcotic analgesics, 254
Narcotic cough suppressants, 250
Nasal sounds, 66
Nasolacrimal duct obstruction, 108
Nasopharyngitis, 103
Nausea and vomiting, 252
Neck
of newborn, 18
in well-child examination, 16
Neglect, risk factors for, 227
*Neisseria gonorrhoeae* conjunctivitis, 107
*Neisseria meningitidis,* 241, 242
Neomycin allergy, 32
Neonatal conjunctivitis, 107–108
Neonatal history, past, 9
Neurocardiogenic syncope, 203
Neuroimaging
for febrile seizures, 212
for headache, 205–206
Neurologic complaints, 203–211. *See also specific conditions*
Neurologic examination
for headache, 205
newborn, 18
in well-child visit, 17
Neurologic referral, 210–211
Neuromusculoskeletal disorders, 193–214. *See also specific disorders*
Neurosurgical consultation, 210–211
Neurosyphilis, 158
Newborn
anticipatory guidance for, 44–45
bedtime behavior in, 273
fever in, 242–243
of HIV-positive mother, 256–259
language development in, 67
metabolic disorder screening in, 21
physical examination in well-child visit, 18
physiologic jaundice of, 143
serious bacterial infections in, 242

Newborn period issues, 8
Nifedipine, 223
Nine-month visit, 19
Nitrofurantoin (Furadantin, Macrodantin)
  dosage guidelines for, 309
  pediatric doses of, 247t
  for urinary tract infections, 155
Nontreponemal test, 157–158
Norplant, 190
Norwalk-like viruses, 133
Nose
  disease of. *See specific disorders*
  of newborn, 18
  in well-child examination, 15
Nucleoside reverse transcriptase inhibitors, 258–259
Nursing personnel, 3
Nutrition, 33
  at 2 months, 46
  at 4 months, 47
  at 6 months, 48
  at 9 months, 49
  at 12 months, 49–50
  at 15 months, 50
  at 18 months, 51–52
  at 2 weeks, 46
  at 2 years, 52
  at 3 years, 53
  at 4 years, 54
  at 5 years, 55
  at 6–10 years, 56
  anticipatory guidance for, 42
  guidelines for first year of life, 35t
  indices for obesity, 182
  for infant of HIV-positive mother, 257–258
  for newborn, 44–45
  in poor growth, 171–172
  prenatal, 44
  RDAs in, 33
  special dietary concerns in, 37–39
  sports and, 39
  with vegetarian diet, 39
Nutritional assessment, 33
Nutritional history, 10
Nutritional requirements
  for adolescent, 36
  first year, 33–36
  with sports activities, 39
  for toddler and child, 36
Nutritional supplements, 37. *See also specific nutrients*
  in first year, 36
Nystatin (Mycostatin), 310

Obesity
  childhood
    body fat measures for, 180
    classification of, 180–181
    consequences of, 181–182
    definitions of, 180
    etiology of, 181
    incidence of, 180
    management of, 183–184
    natural history of, 181
    outpatient approach to, 182–183
  endocrine and genetic, 180–181
  exogenous, 180
  morbidities associated with, 183
  nutritional concerns in, 38
  in school-age children, 279
Ocular infections, 107–109
Office policy, 8
Ofloxacin
  for gonorrhea, 156
  for PID, 159
Ophthalmia neonatorum, 107–108
Opiates, 252
Opportunistic infections, HIV-related, 258
Oral conditions, 110–113
Oral contraceptives
  estrogen-progestogen, 187–188
  progestin-only, 188
Oral examination, infant, 61–62
Oral hygiene, 62
  routines in infant dental health, 61
Oral polio virus vaccination, recommended schedule for, 26t, 27t, 28t
Oral rehydration solution composition, 319
Oral trauma, 112–113
Oral-motor dysfunction, 66
Orthopedic complaints, 193, 196–198, 199–202. *See also specific conditions*
  obesity and, 182
Ortolani test, 196, 197f
Osmotic laxatives, 139–140
Osteomyelitis, 223
Otitis media
  acute, 97
    antibiotics for, 245
    diagnosis of, 97–98
    epidemiology of, 97
    microbiology of, 98
    pathogenesis of, 97
    resolution of, 99
    treatment of, 98–99
  symptomatic therapy for, 251–252
Outpatient care, ethical issues of, 235–237
Ovarian cysts, 165–166
Ovral tablets, 234
Oxycodone, 221
Oxygen
  for bronchiolitis, 121
  for croup, 123
  humidified, for pneumonia, 129
Oxymetazoline, long-acting, 250

Pacifiers, 63
Pain. *See also* Headache
bone, 221–222
chronic abdominal, 136–138
symptomatic therapy for, 253–254
Parainfluenza virus
in pneumonia, 127
in sinusitis, 101
Parasitic infections
medication guidelines for, 314–316
in pneumonia, 127
Parenting
at 2 months, 47
at 4 months, 47
at 6 months, 48
at 9 months, 49
at 12 months, 50
at 15 months, 51
at 18 months, 52
at 2 weeks, 46
at 2 years, 53
at 3 years, 54
at 4 years, 54–55
at 5 years, 55
at 6–10 years, 56
anticipatory guidance for, 43
in early adolescence, 57–58
in late adolescence, 60
in middle adolescence, 59
of newborn, 45
prenatal issues of, 44
Parents
agenda of, 41
child behavior and, 265
concerns of in prenatal interview, 8
eliciting behavioral concerns from, 263
involvement with school, 282–283
Paroxysmal fussing, 145
Partnership, physician-parent, 41
Past medical history, 9–10
in ill-visit interview, 12
Patient
general description of in physical examination, 15
obligation to protect, 236
Pavlik harness, 198f
Pediazole
dosage guidelines for, 310
for otitis media, 98
pediatric doses of, 247t
*Pediculosis capitis*
diagnosis of, 89
epidemiology of, 89
life cycle of, 89
treatment of, 89
Pedulosis pubis infestation, 90
Pelvic examination
for adolescent, 20
for contraception, 187
Pelvic inflammatory disease (PID), 159
antimicrobial drugs for, 313
Pelvic ultrasound examination, 165–166
Pemoline (Cylert), 310
Penicillin
allergy to, 104
bitter taste of, 245
for impetigo of diaper area, 86
cost of, 246
for gonococcal conjunctivitis, 107
interactions of, 246, 248
procaine for neurosyphilis, 158
for sickle cell anemia, 224
Penicillin G
absorption of with food, 246
benzathine, 103, 153, 310
for gonococcal conjunctivitis, 107
for pneumonia, 129
procaine, dosage guidelines for, 310
for syphilis, 158
Penicillin V
pediatric doses of, 247t, 310
for pharyngitis, 103
Pentamidine, 315
Peptic acid disease, 138
Perception, 17
Perinatal history, for HIV-positive mother, 255–256
Peripheral vascular system, 16
Permethrin (Elimite; Nix)
dosage guidelines for, 314
for *Pediculosis capitis,* 89
for scabies, 91
Pertussis, 125
catarrhal, 125
convalescent, 125
epidemiology of, 125
immunization for, 6
laboratory tests for, 125
paroxysmal, 125
in pneumonia, 128
treatment of, 126
Pertussis vaccine
acellular, 29
adverse events occurring after, 29t
Pharyngeal vesicles, 103
Pharyngitis, 103
diagnosis of, 103
treatment of, 103–104
Pharyngoconjunctival fever, 103
Pharynx
disease of. *See specific disorders*
in well-child examination, 15–16
Phenobarbital, 214
Phenol, 251
Phenolphthalein, 253
Phenothiazine
for headache, 210
for nausea and vomiting, 252
Phenylephrine (Neo-Synephrine)
for common cold, 105
short-acting, 250

Phenylketonuria (PKU) screening, 21
Phenytoin (Dilantin), 310
Phonemes, 66
Phototherapy, 143
Phthiriasis palpebrum, 90
*Phthirus pubis,* 90
Physical abuse, 227.
  disposition of, 230
  evaluation of, 229
  follow-up on, 230
  history of, 227
  reporting of, 230
  risk factors for, 227
  specific injuries from, 227–229
  statistics on, 227
Physical activity, 183
Physical aggression, 269
Physical examination
  approach to, 14–15
  for delayed puberty, 168
  for headache, 205
  newborn, 18
  outline of, 15–17
  for pubertal development, 165
  in subsequent visits, 18–20
  well-child, 6
Physical training, 172
Physician
  approach to physical examination, 14
  in contraception, 185
  eliciting behavioral concerns from parents, 263
  in school failure evaluation, 301
  in well-child visit, 3
Physician-parent partnership, 41
Pica, 219
Pickwickian syndrome, 181
Pigeon toes. *See* Intoeing
Playing favorites, 293
*Plesiomonas* gastroenteritis, 133, 135
Plosives, 65–66
*Pneumocystis carinii* pneumonia prophylaxis, 257, 258
Pneumonia
  bacterial, 127
  chlamydial, 128
  etiology of, 127–128
  hospitalization for, 128
  laboratory tests for, 127
  mycoplasma, 128
  pertussis in, 128
  physical examination for, 127
  in sickle cell anemia, 223
  symptoms of, 127
  treatment of, 128–129
  viral, 127
Poliomyelitis vaccination, 6
  active and inactive, 29
  common side effects of, 29
  for infant of HIV-positive mother, 256–257
Polycose, 257–258
Polymerase chain reaction (PCR)
  for HIV testing, 255
  for infant of HIV-positive mother, 256
Polymyxin (Polysporin), 108
Positive reinforcement, 265
Postdischarge visit, well-child, 5–6
Postpartum examination, well-child, 5
Potty training, 290
Prader-Willi syndrome, 181
Praise, 271
Prednisone
  dosage guidelines for, 310
  for tinea capitis, 92
Pregnancy
  prophylaxis for with sexual abuse, 234
  with sexually transmitted disease, 159
  testing for, 187
Premature infant
  growth charts for, 328
  iron deficiency in, 217
  vaccinations for, 24
Premature pubarche, 163
Premature thelarche, 163
Prematurity, 174
Prenatal history
  for HIV-positive mother, 255
  past, 9
Prenatal interview, 8–9
Prenatal visit
  anticipatory guidance during, 43–44
  well-child, 5
Preschoolers
  bedtime behavior in, 275–276
  discipline guidelines for, 268–270
  eating behavior in, 278–279
Prescription medication, 250
Present illness history, 9
Priapism, 222–223
Privileges, removal of, 271
Probenecid
  for neurosyphilis, 158
  for PID, 159
Problem visit
  behavioral, 263–301
  medical, 83–259
Problems
  potential health, 8
  previous, 8
Prochlorperazine (Compazine)
  dosage guidelines for, 310
  for headache, 208t, 210
Promethazine (Phenergan)
  dosage guidelines for, 311
  for headache, 208t
  suppositories for headache, 210
Propranolol (Inderal)
  dosage guidelines for, 311
  for headache, 209t, 210

Protein sources, 34–36
*Proteus* infection
in conjunctivitis, 107
in urinary tract infections, 153
Pseudoephedrine (Sudafed), 105
*Pseudomonas* conjunctivitis, 107
Pseudopuberty, 163
Pseudotumor cerebri, 210
Psychiatric problems, 182
Psychological evaluation, 296
Psychometric testing, 300
Psychopathology, 264
Psychosocial care, 259
Psychosocial issues, 177
in obesity, 182
in prenatal interview, 8–9
Pubarche, precocious, 167
Pubertal development
assessment of variations of, 163–169
clinical stages of, 333
definitions of, 163–164
normal, 164
Puberty
central precocious, 163
delayed
assessment of, 167–168
constitutional, 168–169
definition of, 164
misconceptions about, 164
misconceptions about, 164
normal, 164
onset of, 164
physical change sequence in, 164
precocious
assessment of, 164–166
definition of, 163
history of, 165
increased growth rate with, 173
laboratory tests for, 165
pelvic and abdominal ultrasound for, 165–166
physical examination for, 165
Pubic hair
lice infestation of, 90
misconceptions about, 164
Public Law 1029-119, 71, 300
Pulmonary abnormalities, 181
Punishment. *See also* Discipline
effect of, 265
physical, 268, 269
for school-age children, 271
Purified protein derivative (PPD) test, 21–22
Pyrethrins (A-200, RID)
dosage guidelines for, 314
for *Pediculosis capitis,* 89

Racemic epinephrine, 123
Radiologic evaluation, urinary tract, 154–155
Rape, statutory, 231
Rapid streptococcal antigen test, 103
RBC indices, 217
Recommended dietary allowances (RDAs), 320–321
Rectal examination
for adolescent, 20
for sexual abuse, 234
in well-child visit, 17
Rectum, newborn, 18
Red blood cell distribution width (RDW), 22
in iron deficiency, 218t
in iron-deficiency anemia, 217
Red blood cell indices, 22
Referral
for language development, 69, 70
neurologic, 210–211
for school failure evaluation, 301
for speech therapy, 66
Reflexes
examination in well-child visit, 17
primitive, 72–78
Refractive errors, 22
Rehydration
for diarrhea, 253
for gastroenteritis, 133–134
Religious exemptions, 236
Renal failure, 172
Reporting
of physical abuse, 230
of sexual abuse, 234
Respiratory isolation, 126
Respiratory syncytial virus (RSV)
in bronchiolitis, 120
in pneumonia, 127
prevention of, 121–122
Respiratory tract
lower, disorders of, 117–129
upper, infections of, 101–102. *See also specific conditions*
common cold, 105
Review of systems, 11
Reye's syndrome, 32
Rh incompatibility, 143
Rhinovirus
in bronchiolitis, 120
in pneumonia, 127
in sinusitis, 101
Rhythm method, 190
Ribavirin, 121
Rickets, 193
Rifampin (Rifadin, Rimactane)
dosage guidelines for, 311
interactions of, 246
ROS. *See* Review of systems
Rotavirus, 133
Routine health maintenance supervision, 3–4
Routine visit, well-child care, 4–5
Rubella immunization, 6
Rubeola immunization, 6
Rules, 269

Sabin vaccine, 29
Safety
  at 2 months, 46
  at 4 months, 47
  at 6 months, 48
  at 9 months, 49
  at 12 months, 50
  at 15 months, 51
  at 18 months, 52
  at 2 weeks, 46
  at 2 years, 53
  at 3 years, 53
  at 4 years, 54
  at 5 years, 55
  at 6–10 years, 56
  anticipatory guidance for, 42–43
  in early adolescence, 57
  in late adolescence, 59
  in middle adolescence, 58
  for newborn, 45
  prenatal, 44
Saline nose drops, 251
*Salmonella* gastroenteritis, 133, 134
*Sarcoptes scabiei,* 90–91
Scabies
  diagnosis of, 91
  epidemiology of, 90
  history of, 90
  life cycle of, 90
  pathogenesis of, 90
  physical examination for, 90–91
  treatment of, 91
Scalding injury, 228
Scalp, fungal infection of, 92–93
School
  adolescent behavior in, 12
  performance at, 19
    in early adolescence, 57
    in late adolescence, 59
    in middle adolescence, 58
  performance record for, 299–300
  problems related to, 281–286
  readiness for, 281
  refusal to go to, 283–286
School bully, 284
School failure, 299
  causes of, 299
  evaluation for, 299–301
School-age children
  bedtime behavior in, 276–277
  discipline guidelines for, 271
  eating behavior in, 279–280
  physical examination of, 19
Screening
  for cause of fever in infants, 242
  cholesterol, 38
  in health maintenance supervision, 21–23
  for infant of HIV-positive mother, 257
  for lead poisoning, 219
  for school readiness, 281
  for well-child, 6
Security, teaching child, 268–269
Seizures, febrile, 212–214
Selenium sulfide (Selsun), 93
Senna (Senokot), 140, 253
Sensory system examination, 17
Sentences, 69
Septic arthritis, 223
Septicemia, 223, 224
Serologic testing for syphilis, 257
Sex steroid levels
  in delayed puberty, 168
  excess and increased growth rate, 173
  in precocious puberty, 165
Sexual abuse, 231
  examination for, 232–234
  forensic evidence of, 232
  history of, 231
  nocturnal enuresis and, 151
  presentation of, 231
  reporting of, 234
  statistics on, 231
  STD testing for, 234, 233f
  treatment of, 234
Sexual behavior, adolescent, 11–12, 185–190
Sexual development
  anticipatory guidance for, 42
  in early adolescence, 56–57
  Tanner stage of, 20
Sexual maturity sequence, 334
Sexuality
  in early adolescence, 57
  in late adolescence, 59
  in middle adolescence, 58
Sexually transmitted disease. *See also specific diseases*
  in adolescents, 185
  antimicrobial drugs for, 313
  etiologies for, 156–159
  history of, 185–186
    in HIV-positive mother, 255
  incidence of, 156
  pubic lice, 90
  sexual abuse and, 156
    examination for, 232–234
    prophylaxis for, 234
  symptoms of, 156
  testing for
    algorithm, 233f
    in sexual abuse cases, 234
Shaken baby syndrome, 229
*Shigella* gastroenteritis, 133, 134
Short stature, constitutional, 174
Sibling rivalry, 292
  etiology of, 292
  prevention of, 292–294
Sickle cell anemia
  episodes in, 221–223
  infection with, 223–224
Sickle episodes
  acute splenic sequestration, 223
  aplastic, 223

vaso-occlusive, 221–223
Sinusitis, 101
acute, 101–102
complications of, 102
headache with, 203
subacute and chronic, 102
Six-month visit, 19
Skeletal system
examination of in well-child visit, 17
of newborn, 18
Skin
dry, 83–84
infection, organisms involved in, 245
newborn, 18
superinfection of, 83
in well-child examination, 15
Skinfold thickness (SFT), 180
Sleep
at 6–18 months, 273–275
disturbance of with headache, 204
in newborns, 273
in school-age children, 276–277
in toddlers and preschoolers, 275–276
Sleep apnea, 181
Sleeping
with parents, 276
trouble with, 276
Smoking, 97
Snacks, 36
Snellen charts, 22
Social and environmental history, 11
Social development
in adolescence, 56
in early adolescence, 57
in late adolescence, 59
in middle adolescence, 58
Sodium valproate, 214
Solid foods, 34–36
Spanking, 268
Spectinomycin
for gonorrhea, 156
for STD prophylaxis, 234
Speech. *See also* Articulation; Language
definition of, 64
difficult to understand, 66
milestones in development of, 65t
normal development of, 64–70
Speech-language pathologist, 70
Spermicides, 189
Spinal nerve irritation, 17
Sports activity, 39
Standing ability, 76
Stanford-Binet IV, 72
*Staphylococcus aureus*
fever with, 241
impetigo with, 87
in neonatal conjunctivitis, 107
in otitis media, 98
in pneumonia, 127
skin, 83
*Staphylococcus* conjunctiva, 107
Stature, genetic influence on, 171
Status epilepticus, 213
Stavudine, 258–259
Steam vaporizer, 251
Steroids
for asthma, 118
for croup, 123
nonfluorinated, for diaper dermatitis, 86
sex, 165, 168, 173
topical
for allergic conjunctivitis, 109
for eczema, 83
for scabies, 91
Varicella vaccine and, 32
Stomatitis, 251
Stool softeners
for constipation, 253
for encopresis, 140
*Streptococcus* infection
fever with, 241–242
in pharyngitis, 103
*Streptococcus pneumoniae,* 98, 101, 102
*Streptococcus pyogenes*
in otitis media, 98
in sinusitis, 101
Subarachnoid hemorrhage, 203
Subareolar mass, 164
Sucking, non-nutritive, 61
anticipatory guidance for infants, 63
Sulfacetamide, 108
Sulfadiazine, 315
Sulfisoxazole (Gantrisin)
for chlamydial infection, 157
dosage guidelines for, 311
pediatric doses of, 247t
Sulfonamides
absorption of with food, 246
adverse reactions of, 248
cost of, 246
interactions of, 246
storage of, 246
Superobesity, 180
Surface area nomogram, 336
Swaddling, 273
Symptomatic therapy
advantages and disadvantages of, 249
for congestion, 250–251
for constipation, 253
for cough, 250
definition of, 249
for diarrhea, 252–253
for earache, 251–252
for fever, 254
ideal, 249–250
key, 250
for nausea and vomiting, 252
for pain, 253–254
for sore throat and sore mouth, 251

Syncope, 203
Syntactical errors, 69
Syntax, 68, 69
Syphilis, 157
  antimicrobial drugs for, 313
  congenital, 157–158
  in teen-agers, 158
  testing for infant of HIV-positive mother, 257

Tanner developmental stages, 333
Tattling, 294
Taylor Parent Behavior Rating Scale, 296
Taylor Parent Behavior Scale, 300
TB skin tests, 21–22
Td vaccination recommended schedule, 26t, 27t, 28t
Teeth
  avulsed, 112
  delayed eruption of, 111
  demineralized enamel on, 61
  discoloration of, 111
  ectopic eruption of, 111
  eruption conditions of, 110–111
  eruption hematoma of, 110–111
  fractured, 112
  intruded, 112
  iron stain of, 111
  loose, 112
  natal and neonatal, 110
  number of in infant, 61
  trauma to, 112
    discoloration with, 111
Teething, 110
Temper tantrums, 269
  prevalence of, 287
  prevention of, 287–288
  responding to, 288
Temporomandibular joint dysfunction, 203
Terfenadine, 311
Testosterone, 168
Tetanus immunization, 6
Tetracycline
  absorption of with food, 246
  dental stain with, 111
  dosage guidelines for, 311
  interactions of, 246, 248
  pediatric doses of, 247t
  storage of, 246
  for syphilis, 158
Tetramune, 30
Thalassemia, 223, 224
Thelarche, precocious, 166
Theophylline
  for asthma, 119
  interactions of, 246
Therapeutic privilege, 235
Thiabendazole (Mintezol), 314–315
Thigh fold asymmetry, 196
Thinking patterns, adult, 56
Thorax
  of newborn, 18
  in well-child examination, 16
Thought content, 17
Three-year visit, 19
Throat
  disease of. *See specific disorders*
  sore, 251
Thyroid hormone, excess of, 173
Thyroid-stimulating hormone
  in decreased growth rate, 172
  in delayed puberty, 168
Tibia vara, 193
Time-outs, 270
  declining effectiveness of, 271
  ending, 267
  method of, 267
  pitfalls of, 267
  for problem solving, 267–268
  purpose of, 266
  timing of, 267
Tinea capitis, 92
  clinical presentation and differential diagnosis of, 92
  diagnosis of, 92
  management of, 92–93
Tobramycin, 108
Toddlers
  bedtime behavior in, 275–276
  discipline guidelines for, 268–270
  eating behavior in, 278–279
  nutritional requirements of, 36
Toilet training, 289
  readiness for, 289
  techniques for, 289–290
  use of diapers and training pants in, 290
Tongue tie, 110
Tonsillitis, 103–104
Tonsillopharyngitis, 103
Toothache, 112
Toothpaste, 62–63
TORCH titer, 144
Toxoplasmosis titers, 257, 258
Trace element supplements, 37
Trade name medications, 250
Training pants, 290
Transferrin saturation, 217, 218t
Trauma
  abdominal, from physical abuse, 228
  dental, 111
  oral, 112–113
Treatment, religious exemption from, 236
Trendelenburg's sign, 196
Trichomoniasis, 158–159
*Trichophyton tonsurans,* 92–93
Trimethoprim-sulfamethoxazole (Bactrim, Septra)
  dosage guidelines for, 311, 315
  frequency of administration of, 246

for gastroenteritis, 134, 135
for otitis media, 98, 245
for PCP prophylaxis, 257, 258
pediatric doses of, 247t
for sinusitis, 101
storage of, 246
for urinary tract infections, 155
Tuberculosis
in infant of HIV-positive mother, 258
screening for
for high-risk groups, 22
for low-risk group, 21–22
Twelve-month visit, 19
Two-month visit, 19
Two-week visit, 18–19
Two-year visit, 19
Tympanic membrane
in otitis media, 98
resolution of abnormalities of, 99

Ultrasonography, pelvic and abdominal, 165–166
Underachieving, 299
Urinalysis
for obesity, 182
obtaining sample for, 154
for urinary tract infections, 153–154
in well-child care, 21
Urinary incontinence, 151–152. *See also* Enuresis
Urinary tract infections
clinical presentation of, 153
evaluation for, 153–154
follow-up for, 154–155
incidence of, 153
pathophysiology of, 153
in sickle cell anemia, 223
treatment of, 154
Urine culture
for infant of HIV-positive mother, 257
in well-child care, 21

Vaccination. *See* Immunization
Vaccines, 24
common side effects of, 26–32
licensed in United States, 25t
live, 24
recommended schedule for healthy infants and children, 26t, 27t
suggested schedule for, 28t
Vaginal spermicides, 189
Vaginal sponge, 189–190
Vaginosis, bacterial, 159
Valproic acid, 312
Vancomycin, 312
Varicella vaccination, 6
common side effects of, 31–32
contraindications to, 32
recommended schedule for healthy infants and children, 26t, 27t, 28t
Vaso-occlusive sickle episodes, 221–223
VDRL testing, 158
Vegetables, 34
Vegetarian diet, 39
advantages of, 39
classifications of, 39
Vesicoureteral reflux, 155
Virilization
definition of, 164
in precocious pubarche, 167
with precocious thelarche, 166
Viruses, conjunctivitis, 107–108
Vision testing
beginning of, 19
in well-child care, 22
Visual acuity
testing of, 22
at 3-year visit, 19
Vital signs
of newborn, 18
in well-child examination, 15
Vitamin D
requirements for, 37
supplement of, 37
in first year, 36
Vitamin supplements, 36, 37
Vocabulary development, 68
Voiding cystourethrogram, 155

Waiver, informed consent, 235
Water
fluoridation of, 62
requirements of
with exercise, 39
in first year, 36
in skin hydration, 83–84
sponging with for fever, 254
Water burn, 228
third-degree, length of time to cause, 229t
Wechsler Intelligence Scale for Children, 72, 296, 300
Wechsler Preschool Primary Scale of Intelligence, 72
Weight
concern with, 279–280
as measure of body fat, 180
Well-child care
anticipatory guidance in, 6–7, 41–60
assessment in, 6
dental, infant, 61–63
follow-up in, 7
immunizations in, 6, 24–32
for infant of HIV-positive mother, 256, 257–258
intake visit, 4
for motor and cognitive development, 71–78
nutrition in, 33–40
physical examination, 6
postdischarge visit, 5–6
postpartum examination, 5
routine health maintenance supervision in, 3–4

Well-child care—*continued*
  routine visit, 4–5
  screening tests in, 6, 21–23
  for speech and language development, 64–70
Well-child visit
  history in, 8–12
  physical examination in, 14–20
  routine, 4–5
  time requirements for, 3–4
Western Blot, HIV serology with, 256
Wheezing, 128
Woodcock-Johnson Psychoeducational Battery, 296, 300
Words
  categorizing, 68
  combining, 68–69
  first, 68
  using to delay gratification, 270

*Yersinia* gastroenteritis, 133, 135

Zalcitabine, 258–259
Zidovudine, 258–259
Zinc oxide, 85–86
Zinc protoporphyrin level, 217, 218t